Planning, Implementing, and Evaluating Health Promotion Programs

A Primer

JAMES F. MCKENZIE, Ph.D., M.P.H.
Ball State University

JAN L. JURS, Ph.D.
Lake Hospital System, Painesville, Ohio

Macmillan Publishing Company / New York
Maxwell Macmillan Canada / Toronto
Maxwell Macmillan International / New York   Oxford   Singapore   Sydney

Editor: Ann Castel
Production Editor: Constantina Geldis
Art Coordinator: Peter A. Robison
Artist: Jane Lopez
Text Designer: Anne Flanagan
Cover Designer: Thomas Mack
Production Buyer: Pamela D. Bennett
Electronic Text Management: Ben Ko, Marilyn Wilson Phelps

This book was set in Palatino by Macmillan Publishing Company and was printed and bound by R. R. Donnelley and Sons. The cover was printed by New England Book Company.

Printed in the United States of America

Macmillan Publishing Company
866 Third Avenue
New York, New York 10022

Macmillan Publishing Company is part of the
Maxwell Communication Group of Companies.

Maxwell Macmillan Canada, Inc.
1200 Eglinton Avenue East, Suite 200
Don Mills, Ontario M3C 3N1

Library of Congress Cataloging-in-Publication Data

McKenzie, James F., 1948-
    Planning, implementing, and evaluating health promotion programs : a primer / James F. McKenzie, Jan L. Jurs.
        p.   cm.
    Includes bibliographical references and index.
    ISBN 0-675-22162-5
    1. Health promotion—Planning. 2. Health promotion—Evaluation.
    I. Jurs, Jan L. II. Title.
    [DNLM: 1. Health Education. 2. Health Planning. 3. Health
    Promotion. WA 590 M478p]
    RA427.8M39 1993
    613—dc20
    DNLM/DLC
    for Library of Congress   92-11604
                                                                         CIP

Printing: 3 4 5 6 7 8 9 Year: 5 6 7

This book is dedicated to four special people:

BONNIE, ANNE, HILARY, MIKE

Preface

As its title states, this textbook is a primer and was written for students who are enrolled in their first professional course in health promotion program development. It was designed to help them understand and develop the skills necessary to carry out program development regardless of the setting. The book is unique among the program-planning health textbooks on the market in that it provides readers with both theoretical and practical information. It also provides, under a single cover, material on all three areas of program development—planning, implementing, and evaluating.

Each chapter of the book includes chapter objectives, a list of key terms, presentation of content, chapter summary, review questions, and activities. In addition, many of the key concepts are further explained with information presented in figures, tables, and the appendixes.

> *Chapter objectives.* The chapter objectives identify the content and skills that should be mastered after reading the chapter, answering the end-of-chapter questions, and completing the activities. Most of the objectives are written using the cognitive and psychomotor (behavior) educational domains. For most effective use of the objectives, we suggest that they be reviewed before reading the chapters. This will help readers focus on the major points in each chapter and will facilitate answering the questions and completing the activities at the end.

> *Key terms.* Key terms are introduced in each chapter of the textbook. These terms are important to the understanding of the chapter. The terms are presented in a list at the beginning of each chapter and then are printed boldface at the appropriate points within the chapter. Again, as with the chapter objectives, we suggest that readers skim the list before reading the chapter. Then as the chapter is read, particular attention should be paid to the definition of each term.

Presentation of content. Although each chapter in this book could be expanded—in some cases there are entire books written on topics we have covered in a chapter or less—we believe that each chapter contains the necessary information to help readers understand and develop many of the skills required to be a successful health promotion program planner, implementor, and evaluator.

Chapter summary. At the end of each chapter, readers will find a one- or two-paragraph review of the major concepts contained in the chapter.

Questions. The purpose of the questions at the end of each chapter is to provide readers with some feedback regarding their mastery of the content. We have endeavored to ask questions that would reinforce the chapter objectives and key terms presented in each chapter.

Activities. The final portion of each chapter consists of several activities that will allow readers to put their new knowledge and skills to use. The activities are presented in several different formats for the sake of variety and to appeal to the different learning styles of readers. It should be noted that, depending on the ones selected for completion, activities can build on previous chapter activities and lead to a final product of a completely developed health promotion program.

Readers will find this textbook easy to understand and use. We are confident that, if the chapters are carefully read and an honest effort is put into completing the activities, readers will possess the essential knowledge and skills for program planning, implementation, and evaluation.

ACKNOWLEDGMENTS

A project of this nature could not be completed without the assistance and understanding of many individuals. First, we thank all our past and present students who have had to put up with our "working drafts" of the manuscript.

Second, we are grateful to those professionals who took the time and effort to review and comment on our manuscript. They include: John Sciacca, Northern Arizona University; Kerry Redican, Virginia Tech; Fred Pearson, Ricks College; Susan Cross Lipnickey, Miami University; William K. Spath, Montana Tech; and Vicki Keanz, Eastern Kentucky University.

Third, we thank our friend Robert J. Yonker, Ph.D., professor in the Department of Foundations and Inquiry, Bowling Green State University, for providing valuable feedback on our manuscript.

Fourth, we appreciate the work of several employees of Macmillan Publishing Company for their work: Ann Castel, administrative editor for education/social sciences, College Division, for her initial and continued support of the project; Connie Geldis, manager of electronic text management, for her work as production editor and for keeping us focused; and Jane Lopez, artist, for her finely rendered artwork. We would also like to thank Lys Ann Shore, Ph.D., for her great work as copy editor.

Finally, we want to express our deepest appreciation to our families for their support, encouragement, and understanding of the time that writing takes away from family activities.

James F. McKenzie, Ph.D., M.P.H.
Jan L. Jurs, Ph.D.

Contents

1

Health Education, Health Promotion, Health Educators, and Program Planning   1

Health Education and Health Promotion   3
Health Educators   4
Assumptions of Health Education   6
Program Planning   6

PART I
Planning a Health Promotion Program   9

2

Models for Health Promotion Programming   11

The PRECEDE Framework   12
PRECEDE/PROCEED   14
Model for Health Education Planning (MHEP)   18
Comprehensive Health Education Model (CHEM)   18
Model for Health Education Planning and Resource Development (MHEPRD)   21
Generic Health/Fitness Delivery System (GHFDS)   23

3

Starting the Planning Process   27

Gaining Support of Decision Makers and Executives   28
Identifying a Planning Committee   30
Parameters for Planning   32

4

Assessing Needs   37

What Is a Needs Assessment?   38
Conducting a Needs Assessment   39

Step 1: Determining the Present State of Health of the Target Population   40

Step 2: Determining the Status of Available Health Promotion Programs   47

Step 3: Determining the Need or Measuring the Gaps Between Health Status and Health Promotion and Care   48

Step 4: Dealing with the Problems   49

Step 5: Validating the Need   49

5

Statement of Purpose, Program Goals, and Objectives   53

Statement of Purpose   54
Program Goals   55
Program Objectives   56

Different Levels of Objectives   56

Developing Program Objectives   57

Criteria for Developing Objectives   58

Elements of an Objective   58

Examples of Program Goals and Objectives   60
Goals and Objectives for the Nation   62

6
Theories and Models Commonly Used for Health Promotion Interventions 67

Behavioral Change Theories   69
      Stimulus Response (SR) Theory   69
      Social Cognitive Theory (SCT)   72
      Theory of Reasoned Action (TRA)   74
      Theory of Planned Behavior (TPB)   75
      Theory of Freeing (TF)   77
      Problem-Behavior Theory (PBT)   77
Combination Health Behavior Models   79
      Health Belief Model (HBM)   80
      The Transtheoretical Model (TTM)   81

7
Interventions 87

Macro Versus Micro Interventions   89
Selecting Appropriate Intervention Activities   90
Types of Intervention Activities   92
      Traditional Educational Activities   92
      Behavior Modification Activities   93
      Environmental Change Activities   95
      Regulatory Activities   95
      Community Participation Activities to Influence Public Policy   98
      Activities Affecting Organizational Culture   99
      Communication Activities   99
      Economic and Other Incentives   101
      Social Intervention Activities   102
Designing Health Promotion Interventions   104
      Criteria and Guidelines for Developing a Health Promotion
      Intervention   104
      Ethics and Health Promotion Interventions   106
      A Model for Designing Interventions   107

PART II
Implementing a Health Promotion Program   119

8
Community Organization   121

Community Organization and Its Assumptions   122
The Process of Community Organization   124
   Recognizing the Problem   125
   Making Entry into the Community   125
   Organizing the People   127
   Identifying the Specific Problem to Tackle   128
   Determining Priorities and Setting Goals   130
   Selecting a Solution to the Problem   130
   Final Steps in the Community Organization Process   131
Planned Approach to Community Health (PATCH)   131

9
Identification and Allocation of Resources   135

Personnel   136
Curricula and Other Instructional Resources   138
Space   145
Equipment and Supplies   146
Financial Resources   146
   Participant Fee   146
   Third-Party Support   147
   Organizational Sponsorship   147
   Grants and Gifts   147
   A Combination of Sources   149

10

Marketing: Getting and Keeping People Involved in a Program 151

Market and Marketing   152

Marketing and the Diffusion Theory   154

The Marketing Process and Health Promotion Programs   156

Using Marketing Research to Determine Needs and Desires 156

Developing a Product That Satisfies the Needs and Desires of the Clients   158

Developing Informative and Persuasive Communication Flows and Ensuring That the Product Is Provided in an Appropriate Manner   162

Keeping the Clients Satisfied and Loyal   165

Final Comment on Marketing   171

11

Implementation: Strategies and Associated Concerns 175

Strategies for Implementation   176

First Implementation Model   176

Second Implementation Model (Borg and Gall)   178

First Day of Implementation   180

Dealing with Problems   180

Reporting and Documenting   181

Implementation Timetable   181

Concerns Associated with Planning   182

Legal Concerns   182

Medical Concerns   183

Program Registration and Fee Collection   183

Procedures for Recordkeeping   184

Program Logistics   184

Program Budget   184

Moral and Ethical Concerns   184

Procedural Manual and/or Participant's Manual   186

Training for Facilitators   187

Program Safety   187

☐   PART III
    Evaluating a Health Promotion Program   **189**

12
Evaluation: An Overview   191

Basic Terminology   193
Rationale for Evaluation   194
The Process for Evaluation   195
Practical Problems in Evaluation   196
Evaluation in the Program-Planning Stages   197
Who Will Conduct the Evaluation?   198
Evaluation Results   198

13
Evaluation Models   201

Major Evaluation Approaches   202
    Difficulty in Categorizing Evaluation Models   203
Models Commonly Used in Health Promotion Evaluation   204
    Behavioral Objectives/Goal-Attainment/Goal-Based Model
    204
    Goal-Free Model   207
    Decision-Making Model   208
    Systems Analysis Model   209
    Naturalistic Models   209

14
Evaluation Design   211

Quantitative and Qualitative Approaches   212
Experimental and Control Groups   213
Evaluation Designs   214
Validity   217
    Content Validity   217
    Criterion-Based Validity   217

Construct Validity   218
Internal Validity   218
External Validity   219
Reliability   220
Selecting an Evaluation Design   221

15
Data Collection

Methods of Data Collection   227
Self-Report   227
Direct Observation   233
Existing Records   233
Meetings   234
Sampling   234
Probability Sample   236
Nonprobability Sample   237
Sample Size   237
Pilot Test   237

16
Data Analysis and Reporting

Organization of Data   242
Types of Analyses   243
Descriptive Data Analysis   243
Inferential Data Analysis   244
Interpreting the Results   245
Evaluation Reporting   246
Designing the Written Report   246
Presenting Data   248
How and When to Present the Report   248
Increasing Utilization of the Results   249

Appendixes   253

Appendix A
Responsibilities and Competencies for Entry-Level Health
Educators   254

Appendix B
Health Style: A Self-Test   260

Appendix C
Model Alcohol Policy   267

Appendix D
Indiana Bell Telephone Company Safety Belt Policy   269

Appendix E
Model Ordinance Eliminating Smoking in Workplaces and Enclosed
Public Places   270

Appendix F
Sample Letter for Letter-Writing Campaign   275

Appendix G
Examples of PSAs from the Indiana State Department of Health   277

Appendix H
Code of Practice for Smoking Cessation Programs   280

Appendix I
How to Select the Right Vendor for Your Company's Health Promotion
Program   282

Appendix J
Health Behavior Contract   287

Appendix K
Sample Informed Consent Form   288

Appendix L
Sample Medical Clearance Form   289

Appendix M
Society for Public Health Education Code of Ethics   290

Appendix N
Cost-Benefit and Cost-Effectiveness as a Part of the Evaluation of
Health Promotion Programs   292

References   299

Name Index   310

Subject Index   313

References   299

Name Index   310

Subject Index   313

1

Health Education, Health Promotion, Health Educators, and Program Planning

After reading this chapter and answering the questions at the end, you should be able to:

❑   Explain the relationship between good health behavior, health education, and health promotion.

❑   Write your own definition of health education.

❑   Explain the role of the health educator as defined by the Role Delineation Project.

❑   Explain how the defined role of the health educator is used by the National Council for the Accreditation of Teacher Education (NCATE), the National Commission for Health Education Credentialing, Inc. (NCHEC), and the SOPHE/AAHE Baccalaureate Program Approval Committee (SABPAC).

❑   Identify the assumptions upon which health education is based.

❑   Name the generic components for planning a program.

☐ KEY TERMS

entry-level health educator

health behavior

health education

health educator

health promotion

health promotion and disease
prevention

primary caregivers

primary prevention

Role Delineation Project

secondary prevention

target population

The concern of American people about good health, wellness, and health behavior has reached new heights in recent years, and rightfully so. We now know that better control of behavioral risk factors alone—such as lack of exercise, poor diet, use of tobacco and drugs, and alcohol abuse—could prevent between 40 and 70 percent of all premature deaths, one-third of all acute disabilities, and two-thirds of chronic disabilities (USDHHS, 1990b).

Although many events, research studies, and publications have contributed to this focus on health and **health behavior**, there may be none more important than the government publication, *Healthy People: The Surgeon General's Report on Health Promotion and Disease Prevention* (*Healthy People*, 1979). This document brought together much of what was known about the relationship of personal behavior and health status. The document also presented a "personal responsibility" model that provided Americans with a prescription for reducing their health risks and increasing their chances for good health.

It may have not been the content of *Healthy People* that made the publication so significant, because several publications written before it provided a similar message. *Healthy People* was important because it summarized the research available up to that point, presented it in a very readable format, and made the information available to the general public. The message of *Healthy People* was spread so well that there are few Americans today who do not know the importance of good health behavior.

This focus on health has given many people in the United States a desire to do something about their health. This desire in turn has created a greater need for good health information that can be easily understood by the average person. One only needs to look at the current best-seller list, read the daily newspaper, observe the health advertisements delivered via the mass media, or consider the increase in the number of health-promoting facilities (not illness or sickness facilities) to verify the interest that American consumers have in health. Because of the increased interest in health, health professionals are now faced with the problem of delivering this good health information.

HEALTH EDUCATION AND HEALTH PROMOTION

In the simplest terms **health education** is the process of educating people about health. However, two more formal definitions of health education have been frequently cited in the literature. The first comes from the Joint Committee on Health Education Terminology report (1991, p. 103). The committee defined the health education process as the "continuum of learning which enables people, as individuals and as members of social structures, to voluntarily make decisions, modify behaviors, and change social conditions in ways which are health enhancing." The second definition was proposed by Green, Kreuter, Deeds, and Partridge (1980, p. 7). They defined health education as "any combination of learning experiences designed to facilitate voluntary adaptations of behavior conducive to health." The learning experiences noted in this definition are innumerable, and could be placed on a continuum anchored by self-taught learning experiences on one end and by highly sophisticated, thoroughly planned, multi-activity learning experiences on the other. Obviously, each type of learning experience has the potential for educating the intended **target population** and has its own strengths and weaknesses.

Another term that is closely related to health education, and sometimes incorrectly used in its place, is **health promotion**. Health promotion is a broader term than health education. One of the early definitions of this term stated that health promotion was "any combination of health education and related organizational, political and economic interventions designed to facilitate behavioral environmental adaptations that will improve or protect health" (USDHHS, 1980, p. 1). In this definition, "interventions" refers to systematically planned health promotion programs. A more recent definition of health promotion was offered by Green and Kreuter (1991, p. 4). They simplified the earlier definition to read: "the combination of educational and environmental supports for actions and conditions of living conducive to health." In this definition, "educational" refers to health education, and "environmental" refers to social, political, organizational, policy, economic, and regulatory circumstances bearing on health. A third definition of health promotion was provided in the Joint Committee on Health Education Terminology report (1991, p. 102). The committee defined **health promotion and disease prevention** as "the aggregate of all purposeful activities designed to improve personal and public health through a combination of strategies, including the competent implementation of behavioral change strategies, health education, health protection measures, risk factor detection, health enhancement and health maintenance." According to all three of these definitions of health promotion, health education is an important component of health promotion and firmly implanted in it (Figure 1.1). "Without health education, health promotion would be a manipulative social engineering enterprise" (Green & Kreuter, 1991, p. 14).

The effectiveness of health promotion programs can vary greatly. However, the success of a program can usually be linked to the planning that

Figure 1.1
Relationship of health education
and health promotion

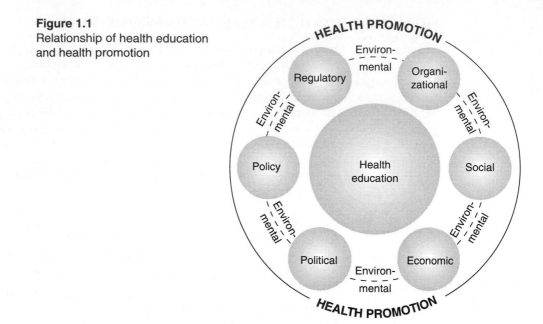

takes place before implementing the program. Programs that have undergone a thorough planning process are usually the most successful.

HEALTH EDUCATORS

The role of the **health educator** has evolved over time based on the need for someone other than the **primary caregivers**—mainly physicians, dentists, other independent practitioners, and nurses—to deliver health information. Before health educators were recognized as contributors to the health care process, the responsibility for delivering health information belonged to the primary caregivers. However, the combination of the heavy workload of the primary caregivers, the lack of formal training in the process of educating others, and the need for public education in the importance of **primary and secondary prevention** created a need for health educators.

Today, health educators can be found working in a variety of settings, including schools, colleges and universities, worksites, community agencies, and sites where primary care is provided, such as hospitals and health maintenance organizations.

Though the need for health educators grew out of the need to deliver health information, their role has expanded over the years so that now health educators are involved in all aspects of health promotion. As the role of health educators has grown, there has been a movement by those in the discipline to clearly define their role so that people inside and outside of the discipline would have a better understanding of what the health educator does. In 1978 the **Role Delineation Project** was begun (National Task Force [on the Preparation and Practice of Health Educators, Inc.], 1985). Through a comprehensive process this project yielded a generic role for the **entry-level health educator** (someone taking a first job). The defined role is generic in that the responsibilities identified are carried out on a regular basis by entry-level health educators regardless of their work setting. The defined role comprises seven major areas of responsibility and several different competencies and subcompetencies, which further delineate the responsibilities. The seven major areas of responsibility identified through the Role Delineation Project include (the entire list of "Responsibilities and Competencies for Entry-Level Health Educators" is presented in Appendix A):

1. Assessing individual and community needs for health education.
2. Planning effective health education programs.
3. Implementing health education programs.
4. Evaluating the effectiveness of health education programs.
5. Coordinating provision of health education services.
6. Acting as a resource person in health education.
7. Communicating health and health education needs, concerns, and resources (National Task Force, 1985, pp. 15–16).

In reviewing the seven areas of responsibility, it is obvious that four of the seven are directly related to program planning, implementation, and evaluation, and that the other three could be associated with programming depending on the type of program being planned. In effect, these responsibilities distinguish health educators from other professionals who try to provide health education experiences.

The importance of the defined role of the health educator is becoming greater as the discipline of health education continues to grow. This is shown by its use in three major professional activities. First, the National Council for the Accreditation of Teacher Education (NCATE) uses the defined role in reviewing and accrediting teacher education programs in institutions of higher education. If a college or university now wants its health education program to have NCATE accreditation, it must show how its curriculum provides opportunities for students to learn the knowledge and skills listed in the defined role.

Second, the defined role is used by the National Commission for Health Education Credentialing, Inc. (NCHEC) for certifying individuals as health educators (Certified Health Education Specialist, or CHES). In 1988, experienced health educators were permitted to apply for charter certification. Now an individual can become certified by passing a national certification examination that is given annually. The first certification examination was given in fall 1990.

Third, the defined role is used by a joint committee of the Society for Public Health Education (SOPHE) and the Association for the Advancement of Health Education (AAHE), known as the SOPHE/AAHE Baccalaureate Program Approval Committee (SABPAC). The committee used the role to develop a process by which colleges and universities could review their undergraduate health education programs. This role is used as part of a self-study and by external reviewers to determine if the program being offered is of high quality.

ASSUMPTIONS OF HEALTH EDUCATION

So far we have discussed the need for health, what health education and health promotion are, and the role health educators play in delivering successful health promotion programs. We have not yet discussed the assumptions that underlie health promotion—all the things that must be in place before the whole process of health promotion begins. In the mid-1980s, Bates and Winder (1984) outlined what they saw as four critical assumptions of health education. We have modified their list by adding several items and referring to them as assumptions of health promotion. We see this expanded list of assumptions as being critical to understanding what we can expect from health promotion programs. Health promotion is by no means the sole answer to the nation's health care problem or, for that matter, the sole means of getting the smoker to stop smoking or the nonexerciser to exercise. Health promotion is an important part of the health care system but it does have limitations. Here are the assumptions:

1. Health status can be changed.
2. Disease occurrence theories and principles can be understood (Bates and Winder, 1984).
3. Appropriate prevention strategies can be developed to deal with the identified health problems (Bates and Winder, 1984).
4. An individual's health is affected by a variety of factors, not just lifestyle. Others include heredity, environment, and the health care system.
5. Changes in individual and societal health behaviors and lifestyles will affect an individual's health status positively (Bates and Winder, 1984).
6. "Individuals, families, small groups, and communities can be taught to assume responsibility for their health, which in turn changes their health behaviors and lifestyles" (Bates and Winder, 1984, p. 2).
7. Individual responsibility should not be viewed as victim blaming.
8. For health behavior change to be permanent, an individual must be motivated and ready to change.

The importance of these assumptions is made clearer if we refer to the definitions of health education presented earlier in the chapter. Implicit in those definitions were a goal of having the participants of health education programs voluntarily adopt health-enhancing behavior. To achieve such a goal, the assumptions must indeed be in place. For health educators to be able to assist people in reaching this goal, they need to have the knowledge and skills to plan, implement, and evaluate appropriate programs.

PROGRAM PLANNING

Since many of health educators' responsibilities are involved in some way with program planning, implementation, and evaluation, they need to become well versed in these processes. "Planning an effective program is more difficult than implementing it. Planning, implementing, and evaluating programs are all inter-related, but good planning skills are prerequisite to programs worthy of evaluation" (Breckon, Harvey, and Lancaster, 1989, p. 95). All three processes are very involved, and much time, effort, practice, and on-the-job training are required to do them well. Even the most experienced health educators find program planning challenging because of the constant changes in settings, resources, and target populations.

Today, it is generally accepted that the process of health promotion can take many different forms. That is, there are many different ways of getting from point A to point B. However, all approaches usually center on a generic set of tasks that include (1) assessing the needs of the target population; (2) identifying the problem(s); (3) developing appropriate goals and objectives; (4) creating an intervention that considers the peculiarities of the setting; (5) implementing the intervention; and (6) evaluating the results. The remaining chapters of this book present a process that health educators can use to plan, implement, and evaluate successful health promotion programs, and will introduce readers to the necessary knowledge and skills to carry out these tasks.

☐ SUMMARY

The increased interest in personal health and the flood of new health information have created a need to provide quality health promotion programs. Individuals are seeking guidance to enable them to make sound decisions about behavior that would be conducive to their health. Those best prepared to help these people are health educators who have received appropriate training. Properly trained health educators are aware of the limitations of the discipline and understand the assumptions on which health promotion is based.

☐ QUESTIONS

1. Explain the role *Healthy People* played in the relationship between the American people and health.
2. How is health education defined by the Joint Committee on Health Education Terminology (1991)?
3. What are the key phrases in the definition of health education presented by Green, Kreuter, Deeds, and Partridge (1980)?
4. What is the relationship between health education and health promotion?
5. Why is there a need for health educators?
6. What is the Role Delineation Project?
7. How is the defined role of the health educator used by NCATE? By NCHEC? By SABPAC?
8. What are the seven major responsibilities of health educators?

9.   What are the assumptions that are critical to health promotion?

10.   What are the generic parts of planning programs?

☐ ACTIVITIES

1.   Based upon what you have read in this chapter and your knowledge of the discipline of health education, write your own definitions for *health, health education, health promotion,* and *health promotion program.*

2.   Write a response indicating what you see as the importance of each of the eight assumptions presented in the chapter. Write no more than one paragraph per assumption.

3.   With your knowledge of health promotion, what other assumptions would you add to the list presented in this chapter? Provide a one-paragraph rationale for each.

4.   If you have recently graduated from college or will be graduating soon, write or call the National Commission for Health Education Credentialing, Inc. (NCHEC), requesting an application for the credentialing process. NCHEC can be contacted in care of Professional Examination Service, 475 Riverside Drive, New York, NY 10115, or by calling (212) 870-3161.

5.   If you have not already done so, go to the government documents section of the library on your campus and read *Healthy People: The Surgeon General's Report on Health Promotion and Disease Prevention (Healthy People,* 1979).

Part I

Planning a Health Promotion Program

2

Models for Health Promotion Programming

After reading this chapter and answering the questions at the end, you should be able to:

❑   Explain the importance of using a model for planning a program.

❑   Identify the models most commonly used in planning health promotion programs and briefly explain each.

❑   Identify the major components of the planning models.

☐ KEY TERMS

administrative diagnosis

behavioral diagnosis

educational diagnosis

enabling factors

epidemiological diagnosis

evaluation

goal setting

implementation

needs assessment

PRECEDE

predisposing factors

PROCEED

reinforcing factors

social diagnosis

As noted in Chapter 1, a major portion of the role of the health educator is associated with health promotion programming—planning, implementing, and evaluating health education programs. Good health promotion programs are not created by chance; they are the product of much effort and should be based on well-developed models. Models are the means by which planners give structure and organization to the programming process. They provide planners with direction and supply a "frame" on which to build. Many different planning models have been developed, some of which are used more frequently than others. Although many of the models have common elements (sometimes with different labels), each has a slightly different perspective. No perfect model yet exists; instead, each has its own strengths and weaknesses.

Most planners find occasions when they do not need to use a model in its entirety or when it is necessary to combine parts of different models to meet specific needs and situations. As Gilmore, Campbell, and Becker (1989, p. 13) have pointed out, "it may not be feasible for every programming effort to use all of the cited considerations at each stage, [but] they do provide prompters for planning committee, and administrative discussions."

The remainder of this chapter will present the models most commonly used in planning health promotion programs. These are tried-and-true models that have been used in a variety of settings with many successes and some failures.

THE PRECEDE FRAMEWORK

Even though the PRECEDE framework, developed by Green, Kreuter, Deeds, and Partridge (1980), has been updated and replaced by the PRECEDE/PROCEED Model (Green & Kreuter, 1991), it is presented here because of its profound impact on health education planning from the day it was developed until its "retirement" in 1991. Many program planners used the PRECEDE framework, either in part or in whole, during its eleven-year "life" and found that it served quite well.

PRECEDE was an acronym for Predisposing, Reinforcing, and Enabling Causes in Educational Diagnosis and Evaluation. It was a framework based on the requirements of four disciplines: epidemiology, social/behavioral sciences, administration, and education. It consisted of seven phases. The first phase of the framework was labeled **social diagnosis** (an assessment of the quality of life). In this phase, planners used appropriate needs assessment techniques to determine the quality of life as defined by social problems in the target population. Examples of social problems that could reflect the quality of life include, but are not limited to, illegitimacy, welfare, unemployment, absenteeism, and crime.

The second phase of the framework was **epidemiological diagnosis**. In this phase, the task for the planners was to use epidemiological data to determine what specific health problems were contributing to the social problems identified in phase 1. Those epidemiological data might include mortality, morbidity, fertility, and disability, and their dimensions (incidence, prevalence, distribution, intensity, and duration). As part of phase 2, the planners were made aware that some nonhealth factors (such as education, race, or gender) can affect the quality of life. Once the health problems were identified, the planners prioritized the problems to determine which one(s) the health education program would address.

Phase 3 of PRECEDE was called **behavioral diagnosis**; its purpose was to identify those specific health-related behaviors that seemed to be associated with the prioritized health problems selected in phase 2. Once again, planners had to establish priorities. This time they needed to determine which behavior(s) the program would address. Priorities could be determined by using a 2 X 2 table, as shown in Figure 2.1. Planners would try to identify behaviors that were both important and changeable. Also in phase 3 planners had to recognize that nonbehavioral factors, such as genetics, economics, and environment, could affect health, in addition to behavioral factors.

Phases 4 and 5 made up the **educational diagnosis**. In phase 4 planners tried to assess the causes of the health behavior by identifying, sorting, and categorizing three classes of factors that have the potential to affect health behavior: predisposing, enabling, and reinforcing factors. **Predisposing factors** included (and still do in the PRECEDE/PROCEED model) many affective traits, such as a

Figure 2.1
Priority decision making

	Important	Less important
Changeable		
Not changeable		

person's attitudes, values, beliefs, and perceptions. These are the factors that can facilitate or hinder a person's motivation to change. Barriers created mainly by societal forces or systems make up the **enabling factors**, which include limited access to health care facilities; inadequate resources, income, or health insurance; and restrictive laws, rules, regulations, and policies. **Reinforcing factors** comprise the different types of feedback that those in the target population receive, which may either encourage or discourage them in changing their behavior (Green et al., 1980).

The second part of the educational diagnosis, phase 5, consisted of deciding which factors would be the focus of the intervention and what educational intervention would be used. The decision was to be made on the importance of the factors and the availability of the resources to influence them.

The sixth phase of the framework was the **administrative diagnosis**, the actual development and implementation of the program. The seventh and final phase of the framework was **evaluation**. Although the developers of the framework listed evaluation as the last phase, they by no means meant to downplay its importance or to imply that evaluation should take place only after the program had been completed. They strongly believed (and this is true for the PRECEDE/PROCEED model as well) that evaluation should begin early in the planning process and be ongoing.

The PRECEDE model was very useful, but the need to use other health promotion activities along with health education necessitated expanding the model to include health promotion planning and evaluation.

PRECEDE/PROCEED

At first glance the revised model looks much like its predecessor, but there are several changes that make it a more useful model. The new title of the model—PRECEDE/PROCEED—summarizes the phases within the model. **PRECEDE** is an acronym for Predisposing, Reinforcing, and Enabling Constructs in Educational/Environmental Diagnosis and Evaluation. **PROCEED** stands for Policy, Regulatory and Organizational Constructs in Educational and Environmental Development (Green & Kreuter, 1991).

As can be seen in Figure 2.2, the new model contains nine phases or steps. It is much more comprehensive than its predecessor and further subdivides the evaluation component. As with the PRECEDE framework, the PRECEDE/PROCEED model begins with the final consequences and works back to the causes. Once again, the first phase in this model is called social diagnosis and seeks to define subjectively the quality of life (problems and priorities) of those in the target population. The designers of this model suggest that this is best accomplished by involving individuals in the target population in a self-study of their own needs. Subjective indicators of the quality of life could include illegitimacy, welfare, discrimination, happiness, and self-esteem.

Phase 2 is the epidemiological diagnosis, in which planners identify and prioritize health goals or problems that may contribute to the needs identified in phase 1. Epidemiological data, together with clinical and investigative data, are used to make these decisions.

PRECEDE

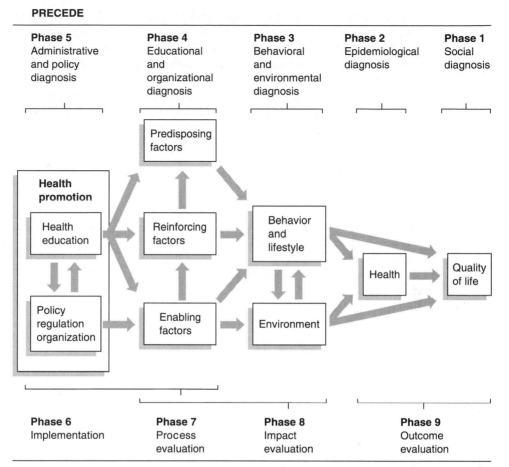

Figure 2.2
The PRECEDE/PROCEED model for health promotion planning and evaluation (From
Health Promotion Planning: An Educational and Environmental Approach [p. 23] by L. W.
Green and M. W. Kreuter, 2nd ed., 1991, Mountain View, CA: Mayfield Publishing.
Copyright 1991 by Mayfield Publishing. Reprinted by permission.)

Phase 3, behavioral and environmental diagnosis, involves determining
and prioritizing the behavioral and environmental risk factors that might be
linked to the health problems in phase 2. Remember, as was mentioned in
Chapter 1, *environmental* refers to the factors outside an individual that have a
bearing on behavior, health, and quality of life. Note that in Figure 2.2 arrows
connect both of the boxes in phase 3 with phases 1 and 2. This suggests that programs attacking specfic risk factors can also have an impact on the social forces.
As with the earlier PRECEDE framework, the prioritization needed in this phase
can be accomplished using the 2 × 2 table presented in Figure 2.1.

Phase 4 of the new model, as of its predecessor, identifies and classifies the predisposing, reinforcing, and enabling factors that have the potential to influence health behavior. These factors can either facilitate or hinder the behavior. Here again, planners must set priorities. The factors identified in this phase become the focus of the intervention that will be planned.

The fifth phase consists of an administrative and policy diagnosis, in which planners determine if the capabilities and resources are available to develop and implement the program. It is between phases 5 and 6 that PRECEDE (the diagnostic portion of the model) ends and PROCEED (implementation and eval-

Table 2.1
Model for Health Education Planning (MHEP)

	Content dimension
Phase 6 **Evaluation**	4. Knowledge of problem and client system 3. Technology of feedback systems 2. Language and systems 1. Nature of evaluation
Phase 5 **Implementation**	4. Writing skills 3. Dynamics of problem solving 2. Knowledge of subject and content Training and Technical Assistance being provided for 1. Knowledge of plan, how it is to work
Phase 4 **Planning/programming**	3. Nature of political process 2. Systems analysis and management science 1. Techniques of planning
Phase 3 **Goal setting**	5. Theory of change 4. Management by Objectives technology 3. Forecasting 2. Nature of policy 1. Role of goals, how to set them, measure
Phase 2 **Needs assessment**	4. Relevance of data 3. Language and systems 2. Data sources 1. Standards and criteria
Phase 1 **Initiate**	3. Power and influence structures, community organization, culture 2. Contract terminology and resources 1. Knowledge of problem and client system

Source: From *Theory and Practice in Health Education* (pp. 214–15) by H. S. Ross and P. R. Mico, 1980. Palo Alto, CA: Mayfield Publishing. Copyright 1980 by Mayfield Publishing and Drs. Helen S. Ross and Paul R. Mico. Reprinted by permission.

uation) begins. However, there is not a clean break between the two phases; they really run together.

The four final phases of the model—phases 6, 7, 8, and 9—comprise the PROCEED portion. In phase 6, with appropriate resources in hand, planners select the methods and strategies of the intervention, and **implementation** begins. Phases 7, 8, and 9 focus on the evaluation and are based on the earlier phases of the model, when program objectives were outlined in the diagnostic process. Whether or not all three of these final phases are used depends on the evaluation requirements of the program. Obviously, the resources needed to con-

Method dimension	Process dimension
4. Redefine problem and standards	4. Consensus of new definitions
3. Feedback to activity, reporting, accountability	3. Communication, threat reduction
2. Data collection and analysis	2. Learning assimilation
1. Clarify evaluation measures	1. Agreement
4. Reporting	4. Communications
3. Problem solving	3. Creativity conflict resolution, win-win
2. Training and technical assistance, consultation	2. Skill development, helping
1. Initiate activity	1. Communications, orientations
3. Negotiate commitments, Memorandums of Agreement	3. Negotiation
2. Design management systems and tools	2. Role clarification, communications
1. Develop implementation plan	1. Understanding and committment
5. Determine strategies for implementation	5. Consensus
4. Select goals and objectives	4. Decision making, consensus
3. Alternative goals statement, force-field analysis	3. Reality testing, creative problem solving
2. Link to policy development	2. Understanding of process and roles
1. Establish criteria for goals	1. Agreement
4. Describe nature and extent of problem	4. Reduce fantasy by fact
3. Data collection and analysis	3. Open communications, sensitivity to data sources
2. Determine data to be collected	2. Agreement
1. Identify and review present criteria	1. Agreement on starting point
3. Organize concerned	3. Involvement, leadership, values clarification
2. Develop initial contract	2. Legitimacy, commitment, trust, readiness
1. Entry or intervention strategy, force-field analysis, interviewing	1. Unfreezing, threat reduction, credibility, awareness of need

duct evaluations of impact (phase 8) and outcome (phase 9) are much greater than those needed to conduct process evaluation (phase 7).

MODEL FOR HEALTH EDUCATION PLANNING (MHEP)

The MHEP (Ross & Mico, 1980), which was first developed by Mico in 1966 and has been periodically updated, analyzes planning through six phases and the dimensions of content (subject matter), method (steps and techniques), and process (interactions). The model is outlined in Table 2.1 (pp. 16–17). Phase 1 is the initiation of the planning activity. To carry out this phase, planners must (1) understand the target population's problem and something about its system; (2) enter into an initial contract; and (3) make the client aware that a problem exists. The second phase of the MHEP involves completing a **needs assessment**. Ross and Mico (1980) suggest that to complete a needs assessment planners should first identify how the problem was measured in the past, determine what data need to be collected now and how best to gather them, collect and analyze the data, and finally describe the nature and extent of the problem.

The third phase of the model deals with **goal setting**. The goals should be based on the problems identified in the needs assessment. They should be appropriate and realistic, and should include input from those who will be affected. Also, in this goal-setting phase planners should develop strategies for implementing the goals. Phase 4, called planning/programming, "converts the agreed-upon strategies into a rational implementation plan or program, designs systems and tools for managing the activity, and negotiates commitments among those involved" (Ross & Mico, 1980, p. 224).

The final two phases of the MHEP are implementation (phase 5) and evaluation (phase 6). In phase 5 planners offer the program, provide any needed assistance to facilitators and participants, and keep track of the progress. Phase 6, as described by Ross and Mico (1980), includes the steps of: (1) clarifying the evaluation measures; (2) collecting and analyzing evaluation data; (3) providing appropriate feedback; and (4) redefining the problem and standards.

COMPREHENSIVE HEALTH EDUCATION MODEL (CHEM)

The CHEM (Sullivan, 1973) comprises six major steps and several suggested procedures within each of the steps (Figure 2.3). The first step is to "involve people." This includes identifying the target population and those needed to carry out the program, determining the roles of those involved, and establishing the necessary relationships among the people.

The second step involves setting the appropriate goals for the program. In the third step, defining the problems, planners determine the gaps between what is and what could be. Once they have identified the problems, planners need to determine what problems to tackle. Next they design the program plans (step 4). This includes identifying the most appropriate approach; setting program objectives; defining a timetable, activities, and resources; conducting a pretest; and developing evaluation procedures. The fifth step consists of obtaining the neces-

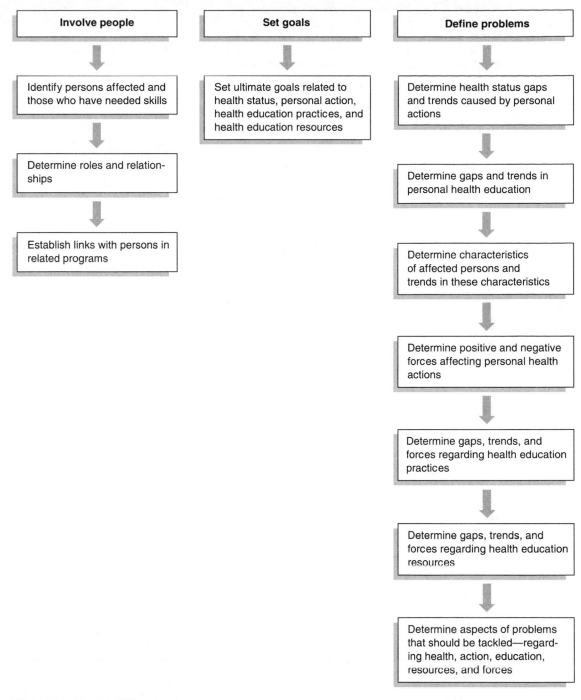

Figure 2.3 (pp. 19–20)
Comprehensive Health Education Model (CHEM) (From "Model for Comprehensive, Systematic Program Development in Health Education" by D. Sullivan, 1973, *Health Education Report, 1*[1], pp. 4–5)

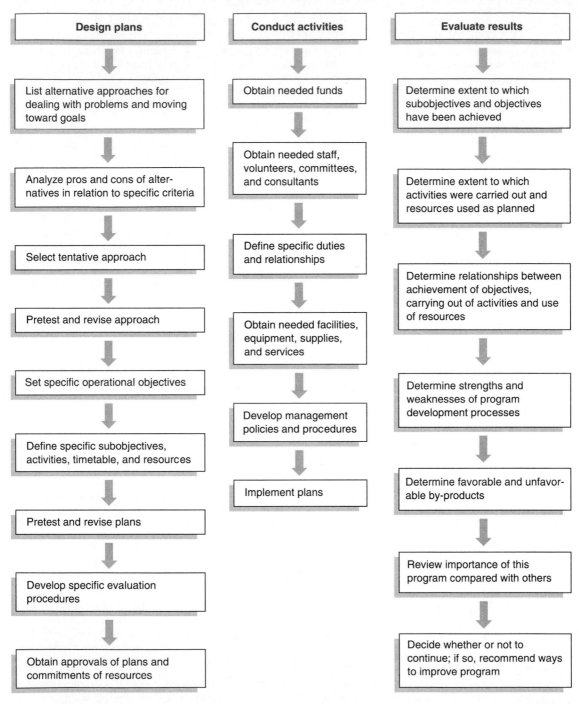

Design plans

List alternative approaches for dealing with problems and moving toward goals

Analyze pros and cons of alternatives in relation to specific criteria

Select tentative approach

Pretest and revise approach

Set specific operational objectives

Define specific subobjectives, activities, timetable, and resources

Pretest and revise plans

Develop specific evaluation procedures

Obtain approvals of plans and commitments of resources

Conduct activities

Obtain needed funds

Obtain needed staff, volunteers, committees, and consultants

Define specific duties and relationships

Obtain needed facilities, equipment, supplies, and services

Develop management policies and procedures

Implement plans

Evaluate results

Determine extent to which subobjectives and objectives have been achieved

Determine extent to which activities were carried out and resources used as planned

Determine relationships between achievement of objectives, carrying out of activities and use of resources

Determine strengths and weaknesses of program development processes

Determine favorable and unfavorable by-products

Review importance of this program compared with others

Decide whether or not to continue; if so, recommend ways to improve program

Figure 2.3, *continued*

sary resources to implement the program, and then implementing it. In the sixth and final step, planners evaluate the program, based on the program objectives. Results of the evaluation then provide data for later decision making regarding the program.

MODEL FOR HEALTH EDUCATION PLANNING AND RESOURCE DEVELOPMENT (MHEPRD)

A less well-known model than those already presented is the MHEPRD introduced by Bates and Winder (1984), shown in Figure 2.4. The creators of this model state that it can be distinguished from others because it separates process from end results, and because of the use of evaluation. Each of the five major components in the MHEPRD—health education plans, demonstration programs, operational programs, research programs, and information and statistics—represents an end result of the planning process. The creators do not see evaluation as a separate phase of the model. Instead it plays an integral part in each phase by testing and validating program assumptions throughout the entire process (Bates & Winder, 1984).

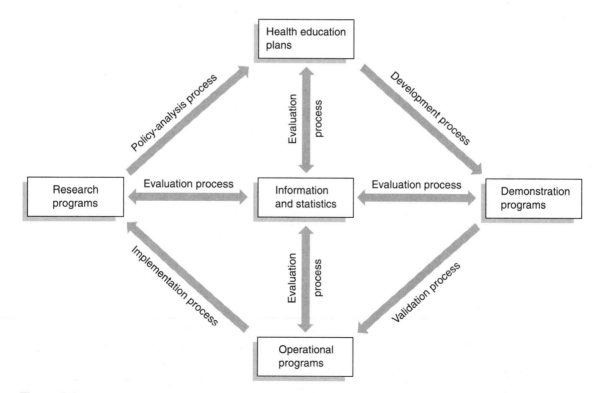

Figure 2.4
A conceptual model for the analysis of Health Education Planning and Resource Development (MHEPRD) (Adapted from *Introduction to Health Education* [p. 103] by I. J. Bates and A. E. Winder, 1984, Palo Alto, CA: Mayfield Publishing)

In the first phase of the model, health education plans are an end result of a needs assessment (or, as Bates and Winder call it, a "policy-analysis process") and ongoing evaluation of information and statistics. The plans developed in phase 1 are treated as hypotheses to be tested in phase 2. To validate their effectiveness, planners create demonstration programs. Phase 3 examines the results of the demonstration programs to determine which should continue and thus become operational programs. This phase also includes the development of an implementation plan that reflects the experiences learned during the demonstration. This process should yield operational programs that are based on a sound rationale of research, planning, and demonstrations.

The fourth phase implements the operational programs. During this phase, steps that are commonly used in a research project are put to use. The problems that surface during implementation provide the basis for research questions for the program planners. The planners in turn formulate possible answers to the questions through appropriate experimentation. The data generated through the experimentation are used for future policy analysis and planning. Thus the planning process becomes cyclic in nature since it always builds on pre-

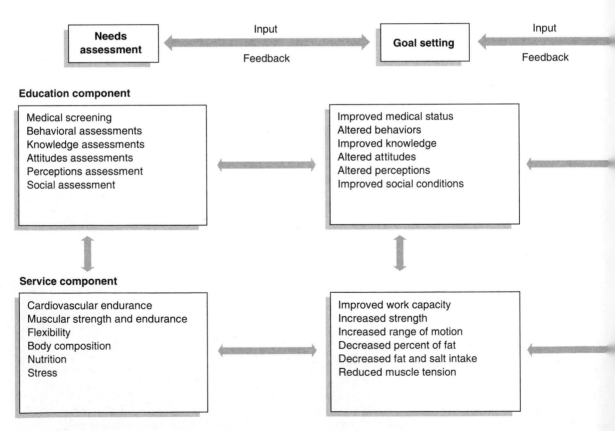

Figure 2.5
Generic Health/Fitness Delivery System (GHFDS) (From *Implementing Health/Fitness Programs* [p. 83] by R. W. Patton, J. M. Corry, L. R. Gettman, and J. S. Graf, 1986, Champaign, IL: Human Kinetics. Copyright 1986 by Human Kinetics. Reprinted by permission.

vious planning. As the process continues, the result should be better organized and more effective health education services (Bates & Winder, 1984).

GENERIC HEALTH/FITNESS DELIVERY SYSTEM (GHFDS)

The final model to be presented in this chapter is the Generic Health/Fitness Delivery System, or GHFDS (Patton, Corry, Gettman, & Graf, 1986). As its name suggests, this model was not developed specifically for health education but can easily be applied to it. This goal-oriented planning model suggests five steps: needs assessment, goal setting, choice of strategies to meet goals, delivery of program, and evaluation. Each of the steps has two components, education and service. The education component provides a cognitive experience in each step, while the service component provides a "hands on" experience. As can be seen in the visual presentation of the model (Figure 2.5), this approach to program planning is dynamic and interactive. It provides constant insight and feedback so as best to meet the needs of those in the target population. Input from a previous step in the GHFDS modifies the approach used in delivering the later steps in the model. Feedback from the later steps becomes most useful in modifying the program delivery (Patton et al., 1986).

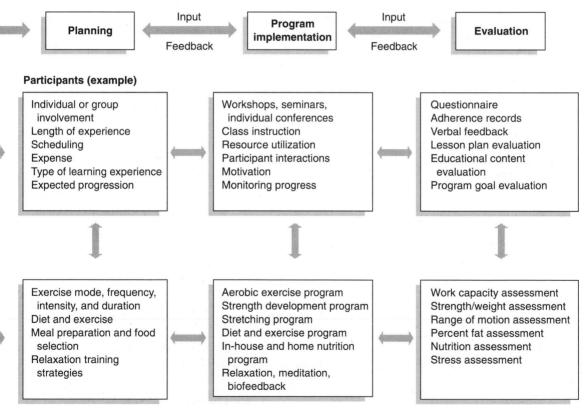

Table 2.2
Summary of health education/promotion planning models

Models (Authors, Year)					
PRECEDE (Green et al., 1980)	PRECEDE/ PROCEED (Green & Kreuter, 1991)	MHEP (Ross & Mico, 1980)	CHEM (Sullivan, 1973)	MHEPRD (Bates & Winder, 1984)	GHFDS (Patton et al., 1986)
Phase 1 Social diagnosis	Phase 1 Social diagnosis	Phase 1 Initiate	Involve people	Health education plans	Needs assessment
Phase 2 Epidem- iological diagnosis	Phase 2 Epidem- iological diagnosis	Phase 2 Needs assessment	Set goals	Demon- stration programs	Goal setting
Phase 3 Behavioral diagnosis	Phase 3 Behavioral & environmental diagnosis	Phase 3 Goal setting	Define problems	Operational programs	Planning
Phase 4–5 Educational diagnosis	Phase 4 Educational & process diagnosis	Phase 4 Planning & programming	Design plans	Research programs	Program implementation
Phase 6 Adminis- trative diagnosis	Phase 5 Administrative & policy diagnosis	Phase 5 Implementation	Conduct activities	Information & statistics	Evaluation
Phase 7 Evaluation	Phase 6 Implementation	Phase 6 Evaluation	Evaluate results	Evaluation process	Educational component
	Phase 7 Process evaluation			Various other processes	Service component
	Phase 8 Impact evaluation				
	Phase 9 Outcome evaluation				

SUMMARY

A model can provide the framework for planning and evaluating a health promotion program. Several different planning models have been developed and revised over the years. The six planning models for health education/promotion presented in this chapter are the following: PRECEDE (Predisposing, Reinforcing, and Enabling Causes in Educational Diagnosis and Evaluation); PRECEDE/PROCEED (Predisposing, Reinforcing, and Enabling Constructs in Educational/Environmental Diagnosis and Evaluation; Policy, Regulatory and Organizational Constructs in Educational and Environmental Development); MHEP (Model for Health Education Planning); CHEM (Comprehensive Health Education Model); MHEPRD (Model for Health Education Planning and Resource Development); and GHFDS (Generic Health/Fitness Delivery System). To date probably the best-known model and the one most often used in health promotion is the original PRECEDE framework; however, the others, with the exception of PRECEDE/PROCEED, have made and continue to make valuable contributions (Table 2.2). Time will tell how useful the PRECEDE/PROCEED model may become.

QUESTIONS

1. Why is it important to use a model when planning?
2. Name the six models presented in this chapter, and list one distinguishing characteristic of each.
3. Of the models presented, which one has been most commonly used? Name the different phases of this model.
4. What five or so components seem to be common to all the models? (Note that the names of the components may not be the same, but the concepts are.)

ACTIVITIES

1. After reviewing the six models presented in this chapter, create your own model by identifying what you think are the common key components of the models. Provide a rationale for including each component. Then draw a diagram of your model and put it on a transparency so that you can share it with the class. Be prepared to explain your model.
2. In a one-page paper, defend what you believe is the best planning model presented in this chapter.

3

Starting the Planning Process

After reading this chapter and answering the questions at the end, you should be able to:

❑   Explain the importance of gaining the support of decision makers.

❑   Give a rationale for planning and implementing a health promotion program.

❑   Identify the individuals who could make up a planning committee.

❑   Explain what program parameters are and the impact they have on program planning.

advisory committee

institutionalizing

organizational culture

parameter

pilot program

planning committee

program ownership

stakeholders

steering committee

vendor

Planning a health promotion program is a multiphase process. "'To plan' is to engage in a process or a procedure to develop a method for achieving an end" (Breckon, Harvey, & Lancaster, 1989, p. 95). At the start of the planning process, program planners need to gain the support of key people in order to ensure that the planning process proceeds as smoothly as possible. This chapter presents the initial steps of obtaining the support of decision makers and executives, identifying those who may be interested in helping to plan the program, and establishing the parameters in which the planners must work.

GAINING SUPPORT OF DECISION MAKERS AND EXECUTIVES

No matter what the setting of a health promotion program—whether a business, an industry, the community, a clinic, a hospital, or a school—it is most important that the program have support from the highest level (the administration, chief executive officer, or board of directors) of the "community" for which the program is being planned. These top-level people in decision-making positions are able to provide the necessary support, moral as well as financial, for the program. There will be times when the idea for, or the motivating force behind, a program comes from the top-level people. When this happens, it is a real boon for the program planners because they do not have to "sell" the idea to these people to gain their support. However, this scenario does not occur frequently.

More often than not, the idea or the big push for a health promotion program comes from someone other than one who is part of the top level of the "community." The idea could start with an employee, an interested parent, a health educator within the organization, or a concerned citizen. The idea might even be generated by an individual outside the "community," such as a **vendor** trying to sell a program to a business. When the scenario begins at a level below the decision makers, those who want to create a program must "sell" it to the decision makers. Without the support of decision makers, it becomes more difficult to plan and implement a program. Behrens (1983) has stated that health promotion programs in business and industry have a greater chance for success if all levels of management including the top, are committed and supportive. This seems to be true of health promotion programs in all settings, not just programs in business and industry.

If they need to gain the support of decision makers, program planners should develop a rationale for the program's existence. Why is it necessary to "sell" something that everyone knows is worthwhile? After all, does anyone doubt the value of trying to help people gain and maintain good health? The answer to these and similar questions is that few people are motivated by health concerns alone. Decisions by top-level management to develop new programs are based on a variety of factors, including finances, policies, public image, and politics, to name a few. Thus, to "sell" the program to those at the top, planners need to develop a rationale that shows how the new program will help those at the top to meet the organization's goals and in turn to carry out its mission. In other words, program planners need to position their program rationale politically, in line with the organization. To do this, planners need to amass as many "political data" (data that help to align the program with the organization's mission) as possible; this will enable them to put together a sound rationale to "sell" program development. There are several different sources of data that can be used in developing a rationale. One source would be the results of a needs assessment showing that such a program is needed and wanted. More than likely, a formal needs assessment will not yet have been completed, since an assessment usually takes place after permission has been given for planning to begin. However, if an assessment has been completed, data from it can be used to help develop the rationale.

The rationale for the program may also be built on the merits common to most health education/promotion programs. These merits include the following: increased awareness and knowledge; change in attitudes, such as improvement of feelings of general well-being and self-concept (Blair, Collingwood, Reynolds, Smith, Hagen, & Sterling, 1984); lowering of health risks (Spilman, Goetz, Schultz, Bellingham, & Johnson, 1986); reduction in health care costs (Bowne, Russell, Morgan, Optenberg & Clarke, 1984; Minter, 1986; Shepard, Corey, Renzland, & Cox, 1982); improvement in workers' job-related attitudes (Spilman et al., 1986); reduction in rates of absenteeism (Blair et al., 1984; Chenoweth, 1987; Cox, Shepard, & Corey, 1981); reduction in employee turnover (Chenoweth, 1987; Cox, Shepard, & Corey, 1981); lowering of health insurance premiums; reduction in numbers of workers' compensation claims (Chenoweth, 1987); fewer hospital admissions and shorter lengths of stay (Bly, Jones, & Richardson, 1986); and better health status and quality of life.

A third source of data is other successful programs that have been conducted in similar settings. For example, planners may know of other successful programs in surrounding communities, companies, or schools; the people associated with those programs may be able to provide data they generated or may be willing to share their thoughts on how they "sold" their program to those at the top. Of course, planners can always refer to successes reported in the professional literature.

A fourth source of information for a rationale is a comparison between the proposed program and the health plan for the nation. Comparing the health needs of the target population with those of other citizens of the state or of all

Table 3.1
Summary of information sources for building a rationale

1. Needs assessment data
2. Merits common to most health education/promotion programs
3. Results of other successful programs in similar settings
4. Compatibility between proposed program and the health plan of a state or the nation
5. Protecting human resources
6. What is best for the stakeholders

Americans, as outlined in the goals and objectives of the nation (USDHHS, 1990a), should enable program planners to show the compatibility between the goals of the program and those of the nation's health plan. A discussion of these national health goals and objectives is presented in Chapter 5.

When preparing a rationale to gain the support of decision makers, program planners should emphasize the importance of people as a resource to any "community." Andrew J.J. Brennan, director of Metropolitan Life Insurance Company's Center for Health Help, sums up this point nicely by stating, "People are our company's single biggest asset. It makes good business sense to invest wisely in our employees' good health" (quoted in Novelli & Ziska, 1982). In addition, planners should be sure their rationale answers the question of what is best for the **stakeholders**—those who have something to gain or lose by having or not having the program.

The sources of information for developing a rationale are summarized in Table 3.1. As a final note about trying to "sell" a program to decision makers, planners must realize that this step is most important in the planning process and should not be taken lightly. Many program ideas have "died" at this stage because the planners were not well prepared. Before making an appeal to decision makers, planners need to be thoroughly prepared. "The 'selling job' should be backed by a soundly researched idea" (McKenzie, 1988, p. 149).

IDENTIFYING A PLANNING COMMITTEE

"One very helpful method to develop a clearer and more comprehensive planning approach is to establish a committee" (Gilmore, Campbell, & Becker, 1989, p. 14). Identifying individuals who would be willing to serve as members of the **planning committee** (sometimes referred to as a **steering committee**) becomes one of the planner's first tasks. The number of individuals on a planning committee can differ depending on the setting for the program and the size of the target population. For example, the size of a planning committee for a safety belt program in a community of 50,000 people would probably be larger than that of a committee planning a similar program for a business with 50 employees. There is no ideal size for a planning committee, but the following guidelines, which have been presented earlier (McKenzie, 1988) and are given here in a modified form, should be helpful in setting up a committee.

1. Select willing individuals who are interested in seeing the program succeed. Select a combination of "doers" and "influencers."

2. Select individuals who represent a variety of groups in the target population. If possible the committee should have representation from all segments of the target population. The greater the number of individuals who are represented by committee members, the greater the chance of the target population developing a feeling of **program ownership**.

3. Ensure that the committee includes an individual who has a key role within the organization sponsoring the program, someone whose support would be most important to ensure a successful program.

4. Include representatives of other stakeholders.

5. Reevaluate committee membership regularly to ensure that the composition lends itself to fulfilling program goals and objectives.

6. Add new individuals periodically to generate new ideas and enthusiasm. It may be helpful to set a term of office for committee members.

7. Be aware of the politics that are always present in an organization or target population.

8. Make sure the committee is large enough to accomplish the work, but small enough to be able to make decisions and reach consensus. If necessary, subcommittees can be formed to handle specific tasks.

The actual means by which the committee members are chosen varies according to the setting. Commonly used techniques include: (1) asking for volunteers by word of mouth, a newsletter, a needs assessment, or other widely distributed publication; (2) holding an election, either community-wide or by subdivisions of the community; (3) inviting people to serve; and (4) having members appointed by a governing group or individual. Figure 3.1 illustrates the composition of a well-chosen planning committee.

Once the planning committee has been formed, someone must be designated to lead it. This is an important step. The leader (chairperson) "should be interested and knowledgeable about health education programs, and be organized, enthusiastic, and creative" (McKenzie, 1988, p. 149). One might think that most program planners, especially health educators, would be perfect for the committee chairperson's job. However, sometimes it is preferable to have someone other than the program planners serve in the leadership capacity. For one thing, it helps to spread out the workload of the committee. Planners who are not good at delegating responsibility may end up with a lot of extra work when they

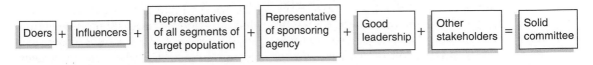

Figure 3.1
Make-up of a solid planning/steering committee

serve as the leaders. Second, having someone else serve as the leader allows the planners to remain objective about the program. And third, the planning committee can act as an **advisory committee** to the planners, if this is considered desirable.

PARAMETERS FOR PLANNING

Once the support of the decision makers has been gained and a planning committee formed, planners must identify the **parameters** within which they can work. There are several questions to which planners should have answers before they become too deeply involved in the planning process. In an earlier work (McKenzie, 1988), six such questions were presented, using the example of school-site health education/promotion programs. The six questions are modified for presentation here. It should be noted, however, that not all of the questions would be appropriate for every program because of the different circumstances of each setting.

1. What is the decision makers' philosophical perspective on health promotion programs? Do they see the programs as something important or as "extras"?

2. What type of commitment to the program are the decision makers willing to make? Are they interested in **institutionalizing** the program by making it a permanent part of the environment, or in providing a one-time or **pilot program**?

3. What type of financial support are the decision makers willing to provide? Does it include personnel for leadership and clerical duties? Released time for managing the program and participation? Space? Equipment? Materials?

4. Are the decision makers willing to consider changing the **organizational culture**? For example, are they interested in "well" days instead of sick days? Would they like to create employee smoking and safety belt policies? Change vending machine selections to more nutritious foods? Set aside an employee room for meditation? Develop a health promotion corner in the organization library?

5. Will all individuals in the target population have an opportunity to take advantage of the program, or will it only be available for certain subgroups?

6. What is the authority of the planning committee? Will it be an advisory group or a programmatic decision-making group? What will be the chain of command for program approval?

After the parameters have been defined, the planning committee should understand how the decision makers view the program, and should know what type and amount of commitment and support to expect. Setting the parameters early will save a great deal of effort and energy for the planning committee throughout the planning process.

☐ SUMMARY

Gaining the support of the decision makers is an important initial step in program planning. Planners should take great care in developing a rationale for "selling" the program idea to these important people. A planning committee can be most useful in helping with some of the planning activities and in helping to "sell" the program to the target population. Therefore, the committee should be composed of interested individuals who are representative of the target population. If the planning committee is to be effective, it will need to be aware of the parameters set for the program by the decision makers.

☐ QUESTIONS

1. Why is the support of the decision makers important in planning a program?
2. What kinds of reasons should be included in a rationale for planning and implementing a health promotion program?
3. How important is "selling" the idea of a program to decision makers?
4. Who should be selected as the members of a planning committee?
5. What are *parameters*? Give a few examples.
6. Why is it important to know the parameters at the beginning of the planning process?

☐ ACTIVITIES

1. Write a two-page rationale for "selling" a program you are planning to decision makers. Tell why the program is needed and what can be gained by having it. The rationale should be documented by citations from the appropriate literature.
2. Write a two-page rationale for beginning an exercise program for a small company with 200 employees. A needs assessment of this target population indicates that the number one cause of lost work time of this cohort is back problems and the number one cause of premature death is heart disease.
3. For a program you are planning, write a two-page description of the individuals (by position/job title, not name) who will be asked to serve on the planning committee, and provide a rationale for asking each to serve.
4. Provide a list (by position/job title, not name) and a rationale for each of the ten individuals you would ask to serve on a community-wide safety belt program. Use the town or city in which your college/university is located as the community.

5.   Below is a rationale to support a new sex education program in a school district. What do you see as the strengths of this rationale? The weaknesses? How would you change the rationale to make it stronger? Be critical. Closely examine the content, reasoning, and references.

A RATIONALE FOR OFFERING A SCHOOL SEX EDUCATION PROGRAM

The issue of sex education programs in the school systems has been debated for years. Some individuals believe they should exist while others do not. In reality, young teens and adults are entitled to and are interested in receiving accurate and effective education about their sexuality, and sexual issues as a whole. Frequently, fingers are pointed as to who should offer the sex education programs; parents to schools, schools to parents, churches to schools, churches to parents, parents to churches, and so forth. As a result of these debates the whole educational experience gets lost "in the system," and youth lose out on valuable information that can influence their entire life. Ideally, the home environment and church could be the best place for sex education to take place, but various problems can be cited with this arrangement. For instance, it can be considered that "like other subjects, sex and sexuality have become far too complex and technical to leave to the typical parent, who is either uninformed or too bashful to share useful sexual information with his child" (Hottois, 1975, p. 6). Additionally, parents and clergy members may be "too emotionally involved with the child to take a calm detached attitude toward the child's values and behaviors or to be an objective educator" (Hottois, 1975, p. 7). Effective school sex education programs can eliminate these problems and provide students with the information they require to permit them to feel comfortable with sexuality.

Appropriate school sex education programs can serve to improve and eliminate a variety of problems. Initially, sex education programs can be successful in reducing the teen pregnancy rates. Evidence shows that teen pregnancy rates can be attributed to the lack of or incorrect use of contraceptives. A study completed in 1975 found "that 70% of sexually active adolescents failed to use birth control because of such faulty assumptions as being too young to get pregnant, having sex too infrequently, or having intercourse during times of the month when fertilization was incorrectly believed to be impossible" (Geer & O'Donohue, 1987, p. 185). When individuals are provided with the correct information, they are more likely to use contraception and use it more responsibly, thus reducing the high teen pregnancy rates.

Providing students with correct and accurate information about sexuality helps them to feel more confident in their behaviors and decision-making processes. It provides them with an opportunity for growth and enables them to realize their own potential as sexual beings. It also provides them with the information they need to resist peer pressure and helps them to realize that their sexuality is their own and not something to be influenced by others.

Finally, sex education programs in the schools can be a wonderful means of creating a comfortable source of sex information to persons requiring it but not knowing where to go to obtain this information. Many teens appreciate having someone "safe" to consult about sexual issues. Parents can be too emotionally involved to provide information about a variety of topics and thus do not always serve well as a source for teens to access. Peers frequently have plenty of "sex education" to share with their friends, but certainly this is not always a reliable source.

Therefore, it is clear that there are many values to the proper sex education programs in school settings. A positive approach to sex education can help to reduce teen pregnancy rates and improve each individual's self-confidence in dealing with sex issues.

References

1.   Geer, J. H., & O'Donohue, W. T. (1987). *Theories of human sexuality*. New York: Plenum Press.

2.   Hottois, J., & Milner, N. A. (1975). *The sex education controversy*. Lexington, MA: D. C. Heath.

This rationale was written by Cathy Nickels while she was an undergraduate health science major in 1990 at Ball State University, Muncie, Indiana. It is used here by permission.

4

Assessing Needs

After reading this chapter and answering the questions at the end, you should be able to:

❑ Explain why a needs assessment must be completed.

❑ Differentiate between primary and secondary sources of target population needs.

❑ Explain how a needs assessment can be completed.

❑ Conduct a needs assessment on a given group of people.

community analysis

community diagnosis

eyeballing the data

needs assessment

networking

opinion leaders

perceived or felt needs

real needs

segmenting

service demands or wants

service needs

target population

Once the planning committee is in place, the next step in the planning process is to identify the need(s) or problem(s) of those to be served—the **target population**. Assessing the needs of the target population may be the most critical step in the planning process. Without determining the needs there is really no way to know whether a program is really warranted. Many fine programs have failed because there was no need for them. An example of such a scenario might be a program planned by a voluntary health agency that has a national goal to offer more smoking cessation programs in the workplace. If we look at the national figures, there may appear to be a need for such a program. Approximately 28% of the adult population in the United States today smokes; that figure is even higher among those who are considered a part of the labor force. So it appears that there is a need on the national level. But it is necessary to consider the local level, where the program must be implemented. What about Blue Earth County, Minnesota? Delaware County, Indiana? Wood County, Ohio? Do 28% of the adults in these counties smoke? What percentage of county residents who work in industry smoke? Do those smokers want to quit? Do employers mind if their employees smoke? Is there really a need for smoking cessation programs in these counties? No one can say for sure until a needs assessment has been completed, and even then the need for such a program may not be clear.

WHAT IS A NEEDS ASSESSMENT?

Up to this point, we have used the term **needs assessment** several different times, without defining it. Now, let's take a closer look at the term and what it means. First, it should be noted that two other terms have been used in a similar context: **community diagnosis** (Green, Kreuter, Deeds, & Partridge, 1980) and **community analysis** (Dignan & Carr, 1987). All these terms are used to describe the process by which those who are planning programs can determine what health problems might exist in any given group of people. Windsor, Baranowski, Clark, and Cutter (1984, p. 54) have defined *needs assessment* "as the process by which the program planner identifies and measures gaps between what is and what ought to be." Some might say this is the difference between a group's health status and the health care needed to improve it. Green and colleagues (1980) have indicated that a needs assessment parallels the first two phases of the PRECEDE process. "Those consist of identifying and ranking the social problems (the social quality of life diagnosis) and health problems (the epidemiological diagnosis) of a given target population" (Green et al., 1980, pp. 145–46). No matter how it is defined, the concept is the same: identifying the health needs of the target population and deciding whether or not these needs are being met.

Although determining the needs of a target population at first seems a straightforward task, planners must ask, Through whose eyes is the need determined or evaluated? Windsor and colleagues (1984) have applied the vocabulary of marketing to the needs assessment process, identifying two types of health needs. The first type is **service needs** or **real needs**. These are the things that "health professionals believe a given population must have or be able to do in order to resolve a health problem." The other type consists of the things that learners (or those in the target population) "say they must have or be able to do in order to resolve a health problem" (Windsor et al., 1984, p. 54). These needs are referred to as **service demands** or **wants** or as **perceived** or **felt needs**.

Both types of needs are important, and if either is ignored the true need of a given target population may not be understood. A program that is based entirely upon service or real needs (from the planners' point of view) may not interest or appeal to the target population even though a serious problem exists that the program could help solve. On the other hand, a program that is planned around service demands/wants or around perceived/felt needs (from the viewpoint of those being served) may not contribute to solving the real health problem. Therefore, it is important for program planners to identify both types of needs. Once this has been done, planners must blend the two to reflect both perspectives.

In addition to identifying the needs of the target population, a needs assessment can also provide valuable information that can help segment the target population according to demographic variables, such as age, gender, or socioeconomic status; behaviors, such as exercisers versus nonexercisers; and attitudes, for example, those who are for or against permitting smoking in public places. Such **segmenting** allows program planners to design programs for a specific subgroup of the target population and thus increases the program's chance of being effective. Further discussion of segmenting will be presented in Chapter 10.

CONDUCTING A NEEDS ASSESSMENT

The process of conducting a needs assessment includes gathering data about the needs of a target population, analyzing the data, and then establishing priorities for the needs, based upon the ability to meet each need and the importance of the need with regard to the health problem.

The data that are gathered can be placed into two major categories—primary data and secondary data. *Primary data* are those that are received firsthand (most likely by the planners or by someone working for them) from the target population, while *secondary data* are those "that are already available from other sources" (Windsor et al., 1984, p. 62). A group planning a worksite health promotion program might collect primary data through a questionnaire distributed to employees or use secondary data from the results of past employee physical examinations. Primary data are usually more expensive and more time consuming to collect, but these data are also the most applicable. This is not to say that primary data are necessarily better than or preferable to secondary data. Indeed, there are times when secondary data are best. There is no need to repeat a data collection process conducted by someone else if good data are already available. Data collection can be expensive, and many health education programs are planned on limited budgets; thus, in most cases the use of secondary data can save money. However, a drawback of using secondary data is that the information might not identify the true needs of the target population—perhaps because of how the data were collected, when they were collected, what variables were considered, or from whom the data were collected. A good rule is to move cautiously and make sure the secondary data are applicable to the immediate situation before using them.

A final point about primary and secondary data is that one does not need to be used exclusively in preference to the other. In most cases, a combination of both will probably provide planners with the clearest picture of the need for a program.

Having explained the general categories of data available, let's consider how a needs assessment is actually conducted. As presented here, the process includes four steps. This is not the only way to conduct a needs assessment, but it will serve to identify and explain the necessary steps. A much more complete explanation of the needs assessment process is provided by Gilmore, Campbell, and Becker (1989); more information about data collection will be presented in Chapter 15.

Step 1: Determining the Present State of Health of the Target Population

The first step in the needs assessment process involves establishing the existing conditions, that is, the present state of health of the target population. To do this, planners must consider sources of data that reflect needs from the viewpoint of the planners and also needs perceived by those in the target population. First, we will discuss data commonly used to express the needs as seen through the eyes of planners.

Service Needs or Real Needs

Epidemiological Data. This type of data describes the distribution and determinants of diseases and injuries in human populations. Planners could collect primary data through either a previously developed instrument or one developed for the specific intent of a given project. Secondary epidemiological data are available from both the federal government (U.S. Department of Health and Human Services [USDHHS]) and state and local health departments. The most common types of epidemiological data collected are figures for morbidity (incidence and prevalence), mortality, disability, and fertility. These secondary data are available free or at very low cost from the various governmental agencies; they are usually broken down for the nation, states, counties, and sometimes cities or towns.

Records of Health and Health Care.   A variety of records concerning a target population's state of health are usually available (secondary data) or can be collected (primary data) if needed and wanted. Clinical indicators, such as blood pressure, height, weight, body composition, or blood analysis, are examples of health status. Also often available are records that deal with the utilization or cost of use of medical services. These data include such items as health insurance claims paid, hospital utilization rates, visits to a doctor's office, disability benefits and insurance premiums paid, and incidental and disability absenteeism.

Health Risk Appraisals (HRA) or Health Hazard Appraisals (HHA).   The HRA/HHA, a relatively recent means of determining an individual's health risks, has also been found useful in helping determine the needs of a target population. The HRA/HHA is an instrument that requires people to answer a number of questions about their health behavior, health history, and the results of a few clinical screenings (height, weight, blood pressure, and total cholesterol count). This information is then entered into a computer that has been programmed to compare the entered data against a data base that contains information from individuals of the same gender, race, and age. The result of such a comparison tells people their risk of dying in the next ten years from the leading causes of death as compared to others of the same gender, race, and age. Most HRA/HHA computer programs are designed to provide not only individual results but also the collective results of any given group of people. The HRA/HHA can therefore provide program planners with valuable needs assessment data. Most of these instruments have been developed to determine overall health risks, but some programs are designed to calculate the risk from a single disease.

    To date several different HRA/HHA instruments have been developed. The most frequently used HRA/HHA computer program is an adaptation of the Canadian health risk appraisal developed by the U.S. Centers for Disease Control; it is now available through the Carter Center of Emory University (Amler, Moriarty, & Hutchins, 1988). It is called Healthier People. Other individuals, organizations, and companies have taken this instrument and adapted it for their own use or to market it to others. In addition to the often used HRA/HHA computer programs, several paper-and-pencil HRA/HHA instruments have been developed. Many of these are made up of relatively few questions and are intended to determine the risk of a specific disease. Some of the most readily

Table 4.1
Selected problem-specific, paper-and-pencil HRA/HHA instruments

Instrument	Available from	Type of instrument
Are You at Risk for Diabetes	American Diabetes Association	Determines risk of diabetes
Cardiovascular Risk Factor Analysis	Arizona Heart Institute	Determines potential risk of cardio-vascular disease
Cancer: Assessing Your Risks	American Cancer Society	Estimates one's risk of getting several types of cancer
Healthstyle	U.S. Department of Health & Human Services (USDHHS)	Helps identify above-normal risks related to alcohol and drugs, lack of exercise, nutrition, safety, and stress
Home Indoor Air Quality Checklist	American Lung Association	Rates the air quality in a home
Message to Teenagers	Alcoholics Anonymous World Services, Inc.	Helps young people determine if they have a drinking problem
Risk Test for Smokers	American Cancer Society Minnesota Division, Inc.	Estimates risk of heart disease, lung cancer, and chronic obstructive lung disease
Risko	American Heart Association	Estimates one's risk of heart disease

available paper-and-pencil HRA/HHA instruments are presented in Table 4.1. One of these instruments was developed to calculate overall risk as opposed to the risk of a specific disease. That instrument, *Healthstyle: A Self-Test* (see Appendix B), was developed by USDHHS (n. d.).

Although this discussion has revolved around the use of HRAs/HHAs as means of providing information for a needs assessment, they have also been used in recent years for other purposes: to help motivate people to act on their health, to increase awareness, to serve as cues to action, and to contribute to program evaluation. However, it should be noted that the instruments were originally developed for physicians to use as an educational tool with their patients. The expanded use of these instruments has prompted several researchers (Alexy, 1985; Best & Milsum, 1978; Elias & Dunton, 1981; Sachs, Krushat, & Newman, 1980; Smith, McKinlay, & McKinlay, 1989) to question the reliability of HRA/HHA data (see Chapter 14 for a discussion of reliability). In general, it has been found that (1) the reliability of HRA/HHA risk scores can vary greatly from one instrument to another; (2) reliability scores decrease when users calculate their own score as opposed to computer scoring; (3) there is a great variance in the self-reporting of specific risk factors and clinical physiologic measurements; and (4) only those HRAs/HHAs for which reliability can be demonstrated should be used for evaluating the effectiveness of health education.

Information from Significant Others.   Another useful means of obtaining data for the needs assessment of a target population is to collect information from the significant others of the target population. Significant others may include family members, friends, community leaders, or religious leaders. Collecting data from the significant others of a group of heart disease patients is a good example. Program planners might find it difficult to persuade the heart disease patients themselves to share information about their outlook on life and living with heart disease. A survey of spouses or other family members might help elicit this information so the program planners could best meet the needs of the heart disease patients.

Examining Current Literature.   Program planners might also be able to identify the needs of a target population by reviewing any available current literature about that target population. An example would be a planner who is developing a health promotion program for individuals infected by the Human Immunodeficiency Virus (HIV). Because of the relative newness and seriousness of this disease and the number of people who have studied and written about it, there is a good chance that present literature could reflect the need of a certain target population.

Service Demands/Wants or Perceived/Felt Needs

The data sources already discussed are commonly used to determine the state of health of the target population as seen through the eyes of the planners. There are also several techniques planners can use to determine the state of health of the community from the viewpoint of those in the target population—in other words, to determine service demands and wants, and perceived or felt needs.

Community Forum.   Put simply, the community forum approach brings together people from the target population to discuss what they see as their group's health problems. It is not uncommon for a community forum to be organized by a group representing the target population, in conjunction with the program planners. Such groups include labor, civic, religious, or service organizations, or groups like the Parent Teacher Association (PTA) or Parent Teacher Organization (PTO). Once people have arrived, a moderator explains the purpose of the meeting and then asks those from the target population to share their concerns. One or several individuals from the organizing group, called recorders, are usually given the responsibility for taking notes or taping the session to ensure that the responses are recorded accurately. However, when moderating a community forum it is important to be aware that the silent majority may not speak out and/or a vocal minority may speak too loudly. For example, an individual parent's view may be wrongly interpreted to be the view of all parents.

　　At a community forum, participants may also be asked to respond in writing (1) by answering specific questions or (2) by completing some type of

Directions: Please rank the need for each program in the community by placing a number in the space to the left of the programs. Use *1* to rank the program of greatest need, *2* for the next greatest need, and so forth, until you have ranked all seven programs. The program with the highest number next to it should be the one that, in your opinion, is least needed. If you feel that a program should not be considered for implementation in our community, please place an *X* in the space to the left of the program instead of a number. Please note that the number you place next to each program represents its need in the community, not necessarily your desire to participate in it. After ranking the program, place an *X* to the right of the program in the column(s) that represents the age group(s) to which you feel the program should be targeted.

Program	All ages	Children 5-12	Teens 13-19	Adults 20-64	Older adults 65+
_____ Alcohol education:	_____	_____	_____	_____	_____
_____ Exercise/fitness:	_____	_____	_____	_____	_____
_____ Nutrition education:	_____	_____	_____	_____	_____
_____ Safety belt use:	_____	_____	_____	_____	_____
_____ Smoking cessation:	_____	_____	_____	_____	_____
_____ Smoking education:	_____	_____	_____	_____	_____
_____ Weight loss:	_____	_____	_____	_____	_____

Figure 4.1
Instrument for ranking program need (Modified from a form developed by Amy Lynn Bernard, a graduate assistant in health science at Ball State University, 1991. Adapted by permission.)

instrument. Figure 4.1 is an example of an instrument that could be used to collect data from a group of people.

Focus Group.   Focus groups are a form of qualitative research that grew out of group therapy. They are used to obtain information about the feelings, opinions, perceptions, insights, beliefs, misconceptions, attitudes, and receptivity of a group of people concerning an idea or issue. Focus groups are rather small compared to community forums and usually include only 8–12 people. If possible, it is best to have a group of people who do not know each other so that their responses are not inhibited by acquaintance. Participation in the group is by invitation. People are invited about one to three weeks in advance of the session. At the time of the invitation, they receive general information about the session but are not given the specifics. This precaution helps ensure that responses will be on target yet spontaneous.

Once assembled, the group is led by a skilled moderator who has the task of obtaining candid responses from the group to a set of predetermined questions. In addition to eliciting reponses to the questions, the moderator may ask the group to prioritize the different responses. As in a community forum, the answers to the questions are recorded either through written notes and/or audio or video recordings, so that at a later date the interested parties can review and interpret the results.

For any one project, it may be necessary to hold several different focus groups to collect the needed information. For example, if planners are using focus groups to find out what the people in the community think about a proposed sex education curriculum, it would be helpful to organize focus groups based on the beliefs of certain subsets within the target population. Otherwise, if liberals were brought together with conservatives or pro-choice advocates were brought together with pro-life people, the focus groups would turn into shouting matches and little would be accomplished. Usually, the more controversial the topic, the greater the need to organize several focus groups with segments of the population.

Focus groups are not easy to conduct. Special care must be given to developing the questions that will be asked. Poorly written questions will yield information that is less than useful. In addition, the facilitator should be one who is skilled in leading a group. As might be surmised, the level of skill needed to conduct a focus group increases as the topic of discussion becomes more controversial.

Although focus groups have been shown to be an effective way of gathering data, they do have one major limitation. Participants in the groups are usually not selected through a random-sampling process. They are generally selected because they possess certain attributes (individuals of low income, city dwellers, parents of disabled children, or chief executive officers of major corporations). Participants are typical, not representative, of the target population. Therefore, the results of the focus group are not generalizable. "Findings [of focus groups] should be interpreted as suggestive and directional rather than as definitive" (Schechter, Vanchieri, & Crofton, 1990, p. 254.)

The steps noted below outline the sequence of events when a focus group, comprising college administrators and student leaders, was organized to determine what topics should be covered in a substance abuse program that was to be conducted on a college campus. The question posed to those in the focus group was, If you were in charge of a drug abuse education and prevention program on a college campus, what would be the specific content areas (or major topics) of the modules? Participants were given 15 minutes to write down their responses (without limit). This was done in silence.

After the people had written down their responses, they were asked to share their responses in a round-robin fashion. The leader (moderator) recorded the responses on a chalkboard. This continued until all responses were shared. No discussion was permitted during this time.

The meaning of the various responses was clarified without participants being able to lobby for a certain response. A preliminary vote of priority was then taken by having the participants rank-order the responses. The leader took the rank ordering and created a priority list. Finally, the results were discussed.

Opinion Leaders' Survey.   In a manner similar to a community forum or a focus group, planners can collect information from a specific subgroup within the target population—the **opinion leaders**. These are the individuals who are well respected in a community and who have an overall view of its needs. These leaders are: (1) active users of the media; (2) demographically similar to the target group; (3) knowledgeable about community issues and concerns; (4) early adopters of innovative behavior (see Chapter 10 for an explanation of these terms); and (5) active in persuading others to become involved in innovative behavior. Opinion leaders include political figures, chief executive officers (CEOs) of companies, union leaders, administrators of local school districts, and other highly respected individuals.

Surveying the Target Population.   Surveying the target population or a representative sample of it may be one of the best means of determining the needs of the target population. However, it can also be one of the most expensive means of collecting information about needs. If appropriate data on a given target population are already available, obviously it would be less expensive to use those data than to collect new data.

The most commonly used means of surveying the target population are by paper-and-pencil questionnaires, telephone interviews, or face-to-face interviews (see Table 15.1 for a comparison of the advantages and disadvantages of these techniques). The means used to collect the data are probably not as important as the specific procedures used. When collecting data, planners must take the necessary steps to ensure that the data collected are representative of the target population. The concept of representativeness will be discussed later (see Chapter 15), but two major questions that must be considered are (1) how the survey sample is chosen, and (2) whether the data collection instrument is valid and reliable. A valid instrument is one that measures what it is supposed to measure. A reliable instrument is one that will provide consistent results in subsequent uses. One other point should be noted here about surveying the target population: it provides an opportunity to obtain answers to marketing questions as well as questions of needs. Marketing questions might be concerned with the best location for the program, the best time of day, and how much participants would be willing to pay to participate.

Fieldwork and Observation.   Another means by which program planners can collect needs information "through the eyes of the consumer" is by actually watching the target population. The planners or their workers can become a part of the day-to-day events where the health problems may occur, so that they can observe the actions of the target population. Examples of such fieldwork may include watching the eating patterns of teachers in a school lunchroom, observing to see if the workers on an assembly line are wearing their protective glasses, checking the smoking behavior of employees on break, and observing community members for safety belt use.

Although each needs assessment is different, the types of information usually generated from this first step of determining the present state of health of

Table 4.2
Sources of needs assessment data

Service Needs or Real Needs: Through the Eyes of the Planners

1. Epidemiological data
2. Records of health and health care
3. Health risk appraisals/health hazard appraisals (HRAs/HHAs)
4. Information from significant others
5. Examination of current literature

Service Demands/Wants or Perceived/Felt Needs: Through the Eyes of the Target Population

1. Community forum
2. Focus group
3. Opinion leaders' survey
4. Survey of target population
5. Fieldwork and observation

the target population could include data describing: demographics, disease incidence, disease prevalence, health awareness, health attitudes, health knowledge, health skills, health behavior, health risks, health interests, health history, and marketing information. With these data, planners would be in a good position to segment the target population (Table 4.2).

Step 2: Determining the Status of Available Health Promotion Programs

The second step of the needs assessment process must be completed in order to avoid duplication of existing programs. This step of the process, like the first, is also an information-seeking procedure. In this step, program planners seek to determine the status of existing health promotion programs by trying to answer as many questions as possible from the following list:

1. What health promotion programs are presently available to the target population?
2. Are the programs being utilized? If not, why not?
3. How effective are the programs? Are they meeting their stated goals and objectives?
4. How were the needs for these programs determined?
5. Are the programs accessible to the target population? Where are they located? When are they offered? Are there any qualifying criteria that people must meet to enroll? Can the target population get to the programs? Can the target population afford the programs?
6. Are the needs of the target population being met?

There are several ways to seek answers to these questions. Probably the most common way is through **networking** with other people working in health promotion and the health care system—that is, communicating with others who may know about existing programs. (See Chapter 8 for a more detailed discussion of networking.) These people may be located in the local or state health department, in voluntary health agencies, or in health care facilities, such as hospitals, clinics, nursing homes, extended care facilities, or Health Maintenance Organizations (HMOs).

Planners might also find information about existing programs by checking with someone in an organization that serves as a clearinghouse for health promotion programs or by using a community resource guide. The local or state health department, a local chamber of commerce, a coalition, the local medical/dental societies, a community task force, or a community health center may serve as a clearinghouse or produce such a guide. Another avenue is to talk with people in the target population. Although they may not know about all existing programs, they may be able to share information on the effectiveness and accessibility of some of the programs. Finally, some of the information could be collected in step 1 through separate community forums, focus groups, or surveys.

Step 3: Determining the Need or Measuring the Gaps Between Health Status and Health Promotion and Care

At this point in the needs assessment process, the planners must analyze all the data collected in steps 1 and 2. The analysis of the data may be formal or informal. The approach used would depend upon what data were collected and how exact the planners wanted to be. Formal analysis would consist of some type of statistical analysis. This approach could only be used when appropriate statistical criteria (see any introductory statistics book) have been met. Much of the time, a less formal means of analyzing the data is used. This approach is commonly referred to as **eyeballing the data**—that is, looking at the data for obvious differences between health status, and health promotion and care. As Windsor and colleagues (1984, p. 54) have stated, eyeballing the data means looking for differences between "what is and what ought to be."

Sometimes this third step in the needs assessment process is not very complicated because the need is obvious. For example, breast cancer rates may have risen in a given community, the number of breast screenings may be low, and the consumers may recognize this. Or, in another setting, the planners may find a direct correlation between the health status of a community and the lack of health care. However, not all needs assessments yield an obvious problem. The data may be mixed or confusing. In such cases it is probably a good idea to see if additional data might be collected to paint a clearer picture. If obtaining additional data does not help, then asking other professionals for their opinions or relying on one's own "gut reactions" may aid in reaching a conclusion.

What conclusion should planners be looking for? At the end of step 3, the planners should be able to list the problems, with a description of the nature and extent of each.

Step 4: Dealing with the Problems

This fourth step in the needs assessment process will set the program direction. Step 3 identified the problems; step 4 is the stage at which planners will prioritize them. With limited funding it is unlikely that all exposed problems can be dealt with, so planners need to see how the health promotion dollar can best be used. Therefore, in setting priorities, the planners should seek answers to these questions: (1) What is the most pressing need? (2) Are there resources adequate to deal with the problem? (3) Can the problem best be solved by a health promotion intervention, or could it be handled better through administration, politics, or changes in the economy? (4) Can the problem be solved in a reasonable amount of time?

After answering these questions, the planners should be able to prioritize the identified problems. If help is needed, planners may want to turn to the target population or key people from the community to rank-order the identified needs.

Step 5: Validating the Need

The final step in the needs assessment process is to validate the identified need(s). By *validate*, we mean to confirm that the need that was identified is the need that should be addressed. Obviously, if great care was taken in the needs assessment process, validation should be a perfunctory step. However, there have been times when a need was not properly validated; much energy and many resources have thereby been wasted on unnecessary programs.

Validation amounts to "double checking" or making sure that an identified need is the real need. Any means available can be used, such as (1) rechecking the steps followed in the needs assessment to eliminate any bias; (2) conducting a focus group with some individuals from the target population to determine their reaction to the identified need (if a focus group was not used earlier to gather the data); and (3) getting a "second opinion" from other health professionals.

☐ SUMMARY

Presented in this chapter is a five-step approach that health planners can follow in conducting a needs assessment on a given group of people. It is by no means the only way of conducting an assessment, but it is workable.

No matter what procedure is used to conduct a needs assessment, the end result should be the same. Planners should finish with a list of clearly defined, prioritized problems of the target population.

☐ QUESTIONS

1. What does *needs assessment* mean?
2. Why must a needs assessment be viewed through the eyes of both the planners and the consumers?
3. What is a health risk appraisal/health hazard appraisal (HRA/HHA)?
4. What advice might you give to someone who is interested in using previously collected data (secondary data) for a needs assessment?
5. What are the five steps in the needs assessment process, as identified in the chapter?
6. Explain the difference between a community forum and a focus group.

☐ ACTIVITIES

1. Assume that you have been hired by the board of trustees of your college or university to conduct a needs assessment on the student body for the possibility of developing a health promotion program. Assume that there are few existing data on this group of people, other than national norms for college students. You could conduct a "university forum" or hold a series of focus groups, but instead you have decided to survey a random sample of the population with a paper-and-pencil instrument. Your task now is to develop a needs assessment instrument. When developing the instrument, use questions that will collect data that are reflective of your target population's awareness of health, attitudes about health, knowledge of health, health behavior, health interests, and demographics, as well as marketing possibilities. After completing the instrument, pilot test it on 10 students (for the purposes of this assignment, this does not need to be a random group). Use the results of the pilot test to complete steps 3 and 4 in the needs assessment process.

2. Develop a needs assessment instrument for a program you will be planning. Collect the same type of data noted in activity 1, administer the instrument to a small group of people, then complete steps 3 and 4 in the needs assessment process.

3. Using previously collected data provided by your instructor (such as data from a Behavioral Risk Factor Survey, state or local secondary data, or data from the National Center for Health Statistics), analyze the data and determine the needs of the target population. Finally, prioritize the needs using the criteria noted in step 4 of the needs assessment process.

4. Administer an HHA/HRA to a group of 25–30 people. Using the data generated, identify and prioritize a collective list of health problems of the group.

5. Plan and conduct a focus group on an identified health problem on your campus. Develop a set of questions to be used, identify and invite people

to participate in the group, facilitate the process, and then write up a summary of the results based upon your written notes and an audio tape of the session.

6.   Using the data (paper-and-pencil instruments, clinical tests, and health histories) generated from a local health fair, identify and prioritize a collective list of health problems of those who participated.

5

Statement of Purpose, Program Goals, and Objectives

After reading this chapter and answering the questions at the end, you should be able to:

❑   Explain what is meant by the term *statement of purpose*.

❑   Define goals and objectives, and distinguish between the two.

❑   Identify the different levels of objectives as presented in the chapter.

❑   State the necessary elements of an objective as presented in the chapter.

❑   Specify appropriate criteria for objectives.

❑   Write program goals and objectives.

KEY TERMS

attitudes   objectives

awareness   outcomes

behavior   risk reduction

conditions   skill development

criteria   statement of purpose

goal   target population

knowledge

To plan, implement, and evaluate effective health promotion programs, planners must have a solid foundation in place to guide them through their work. The statement of purpose, goals, and objectives of a program can provide such a foundation. If prepared properly, a statement of purpose, goals, and objectives should not only give the necessary direction to a program but also provide the groundwork for the eventual program evaluation. There are two old sayings that help express the need for a statement of purpose, goals, and objectives. The first is, If you do not know where you are going, then any road will do—and you will end up someplace where you do not want to be. The second is, If you do not know where you are going, how will you know when you have arrived? Without a statement of purpose, goals, and objectives, a program may lack direction, and at best it will be difficult to evaluate. Figure 5.1 shows the relationship between a statement of purpose, goals, and objectives.

STATEMENT OF PURPOSE

Sometimes referred to as a program overview or program aim, a **statement of purpose** is a short narrative that describes the general focus of the program. The statement not only describes the intent of a program but also may reflect the philosophy behind it. The statement of purpose also helps to guide program planners in the development of program goals and objectives. Table 5.1 presents examples of statements of purpose for several different settings.

Figure 5.1
Relationship of statement of
purpose, goals, and objectives

Table 5.1
Examples of statements of purpose

Clinical Setting

This program is aimed at helping patients and their families to understand and cope with physical and emotional changes associated with recovery following cancer surgery.

School Setting

School District #77 wants happy and healthy students. To that end the district's personnel strives, through a comprehensive school health program, to provide students with experiences that are designed to motivate and enable them to maintain and improve their health.

Worksite Setting

The purpose of the employee health promotion program is to develop high employee morale. This is to be accomplished by providing employees with a working environment that is conducive to good health and by providing an opportunity for employees to engage in behavior that will improve and maintain good health.

PROGRAM GOALS

Although some individuals use the terms *goals* and *objectives* synonymously, there are important differences between them. Ross and Mico (1980, p. 219) have stated that "a goal is a future event toward which a committed endeavor is directed; objectives are the steps to be taken in pursuit of a goal." In comparison to objectives, a **goal** is an expectation that (1) is much more encompassing, or global; (2) is written to include all aspects or components of a program; (3) provides overall direction for a program; (4) is more general in nature; (5) usually takes longer to complete (weeks, months, or even years); (6) usually is not observed, but rather must be inferred because it includes words like *evaluate, know, improve,* and *understand* (Jacobsen, Eggen & Kauchak, 1989); and (7) is often not measurable in exact terms.

Goals state what should happen as a result of the program. In other words, a goal should state what will be accomplished. Program goals are not difficult to write and need not be written as complete sentences. They should, however, be simple and concise, and should include two basic components: who will be affected, and what will change as a result of the program. A program need not have a set number of stated goals. It is not uncommon for some programs to have a single goal while others have several. Here are some examples of goals for health promotion programs.

1. To improve the health status of the employees of the Smith Company.

2. Those in the target population will understand the importance of good health.

3. Program participants will appreciate the rights of both smokers and non-smokers.

4.   The technicians will know how to handle emergency situations.

5.   The patients will be able to apply principles of good nutrition.

PROGRAM OBJECTIVES

As Ross and Mico (1980) have indicated, program **objectives** are more precise and represent smaller steps than program goals—steps that, if completed, will lead to reaching the program goal(s). Program objectives outline the specific changes that will occur in the target population as a result of exposure to the program. Objectives can be thought of as the bridge between needs assessment and a planned intervention. Knowing how to construct objectives for a program is a most important skill for program planners.

Different Levels of Objectives

The projected **outcomes**—the objectives—of any program depend upon several variables. These include, but are not limited to: the purpose of the program, the target population being served, the availability of other programs that have similar purposes, and the availability of appropriate program resources. For example, some programs are planned just to raise awareness, while others are aimed at trying to help individuals change their behavior, and still others are intended to improve access to health care. It is reasonable to expect that the amount of effort and resources necessary to increase people's awareness would almost always be less than that required to help change behavior. The objectives for the two kinds of programs would take different foci.

To deal with these different program foci, a group of health educators (Parkinson & Associates, 1982) developed a framework or hierarchy of program objectives or outcomes. This hierarchy includes six different levels of program objectives, beginning with the least complex and moving toward the most complex. Complexity is defined in terms of time and resources needed to reach the objective. The six levels include: (1) increase in awareness; (2) increase in knowledge; (3) change in attitudes; (4) change in behavior; (5) reduction in risk; and (6) reduction in morbidity and mortality. Although we believe this is a valid hierarchy, our experience would suggest that two more levels should be added, and that the sixth level, reduction in morbidity and mortality, should be renamed and called health status. We believe that the new levels should be added to the hierarchy between level 3, change in attitudes, and level 4, change in behavior. The first level to be added is the development of health skills. This is an important level, and one that is often forgotten in health promotion programs. For a target population to move through this hierarchy and change their behavior, individuals need more than just awareness, knowledge, and a positive attitude; they also need the appropriate skills. It is our belief that this holds true for any health behavior (managing stress, stopping smoking, eating right, taking insulin injections, losing weight, or wearing safety belts).

The second level to be added, which should come right after development of health skills and before change in behavior, is available health services. Those in the target population may be aware and may possess the necessary knowledge, the right attitudes, and the necessary skills, but if needed health services are not available to them they cannot behave in a "healthy" manner. In view of these additions, we present here a modified hierarchy with an explanation of each of its levels.

1. Increase in **awareness**—making those in the target population aware or more aware of what is appropriate health behavior.

2. Increase in **knowledge**—providing people with more information for the purpose of expanding their understanding of a health concern.

3. Change in **attitudes**—helping people attain and maintain a positive attitude toward healthy behavior.

4. Development of health skills—developing the skills necessary for behavior change and improvement of health status. Examples of **skill development** are measurement of blood pressure, self-examination of breasts or testicles, the ability to put together a balanced meal, or application of the principles of aerobic exercise.

5. Available health services—providing access to the necessary health services, whether prevention, diagnosis, care/treatment, or rehabilitation.

6. Change in **behavior**—participating in health behavior that can lead to better health.

7. Reduction in risk—lowering individual risk to a certain disease or illness by engaging in specific **risk reduction** behaviors.

8. Improving health status—changing health status because of reduction of risk (often measured in clinical terms).

Developing Program Objectives

Does every program require objectives from each of the eight levels described here? The answer is no. Most successful programs, however, will have multiple program objectives. Too often, health promotion programs have too few objectives, all of which fall into one or two levels of the hierarchy. Many planners have developed programs hoping solely to change the health behavior of a target population. For example, a smoking cessation program may have an objective of getting 30% of the participants to stop smoking. Perhaps this program is offered, and only 10% of the participants quit smoking. Is the program a failure? If the program has a single objective of changing behavior, its sponsors would have a good case for saying the program was not effective. However, it is quite possible that as a result of participating in the smoking cessation program, the participants increased their awareness of the dangers of smoking. They probably also increased their knowledge, changed their attitudes, and developed skills for quitting or cutting back on the number of cigarettes they smoke each day. These are all very positive outcomes—and they could be overlooked when the program is evaluated, if the planner did not write program objectives that cover a variety of levels of the hierarchy.

Criteria for Developing Objectives

In addition to making sure that the objectives are written in an appropriate manner, planners also need to be realistic with regard to the other parameters of the program. These are some of the questions that program planners should consider when writing objectives.

1. Can the objective be realized during the life of the program or within a reasonable time thereafter? It would be quite realistic to assume that a certain number of people will not be smoking one year after they have completed a smoking cessation program, but it would not be realistic to assume that a group of elementary school students could be followed for life to determine how many of them die prematurely due to inactivity.

2. Can the objective realistically be achieved? It is probably realistic to assume that 30% of any smoking cessation class will stop smoking within one year after the program has ended, but it is not realistic to assume that 100% of the employees of a company will participate in its fitness program.

3. Does the program have enough resources (personnel, money, and space) to obtain a specific objective? It would be ideal to be able to reach all individuals in the target population, but generally there are not sufficient resources to do so.

4. Are the objectives consistent with the policies and procedures of the sponsoring agency? It would not be realistic to expect to incorporate a no-smoking policy in a tobacco company.

5. Do the objectives violate any of the rights of those who are involved (participants or planners)? Right-to-know laws make it illegal to withhold information that could cause harm to a target population.

Elements of an Objective

For an objective to provide direction and to be useful in the evaluation process, it must be written in such a way that it can be clearly understood, states what is to be accomplished, and is measurable. To ensure that an objective is indeed useful it should include the following elements: (1) the outcome to be achieved; (2) the conditions under which the outcome will be observed; (3) the criteria for deciding whether the outcome has been achieved; and (4) the target population. The first element, the **outcome**, is defined as the action or behavior that will occur as a result of the program. In a written objective, the outcome is usually identified as the verb of the sentence. Thus words such as *apply, argue, build, compare, demonstrate, evaluate, exhibit, judge, perform, recall, spend, state,* and *test* would be considered outcomes (see Table 5.2 for a more comprehensive listing of appropriate outcome words). It should be noted that not all verbs would be considered appropriate outcomes for an objective; the verb must be measurable and observable. Words such as *know* or *understand* by themselves are not measurable and observable, and therefore they are not good choices for outcomes.

Table 5.2
Outcome verbs for program objectives

abstract	copy	form	observe	round
accept	count	gather	offer	score
adjust	create	(information)	order	seek
adopt	criticize	generalize	organize	select
advocate	deduce	generate	pair	separate
analyze	defend	group	participate	share
annotate	define	guess	partition	show
apply	delay	hypothesize	perform	simplicity
approximate	(response)	identify	persist	simulate
argue	demonstrate	illustrate	plan	solve
(a position)	derive	imitate	practice	spend
ask	describe	improve	praise	(money)
associate	design	infer	predict	state
attempt	determine	initiate	prepare	structure
balance	develop	inquire	preserve	submit
build	differentiate	integrate	produce	subscribe
calculate	discover	interpolate	propose	substitute
categorize	discriminate	interpret	prove	suggest
cause	dispute	invent	qualify	summarize
challenge	distinguish	investigate	query	supply
change	effect	join	question	support
choose	eliminate	judge	recall	symbolize
clarify	enumerate	justify	recite	synthesize
classify	estimate	keep	recognize	tabulate
collect	evaluate	label	recommend	tally
combine	examine	list	record	test
compare	exemplify	locate	regulate	theorize
complete	exhibit	manipulate	reject	translate
compute	experiment	map	relate	try
conceptualize	explain	match	reorganize	unite
connect	express	measure	repeat	visit
construct	extend	name	replace	volunteer
consult	extract	obey	represent	weigh
contrast	extrapolate	object	reproduce	write
convert	find	(to an idea)	restructure	

The second element of an objective is the **conditions** under which the outcome will be observed. That is, when, where, or how will the outcome be observed? "Typical" conditions found in objectives might be "upon completion of the exercise class," "as a result of participation," "after reading the pamphlets and brochures," "orally in class," "when asked to respond by the facilitator," "one year after the program," or "during the class session."

The third element of an objective is the **criteria** for deciding when the outcome has been achieved. The purpose of this element is to provide a standard by which the program planners/evaluators can determine if an outcome has been performed in an appropriate and/or successful manner. Examples might include

Figure 5.2
Elements of a well-written objective

"with a 100% accuracy," "as presented in the lecture," "according to the criteria developed by the American Heart Association," or "using the technique outlined in the American Cancer Society's pamphlet."

The last element that needs to be included in an objective is mention of the **target population** for whom the outcome is intended. Examples are "1,000 teachers," "all employees of the company," and "those residing in the Muncie and Bowling Green areas." Figure 5.2 summarizes the key elements in an objective.

EXAMPLES OF PROGRAM GOALS AND OBJECTIVES

It might be helpful at this point to review some objectives that have been written to support a typical program goal. The objectives presented here include the four basic elements and have been written so as to cover the eight levels in our modified hierarchy. The program goal is to provide a company's employees with the opportunity to become more knowledgeable about cardiovascular health and to participate in a regular exercise program.

❑   *Objective for the awareness level:* After the American Heart Association's pamphlet on cardiovascular health risk factors has been distributed along with payroll checks, at least 50% of the employees will be able to identify their own risk factors.

Outcome: Identify their own risk factors.

Conditions: After distribution of the pamphlet.

Criteria: 50%.

Target population: The employees.

❑   *Objective for the knowledge level:* When asked in class, those employees attending "brown bag" lunch sessions will be able to explain the four principles of cardiovascular conditioning with 100% accuracy.

Outcome: Explain the four principles of cardiovascular conditioning.

Conditions: When asked in class.

Criteria: 100% accuracy.

Target population: Those employees attending the "brown bag" lunch sessions.

❑   *Objective for the attitude level:* During one of the class lectures, the participants will be asked to defend their views about the importance of aerobic exercise using facts learned in previous class sessions.

Outcome: Defend their feelings.

Conditions: During one of the class sessions.

Criteria: Using facts learned in previous class sessions.

Target population: The class participants.

❑ *Objective for the skill development level:* After the orientation session, "How to Exercise," those participating will be able to find and count their pulse for 60 seconds each time they are asked to do so.

Outcome: Find and count their pulse for 60 seconds.

Conditions: After the orientation session, "How to exercise."

Criteria: Each time they are asked to do so.

Target population: Those participating.

❑ *Objective for available health services level:* Within two weeks of the blood cholesterol awareness campaign, the employer will sponsor at least one additional blood cholesterol screening session for its employees.

Outcome: Sponsor blood cholesterol screening.

Conditions: Within two weeks of the blood cholesterol awareness campaign.

Criteria: At least one additional session.

Target population: Employees.

❑ *Objective for the behavior level:* One year after the formal exercise classes have been completed, 40% of those who completed 80% of the classes will still be involved in a regular aerobic exercise program as defined in class.

Outcome: Will still be involved in a regular aerobic exercise program.

Conditions: One year after the formal exercise classes have been completed.

Criteria: 40% and as defined in class.

Target population: Those who completed 80% of the classes.

❑ *Objective for the risk reduction level:* Half of all those employees who complete a regular, aerobic, 12-month exercise program will reduce their "risk age" on their follow-up health risk appraisal by a minimum of two years as compared to the results of their preprogram health risk appraisal.

Outcome: Will reduce their "risk age" on their follow-up health risk appraisal.

Conditions: After completion of a regular, aerobic, 12-month exercise program.

Criteria: As compared to the results of their preprogram health risk appraisal.

Target population: Employees.

❑ *Objective for health status:* Those employees who participate in the formal exercise and fitness program will use 10% fewer sick days during the life of the program than those employees who do not participate.

Outcome: Use fewer sick days.

Conditions: During the life of the program.

Criteria: 10% fewer sick days than those who do not participate.

Target population: Employees.

GOALS AND OBJECTIVES FOR THE NATION

A chapter on goals and objectives would not be complete without at least a short discussion of the health goals and objectives of the nation. These goals and objectives have been most helpful to program planners throughout the United States.

The U.S. government is very interested in improving the health status of Americans. It is concerned about individuals and the population as a whole. The country is facing many problems and issues that revolve around health; the cost of ill health is the most obvious. Therefore, for at least some parts of the federal government, there is a goal to improve the health status of the public. Objectives have been developed to guide the work of reaching this goal. Some people have referred to these statements of objectives as the health plan for the United States.

The first set of objectives was developed by many health professionals throughout the country; it was published in 1980 under the title, *Promoting Health/Preventing Disease: Objectives for the Nation* (USDHHS, 1980). This volume was divided into three main areas: preventive services, health protection, and health promotion. Each of these contained 5 focus areas, or 15 in all. From these 15 areas came a total of 226 objectives. These objectives, which were based upon the data collected for the U.S. surgeon general's report *Healthy People* (1979), were the basis for health promotion and disease prevention planning during the 1980s.

Data for 1987 give evidence that nearly half of those objectives had been achieved or were likely to be achieved by 1990, while about a quarter were unlikely to be achieved; the status of the remaining quarter was in doubt because tracking data were not available. Progress was slow for some of the 15 priorities identified in 1980, such as pregnancy and infant health, nutrition, physical fitness and exercise, family planning, sexually transmitted diseases, and occupational safety and health. Substantial progress was made, however, in high blood pressure control, immunization, unintentional injury prevention and control, control of infectious diseases, smoking, and alcohol and drugs (Mason & McGinnis, 1990, p. 442).

As the 1980s came to a close, it was obvious from the evaluation conducted on these national goals and objectives (USDHHS, 1986) that there was a need to develop new goals and objectives to guide the country through the 1990s. Therefore, a second set of goals and objectives (USDHHS, 1990a) was developed. The newest set is much more detailed than the first and should be more useful to all program planners. The three broad goals for public health over the next 10 years are: (1) increase the span of healthy life for Americans; (2) reduce health disparities among Americans; and (3) achieve access to preventive services for all Americans (Mason & McGinnis, 1990). As in the previous version, the new objectives are still divided into 3 categories—preventive services, health protection, and health promotion—but now there are 22 priority areas and approximately 300 objectives to chart the direction of public health over the decade (Mason & McGinnis, 1990). Within the 22 priority areas are guidelines for surveillance and data systems and suggested actions that individuals and community organizations should take in pursuit of these goals and objectives. Table 5.3 lists the 22 priority areas and the lead governmental agency or agencies responsible for working toward the accomplishment of the objective. In addition, a companion document, *Healthy Communities 2000: Model Standards,* has been prepared jointly by the American Public Health Association, American Society of State and Territorial Health Officers, National Association of County Health Officers, U.S. Conference of Local Health Officers, and the Association of Schools of Public Health (1991), in

Table 5.3
Twenty-two priority areas of the national health objectives and the lead governmental agencies responsible for each

1. Physical activity and fitness—President's Council on Physical Fitness and Sports.
2. Nutrition—Food and Drug Administration; National Institutes of Health.
3. Tobacco—Centers for Disease Control.
4. Alcohol and other drugs—Alcohol, Drug Abuse, and Mental Health Administration.
5. Family planning—Office of Population Affairs.
6. Mental health—Alcohol, Drug Abuse, and Mental Health Administration.
7. Violent and abusive behavior—Centers for Disease Control.
8. Educational and community-based programs—Centers for Disease Control; Health Resources and Services Administration.
9. Unintentional injuries—Centers for Disease Control.
10. Occupational safety and health—Centers for Disease Control.
11. Environmental health—Centers for Disease Control; National Institutes of Health.
12. Food and drug safety—Food and Drug Administration.
13. Oral health—Centers for Disease Control; National Institutes of Health.
14. Maternal and infant health—Health Resources and Services Administration.
15. Heart disease and stroke—National Institutes of Health.
16. Cancer—National Institutes of Health.
17. Diabetes and chronic disabling conditions—Centers for Disease Control; National Institutes of Health.
18. HIV infection—National AIDS Program Office.
19. Sexually transmitted diseases—Centers for Disease Control.
20. Immunization and infectious diseases—Centers for Disease Control.
21. Clinical preventive services—Centers for Disease Control; Health Resources and Services Administration.
22. Surveillance and data systems—Centers for Disease Control.

Source: From *Healthy People 2000: National Health Promotion Disease Prevention Objectives* by U.S. Department of Health and Human Services (USDHHS), DHHS Publication (PHS) 90-50212, Washington, DC: U.S. Government Printing Office.

conjunction with the Centers for Disease Control to assist states and localities in putting the new objectives into practice.

As has been noted, these two sets of objectives have been important components in the process of health promotion planning since 1980. We highly recommend that planners review these objectives before developing goals and objectives for programs. The national objectives may be helpful in providing a rationale for a program and in focusing program goals and objectives toward the areas of greatest need, as planners work toward the year 2000.

SUMMARY

The statement of purpose provides an overview of a program and is most useful in the development of goals and objectives. The terms *program goals* and *program objectives* are sometimes used synonymously, but they are quite different. Together the two provide a foundation for program planning and evaluation. Goals are more global in nature and often are not measurable in exact terms, while objectives are more specific and consist of the steps used to reach the program goals. Program objectives can and should be written for several different levels. For objectives to be useful, they should be written so as to be observable and measurable. At a minimum, an objective should include the following elements: a stated outcome, conditions under which the outcome will be observed, criteria for considering that the outcome has been achieved, and mention of the target population.

QUESTIONS

1. Why is a statement of purpose important?
2. What is (are) the difference(s) between a program goal and a program objective?
3. What is the purpose of program goals and objectives?
4. What are the eight different levels of program objectives? (Note that six are from Parkinson and Associates and two are from this volume.)
5. What are the necessary elements of a program objective?
6. What are the goals and objectives for the nation? How can they be used by program planners?

ACTIVITIES

1. Write a statement of purpose, a goal, and eight supporting objectives (one at each level) for a program you are planning.
2. Identify which of the following objectives include all four elements necessary for a complete objective; revise those objectives that do not include all the elements.

    a.   After the class on objective writing, the student will know the difference between a goal and an objective.

    b.   The student knows how a skinfold caliper works.

    c.   After completing this chapter, the student will be able to write program objectives based on the four elements outlined in the chapter.

    d.   Given appropriate instruction, the employees will be able to take blood pressure readings of fellow employees.

    e.   Program participants will be able to list the reasons why people do not exercise.

3.   Write a statement of purpose, a goal, and eight supporting objectives (one at each level) for a workshop on responsible use of alcohol by college students.

6

Theories and Models Commonly Used for Health Promotion Interventions

After reading this chapter and answering the questions at the end, you should be able to:

❑ Define *theory, model*, and *construct*.

❑ Explain why health promotion interventions should be planned using theoretical frameworks.

❑ Briefly explain the theories and models identified in the chapter.

❑ List and briefly explain the constructs of the social cognitive theory.

❑ Identify the major components of the Health Belief Model.

☐ KEY TERMS

aversive stimulus

behavioral capability

construct

efficacy expectations

emotional-coping responses

expectancies

expectations

health belief model

model

negative punishment

negative reinforcement

outcome expectations

perceived barriers

perceived benefits

perceived seriousness

perceived susceptibility

perceived threat

positive punishment

positive reinforcement

punishment

reciprocal determinism

reinforcement

self-control

self-efficacy

self-management

theory

vicarious

Whenever there is a discussion about the theoretical bases for health education and health promotion, we often find the terms *theory* and *model* used. Some use the terms correctly, while others either use them synonymously or confuse their meaning. We begin this chapter with a brief explanation of these terms, to establish a common understanding of their meaning.

According to one definition, a **theory** is "an integrated set of propositions that serves as an explanation for a class of phenomena. In general, theories are introduced into a science only after a class of phenomena has already revealed a systematic set of uniformities" (Chaplin & Krawiec, 1979, p. 67). "A theory is then intended to provide deeper understanding by presenting those phenomena as manifestations of certain underlying processes, governed by characteristic laws which account for, and usually correct and refine, the previously established generalizations" (Hempel, 1977, p. 244). In other words, a theory is a systematic arrangement of fundamental principles that provide a basis for explaining certain happenings of life.

In comparison, a **model** is a subclass of a theory. It provides researchers with a plan for investigating the phenomena. Unlike theories, a model "does not attempt to explain the processes underlying learning, but only to represent them" (Chaplin & Krawiec, 1979, p. 68).

Based upon these descriptions, it seems logical to think of theories as the backbone of the processes used to plan and evaluate health promotion interventions. Theories provide planners with a framework for identifying the necessary components in each of the processes. For example, developmental theories can be used to ensure that the goals and objectives of programs are consistent with the participants' developmental stages and abilities. Theories also can guide program planners in selecting the types of interventions that are needed to accomplish the stated goals and objectives. Appropriate use of learning and behavioral theories can help to ensure congruence between the planned interventions and expected outcomes. In addition, theoretical frameworks can alert planners to consider important influences outside the teaching-learning process, such as social support and environment, that have an impact on targeted program outcomes (Parcel, 1983). Models provide the vehicle for applying the theories.

All health promotion interventions should be planned and evaluated based upon proven theories, and not because they are someone's "good idea" or because "it's something I think will work." However, this is not to say that a theory cannot be modified or expanded to include a logically valid idea or parts of other theories. "In fact, it is well understood that working with a theory has certain disadvantages; one of which is leaving out or ignoring factors that happen not to be theoretically relevant, even though they may be empirically significant" (Jessor & Jessor, 1977).

The importance of theory in planning health promotion interventions is best shown by the large number of health promotion programs that are designed to help facilitate health behavior change in the target population. Getting people to engage in health behavior change is a complicated process that is very difficult under the best of conditions. Without the direction that theories provide, planners can easily waste valuable resources in trying to achieve the desired behavior change. Therefore, program planners should ground their programming process in the theories that have been the foundation of other successful health promotion efforts. An article by Shea and Basch (1990) provides a good review and rationale of the theories behind and the models used in some of the most successful health promotion programs: the North Karelia Project, the Stanford Three Community Study, the Stanford Five-City Project, the Minnesota Heart Health Program, and the Pawtucket Heart Health Program. Table 6.1 summarizes the theories and models used in these programs, based on the information provided by Shea and Basch (1990). As can be seen by the information presented in the table, each of these programs is well grounded in theory.

Essentially, the principles and practices of health education are "derived from the egalitarian spirit and progressive theories of education and the fundamental theories of the behavioral sciences" (National Task Force, 1985, p. vii). The remaining sections of this chapter present an overview of the theories and models that are most often used in planning and evaluating health promotion interventions.

BEHAVIORAL CHANGE THEORIES

Stimulus Response (SR) Theory

One of the theories used to explain and modify behavior today is the stimulus response, or SR, theory (Thorndike, 1898; Watson, 1925; Hall, 1943). This theory

Table 6.1
Theories and models used in five community-based cardiovascular disease prevention programs

Program	Year Begun	Theories and Models Used
Minnesota Heart Health Program	1980	• Social learning theory [a] • Communication–persuasion model [b] • Model of innovation diffusion [d] • Community development [c] • Problem behavior theory [a]
North Karelia Project	Late 1950s	• Social learning theory [a] • Theory of reasoned action [a] • Communication–persuasion model [b] • Model of innovative diffusion [d] • Community organization model [c]
Pawtucket Heart Health Program	1980	• Community organization model [c] • Social behavioral community psychology theory [a]
Stanford Five-City Project	1978	• Social learning theory [a] • Theory of reasoned action [a] • Communication–persuasion model [b] • Model of innovative diffusion [d]
Stanford Three Community Study	1972	• Social learning theory [a]

[a] = Discussed in Chapter 6
[b] = Discussed in Chapter 7
[c] = Discussed in Chapter 8
[d] = Discussed in Chapter 10

reflects the combination of classical conditioning (Pavlov, 1927) and instrumental conditioning (Thorndike, 1898) theories. These early conditioning theories explain learning based upon the associations among stimulus, response, and reinforcement (Parcel & Baranowski, 1981; Parcel, 1983). "In simplest terms, the SR theorists believe that learning results from events (termed `reinforcements') which reduce physiological drives that activate behavior" (Rosenstock, Strecher & Becker, 1988, p. 175). The behaviorist B. F. Skinner believed that the frequency of a behavior was determined by the reinforcements that followed that behavior.

In Skinner's view, the mere temporal association between a behavior and an immediately following reward is sufficient to increase the probability that the behavior will be repeated. Such behaviors are called operants; they operate on the environment to bring about changes resulting in reward or reinforcement (Rosenstock et al., 1988, p. 176). Stated another way, operant behaviors are behaviors that act on the environment to produce consequences. These consequences in turn either reinforce or do not reinforce the behavior that preceded.

The consequences of a behavior can come as either **reinforcement** or **punishment**. Individuals can learn from both. Reinforcement has been defined by Skinner (1953) as any event that follows a behavior, which in turn increases the probability that the same behavior will be repeated in the future. Behavior has a greater probability of occurring in the future (1) if reinforcement is frequent, and (2) if reinforcement is provided soon after the desired behavior. This immediacy clarifies the relationship between the reinforcement and appropriate behavior (Skinner, 1953). If a behavior is complex in nature, smaller steps working toward the desired behavior with appropriate reinforcement will help to shape the desired behavior. This was found to be true in getting pigeons to play ping-pong, and it can be useful in trying to change a complex health behavior like smoking or exercise. While reinforcement will increase the frequency of a behavior, punishment will decrease the frequency of a behavior. However, both reinforcement and punishment can be either positive or negative. The terms *positive* and *negative* in this context do not mean good and bad; rather, *positive* means adding something (effective of the stimulus) to a situation while *negative* means taking something away (removal or reduction of the effects of the stimulus) from the situation.

If individuals act in a certain way to produce a consequence that makes them feel good or that is enjoyable, it is labeled **positive reinforcement**. Examples of this would be an individual who is involved in an exercise program and "feels good" at the end of the workout, or one who participates in a weight loss program and receives verbal encouragement from the facilitator, again making that person "feel good." SR theorists would note that in both of these situations the pleasant experiences (internal feelings and verbal encouragement, respectively) occur right after the behavior, which in turn increases the chances that the frequency of the behavior will increase.

While positive reinforcement helps individuals learn by shaping behavior, behavior that avoids punishment is also learned because it reduces the tension that precedes the punishment (Rosenstock et al., 1988). "When this happens, we are being conditioned by *negative reinforcement*: A response is strengthened by the *removal* of something from the situation. In such cases, the `something' that is removed is referred to as a *negative reinforcer* or *aversive stimulus* (these two phrases are synonymous)" (Nye, 1979, p. 33). A good example of **negative reinforcement** is a weight loss program that requires weekly dues. When participants stop paying dues because they have met their goal weight, this removal of an obligation should increase frequency of the desired behavior (weight maintenance).

Some people think of negative reinforcement as a form of punishment, but it is not. While negative reinforcement increases the likelihood that a behavior will be repeated, punishment typically suppresses behavior. "Skinner suggests two ways in which a response can be punished: by *removing a positive reinforcer* or by *presenting a negative reinforcer* (aversive stimulus) as a consequence of the response" (Nye, 1979, p. 43). Punishment is usually linked to some uncomfortable (physical, mental, or otherwise) experience and decreases the frequency of a behavior. An aversive smoking cessation program that circulates cigarette smoke around those enrolled in the program as they smoke is an example of **pos-**

Figure 6.1
2 × 2 table of the stimulus
response theory

		Consequences	
		Positive (adding to)	Negative (taking away)
Behavior	Increase in frequency	Positive reinforcement	Negative reinforcement
	Decrease in frequency	Positive punishment	Negative punishment

itive punishment. It decreases the frequency of smoking by presenting (adding) a negative reinforcer or **aversive stimulus** (smoke) as a consequence of the response. An example of **negative punishment** (removing a positive reinforcer) would be not allowing teachers to use the teacher's lounge if they continue to smoke while using it. SR theorists would note that taking away the privilege of using the teacher's lounge would cause a decrease in frequency of smoking among the teachers. Figure 6.1 illustrates the relationship between reinforcement and punishment.

Finally, if reinforcement is withheld—or, stating it another way, if the behavior is ignored—the behavior will become less frequent and eventually will not be repeated. Skinner (1953) refers to this as extinction. Teachers frequently use this technique with disruptive children in the classroom. If a child is acting up in class, the teacher may choose to ignore the behavior in hopes that the non-reinforced behavior will go away.

Social Cognitive Theory (SCT)

The social learning theories (SLT) of Rotter (1954) and Bandura (1977b)—or, as Bandura (1986) recently relabeled them, the social cognitive theory (SCT)—combine SR theory and cognitive theories. SR theorists emphasize the role of reinforcement in shaping behavior and believe that no "thinking" or "reasoning" is needed to explain behavior. Those who espouse SCT believe that reinforcement is an integral part of learning, but emphasize the role of subjective hypotheses or **expectations** held by the individual (Rosenstock et al., 1988). In other words, reinforcement contributes to learning, but reinforcement along with an individual's expectations of the consequences of behavior determine the behavior. "Behavior, in this perspective, is a function of the subjective value of an outcome and the subjective probability (or `expectation') that a particular action will achieve that outcome. Such formulations are generally termed `value-expectancy' theories" (Rosenstock et al., 1988, p. 176). In brief, SCT describes learning as a reciprocal interaction between the individual's environment, cognitive processes, and behavior (Parcel, 1983). SCT explains learning through **constructs** (synthesized thoughts). Those that have been most often used in designing health education/promotion interventions will be presented here.

Parcel and Baranowski (1981) have provided an explanation of several constructs of SCT and health education, starting with reinforcement. As already noted, reinforcement is an important component of SCT. According to SCT, reinforcement can be accomplished in one of three ways: directly, vicariously, or through **self-management**. An example of direct reinforcement is a group facilitator who provides verbal feedback to participants for a job well done. **Vicarious reinforcement** is having the participants observe someone else being reinforced for behaving in an appropriate manner. This is often referred to as social modeling. In a system of reinforcement by self-management, the participants would keep records of their own behavior, and when the behavior was performed in an appropriate manner they would reinforce or reward themselves.

In addition to the constructs dealing with reinforcement, SCT has other constructs applicable to health promotion. Although there may be some situations where more than one construct will be applicable to a learning situation, program planners will find that certain constructs will be more useful than others, depending on the type of learning taking place. Those constructs identified by Parcel and Baranowski (1981) include behavioral capability, expectations, expectancies, self-control, self-efficacy, emotional-coping responses, and reciprocal determinism.

If individuals are to perform specific behaviors, they must know first what the behaviors are and then how to perform them. This is referred to as **behavioral capability**. For example, if people are to exercise aerobically, they first must know that aerobic exercise exists, and second, they need to know how to do it properly. Many people begin exercise programs only to quit within the first six months (Dishman, Sallis & Orenstein, 1985), and some of those people quit because they do not know how to exercise properly. They know they should exercise so they decide to run a few miles, have sore muscles the next day, and quit. The construct of **expectations** refers to the ability of human beings to think and thus to expect certain things to happen in certain situations. For example, if people are enrolled in a weight loss program and follow the directions of the group facilitator, they will expect to lose weight. **Expectancies**, not to be confused with expectations, are the values that individuals place on an expected outcome. If people value an expected outcome, they are more likely to perform the necessary behavior to yield the outcome. Someone who enjoys the feeling of not smoking more than that of smoking is more likely to try to do the things necessary to stop. The construct of **self-control** states that individuals may gain control of their own behavior through monitoring it. When helping individuals to change their behavior, it is a common practice to have them monitor their behavior over a period of time, through 24-hour diet or smoking records or exercise diaries, and then to have them reward (reinforce) themselves based upon their monitored performance.

One construct of SCT that has received special attention in health promotion programs is **self-efficacy** (Strecher, DeVellis, Becker & Rosenstock, 1986). Self-efficacy refers to the internal state that individuals experience as "competence" to perform certain desired tasks or behavior. This state is situation specific, that is, someone may be self-efficacious when it comes to aerobic exercise but

Figure 6.2
Diagrammatic representation of the difference between efficacy and outcome expectations (From *Social Learning Theory* [p. 79] by Albert Bandura, 1977, Englewood Cliffs, NJ: Prentice-Hall. Copyright 1977. Reprinted by permission of Prentice-Hall.)

not so when faced with reducing the amount of fat in her diet. People's competency feelings have been referred to as **efficacy expectations**. Thus, someone who thinks she can exercise on a regular basis no matter what the circumstances has efficacy expectations. Even though people have efficacy expectations, they still may not want to engage in a behavior because they may not think the outcomes of that behavior would be beneficial to them. Stated another way, they may not feel the reward (reinforcement) of performing the behavior is great enough for them. These beliefs are called **outcome expectations**. For example, in order for a person to quit smoking for health reasons (behavior) she must believe both that she is capable of quitting (efficacy expectation) and that cessation will benefit her health (outcome expectation) (I. M. Rosenstock, personal communication, April 1986). Figure 6.2 (Bandura, 1977a) illustrates efficacy and outcome expectations.

Individuals become self-efficacious in four main ways: (1) through performance attainments (personal mastery of a task); (2) through vicarious experience (observing the performance of others); (3) as a result of verbal persuasion (receiving suggestions from others); and (4) through emotional arousal (interpreting one's emotional state).

The construct of **emotional-coping responses** states that for a person to learn, she must be able to deal with the sources of anxiety that may surround a behavior. For example, fear is an emotion that can be involved in learning; according to this construct, participants would have to deal with the fear before they could learn the behavior.

The final construct to be mentioned here is that of **reciprocal determinism**. Reciprocal determinism states, unlike SR theory, that there is an interaction among the person, the behavior, and the environment, and that the person can shape the environment as well as the environment shaping the person. All these relationships are dynamic.

Theory of Reasoned Action (TRA)

Another theory that has received considerable attention in the literature of health behavior change is Fishbein's theory of reasoned action (TRA) (Fishbein & Ajzen, 1975). Like the theories already discussed, this theory was developed to explain not just health behavior but all volitional behaviors. However, while the theories discussed earlier in this chapter were directly concerned with behavior, this one provides a framework to study attitudes toward behaviors.

Fishbein and Ajzen distinguish among attitude, belief, behavioral intention, and behavior, and they present a conceptual framework for the study of the relationship among these four constructs. According to the model, an individual's intention to perform a given behavior is a function of her attitude toward performing the behavior, and normative beliefs about what relevant others think she should do, weighted by motivation to comply with those others. Behavioral intention is viewed as a special type of belief and is indicated by the person's subjective perception and report of the probability that she will perform the behavior (Parcel, 1983, p. 41).

In our opinion, this theory has one element that distinguishes it from other theories that try to explain human behavior: this is the construct that deals with the normative beliefs about what relevant others think the person should do. This construct states that individuals' intent to perform a given behavior is dependent partly on their belief that others (individuals or groups) think they should do so, and partly on the fact that they care about what these others think. This construct is often referred to as the subjective norm. An example of this construct applied to health promotion is the employee who intends to participate in the company's exercise program because she believes her boss thinks she should engage in exercise. For many behaviors the relevant others may include a person's parents, spouse, close friends, and coworkers, as well as experts or professionals like physicians or lawyers. Figure 6.3 shows the major elements of TRA.

Theory of Planned Behavior (TPB)

TRA has proven to be most successful when dealing with purely volitional behaviors, but complications are encountered when the theory is applied to behaviors that are not fully under volitional control. A good example of this is a smoker who intends to quit but fails to do so. Even though intent is high, nonmotivational factors, such as lack of requisite opportunities and resources, could prevent success (Ajzen, 1988).

The theory of planned behavior (TPB) (see Figure 6.4) is an extension of the theory of reasoned action that addresses the problem of incomplete volitional control. The major difference between TPB and TRA is the addition of a third,

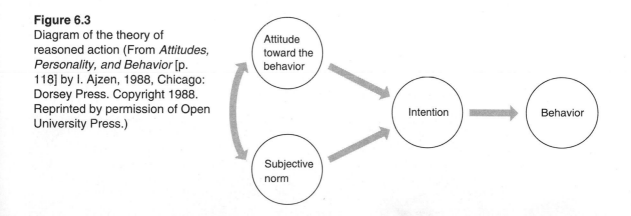

Figure 6.3
Diagram of the theory of reasoned action (From *Attitudes, Personality, and Behavior* [p. 118] by I. Ajzen, 1988, Chicago: Dorsey Press. Copyright 1988. Reprinted by permission of Open University Press.)

Figure 6.4

Diagram of the theory of planned
behavior (From *Attitudes,
Personality, and Behavior* [p.
135] by I. Ajzen, 1988, Chicago:
Dorsey Press. Copyright 1988.
Reprinted by permission of Open
University Press.)

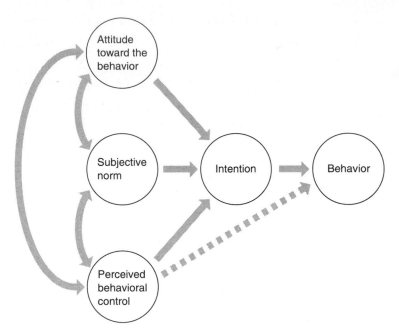

conceptually independent determinant of intention. Like TRA, TPB includes attitude toward the behavior and subjective norm, but it has added the concept of
perceived behavioral control. This refers to the perceived ease or difficulty of
performing the behavior and is assumed to reflect past experience as well as
anticipated impediments and obstacles. As a general rule, the more favorable the
attitude and subjective norm with respect to a behavior, and the greater the perceived behavioral control, the stronger should be the individual's intentions to
perform the behavior under consideration (Ajzen, 1988, pp. 132–33).

Figure 6.4 illustrates two important features of this theory. First, perceived
behavioral control has motivational implications for intentions. That is, without
perceived control, intentions could be minimal even if attitudes toward the
behavior and subjective norm were strong. Second, there may be a direct link
between perceived behavioral control and behavior. Behavior depends not only
on motivation but also on adequate control. Thus, it stands to reason that perceived behavioral control can help predict goal attainment independent of
behavioral intention (Ajzen, 1988). To use the example of smoking once again as
a behavior not fully under volitional control, TPB predicts that a person will give
up smoking if she (1) has a positive attitude toward quitting; (2) thinks others
whom she values believe it would be good for her to quit; and (3) perceives that
she has control over whether or not she quits.

Because this theory is comparatively new, there have been few references
to it in the health promotion literature. However, an article by Murphy and
Brubaker (1990) very nicely explains the application of this theory to testicular
self-examination in high school males. We believe this theory will have a significant impact on the development of future health promotion interventions.

Theory of Freeing (TF)

A theory that takes a much different approach from the other theories presented is the theory of freeing (TF) (Freire, 1973, 1974). Like the others, it is not specific to health promotion, but it does have application to health promotion. One of the first to apply this theory to health promotion was Greenberg. He stated (1978, p. 20) that the task of health education should be to "free people so they may make health-related decisions based upon their needs and interests as long as these needs and interests do not adversely affect others." In essence, Freire's concept of freeing contrasts "being free with being oppressed" (Walker & Bibeau, 1985/1986, p. 5). People become free by being critically conscious.

The underlying concept of this theory is that critical consciousness is determined by the interaction with culture. Consciousness is influenced by and influences the culture. Oppressed people are "of the world," and their consciousness is a product of the culture. Being "of the world" is defined by the lack of the person's ability to perceive, respond, and act with power to change concrete reality (Walker & Bibeau, 1985/1986). Free people are "in the world," and their consciousness is a producer of culture.

Education is the key to becoming critically conscious. However, the education that is meant here is not education in the traditional sense. Education occurs through dialogue, not through lecture. People who use dialogue are teachers, while those who just talk are lecturers. And in this type of education participants replace pupils. All those involved in the educational process learn from each other.

In applying TF to health promotion, one could say that for people to become health educated they need to be free. Program participants should not be pupils or listeners; rather, they should be actively involved in the teaching-learning process.

Problem-Behavior Theory (PBT)

Because many health promotion programs focus on problem behaviors, program planners have found problem-behavior theory (PBT) to be a useful framework for guiding program development. This theory rests upon the social-psychological relationships that occur within and among the three major systems of personality, perceived environment, and behavior. Each of these systems includes a variety of variables that are interrelated and organized in such a manner as to generate a greater or lesser likelihood of occurrence of problem behavior (Jessor & Jessor, 1977).

The logic and rationale of the original formulation of PBT were presented by Jessor, Graves, Hanson, and Jessor (1968), while the present content and structure of the framework were presented in detail by Jessor and Jessor (1977). This later presentation of the theory was based upon the study of adolescence and youth in American society in the late 1960s and early 1970s. As such, the theory is designed to account for problem behaviors that organize the daily lives of young people (Jessor & Jessor, 1977). A schematic representation of this theory is presented in Figure 6.5.

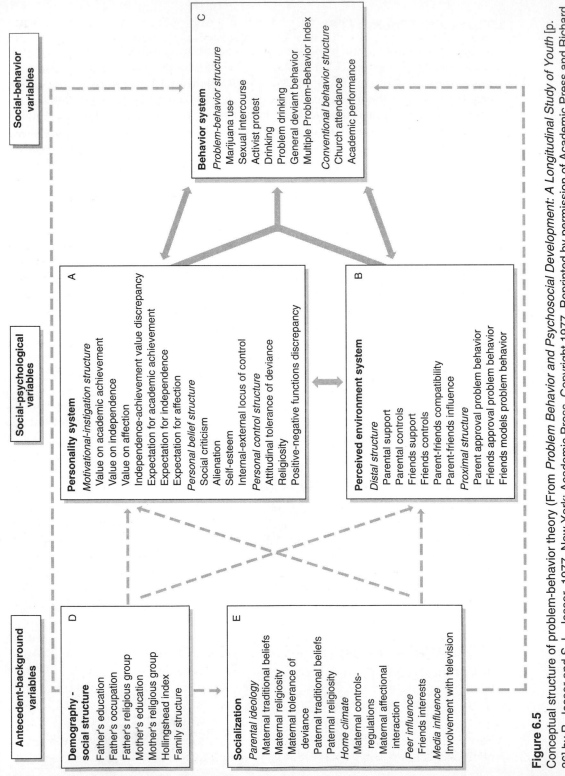

Figure 6.5

Conceptual structure of problem-behavior theory (From *Problem Behavior and Psychosocial Development: A Longitudinal Study of Youth* [p. 36] by R. Jessor and S. L. Jessor, 1977, New York: Academic Press. Copyright 1977. Reprinted by permission of Academic Press and Richard Jessor.)

Antecedent-background variables

D

Demography - social structure
Father's education
Father's occupation
Father's religious group
Mother's education
Mother's religious group
Hollingshead index
Family structure

E

Socialization
Parental ideology
Maternal traditional beliefs
Maternal religiosity
Maternal tolerance of deviance
Paternal traditional beliefs
Paternal religiosity
Home climate
Maternal controls-regulations
Maternal affectional interaction
Peer influence
Friends interests
Media influence
Involvement with television

Social-psychological variables

A

Personality system
Motivational-instigation structure
Value on academic achievement
Value on independence
Value on affection
Independence-achievement value discrepancy
Expectation for academic achievement
Expectation for independence
Expectation for affection
Personal belief structure
Social criticism
Alienation
Self-esteem
Internal-external locus of control
Personal control structure
Attitudinal tolerance of deviance
Religiosity
Positive-negative functions discrepancy

B

Perceived environment system
Distal structure
Parental support
Parental controls
Friends support
Friends controls
Parent-friends compatibility
Parent-friends influence
Proximal structure
Parent approval problem behavior
Friends approval problem behavior
Friends models problem behavior

Social-behavior variables

C

Behavior system
Problem-behavior structure
Marijuana use
Sexual intercourse
Activist protest
Drinking
Problem drinking
General deviant behavior
Multiple Problem-Behavior Index
Conventional behavior structure
Church attendance
Academic performance

The personality system found in box A of the schematic diagram in Figure 6.5 contains three major structures: motivational-instigation, personal belief, and personal control. The interaction of these three structures determines a person's personality as it relates to a problem behavior. The motivational-instigation structure is concerned with the directional orientation of action or goals (not directly related to problem behavior) toward which the individual strives and the motivation to begin behaviors to work toward the goals. The greater the value placed on a goal, the greater the likelihood of action directed toward the goal. The personal belief structure deals with the cognitive controls exerted against the occurrence of a problem behavior. There are four variables in this structure: social criticism, alienation, self-esteem, and locus of control. The third structure in this system, personal control, includes variables that are directly linked to the problem behaviors.

The second system in this theory is the perceived environment system (box B), which Jessor and Jessor describe as "the environment that is contributed by the actor from his experience with it" (1977, p. 27). This structure includes both distal variables (those that are remote from the causal chain) and proximal variables (those obviously related to the occurrence of problem behavior). Both types of variables deal with the individual's interactions with friends and parents/family. The distal variables can be thought of as the social content in which a person is located, while the proximal variables determine the degree to which the person is located in the social content.

The third system of the theory is the behavior system, represented by box C. This component contains two major areas: problem behavior and conventional behavior. *Problem behavior* refers to behavior that is undesirable by the norms of society and needs some type of social control, while conventional behavior includes what is seen as desirable behaviors by society.

Two other boxes (D and E) shown in Figure 6.5 contain antecedent and background variables, mainly demography/social structure and socialization. These variables affect both the personality and perceived environment systems, but the amount of impact is hard to measure.

In applying this theory to health promotion programs, we would refer to a problem behavior as one that is detrimental to good health. This detrimental health behavior is thus related to the personality and perceived environment systems, which in turn are affected by social structure and socialization of a person. In other words, if a person is an overeater or a nonexerciser, there are many variables that could lead to this behavior and would need to be examined if these behaviors are to be changed.

COMBINATION HEALTH BEHAVIOR MODELS

Several models have been developed (Becker & Maiman, 1983) to explain the various types of health behavior. Several of these models are based upon parts of theories that have been discussed earlier in this chapter. This section presents the best known of these models, the health belief model, and a lesser known model, the transtheoretical model. Both of these models should provide program planners with frameworks for developing appropriate interventions.

Health Belief Model (HBM)

The **health belief model (HBM)**, which is probably the one most frequently used in health behavior applications, was developed in the 1950s by a group of psychologists to help explain why people would or would not use health services (Rosenstock, 1966). The HBM is based upon Lewin's decision-making model (Lewin, 1935, 1936; Lewin, Dembo, Festinger & Sears, 1944). Since its creation the HBM has been used to help explain a variety of health behaviors (Janz & Becker, 1984).

The HBM hypothesizes that health-related action depends upon the simultaneous occurrence of three classes of factors:

1.   The existence of sufficient motivation (or health concern) to make health issues salient or relevant.

2.   The belief that one is susceptible (vulnerable) to a serious health problem or to the sequelae of that illness or condition. This is often termed **perceived threat**.

3.   The belief that following a particular health recommendation would be beneficial in reducing the perceived threat, and at a subjectively acceptable cost. Cost refers to the **perceived barriers** that must be overcome in order to follow the health recommendation; it includes, but is not restricted to, financial outlays (Rosenstock et al., 1988, p. 177).

Figure 6.6 provides a diagram of the HBM as presented by Becker, Drachman, and Kirscht (1974).

As noted, the HBM has been applied to all types of health behavior. Here is an example of the HBM applied to exercise. Someone watching television sees an advertisement about exercise. This is a cue to action that starts her thinking about her own need to exercise. There may be some variables (demographic, sociopsychological, and structural) that cause her to think about it a bit more. She remembers her college health course that included information about heart disease and the importance of staying active. She knows she has a higher than normal risk for heart disease because of family history, poor diet, and slightly elevated blood pressure. Therefore, she comes to the conclusion that she is susceptible to heart disease (**perceived susceptibility**). She also knows that if she develops heart disease it can be very serious (**perceived seriousness**/severity). Based upon these factors, she thinks there is reason to be concerned about heart disease (perceived threat). She knows that exercise can help delay the onset of heart disease and can increase the chances of surviving a heart attack if one should occur (**perceived benefits**). But exercise takes time from an already busy day, and it is not easy to exercise in the variety of settings in which she typically finds herself, especially during bad weather (perceived barriers). She must now weigh the threat of the disease against the difference between benefits and barriers. This decision will then result in a likelihood of exercising or not exercising (likelihood of taking recommended preventive health action).

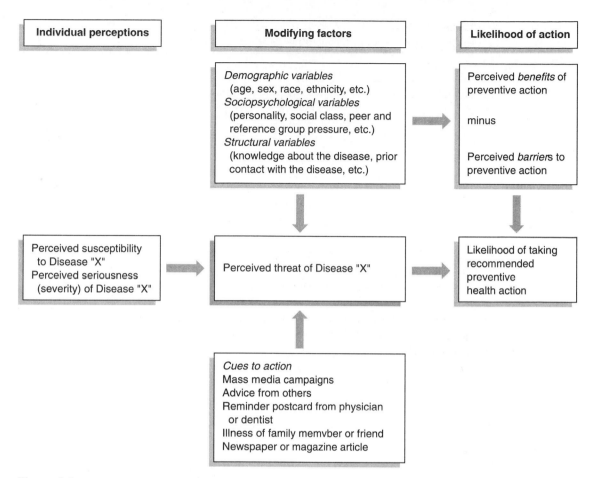

Figure 6.6
The HBM as a predictor of preventive health behavior (From "A New Approach to Explaining Sick Role Behavior in Low Income Populations" by M. H. Becker, R. H. Drachman, and J. P. Kirscht, 1974, *American Journal of Public Health*, 64 (March), pp. 205–16. Copyright 1974. Reprinted by permission of APHA and Marshall H. Becker.)

The Transtheoretical Model (TTM)

The transtheoretical model, or TTM (summarized in Table 6.2), helps to explain the stages that a majority of people experience as they attempt to change their health behavior over time. The model has its roots in psychotherapy and was developed by Prochaska (1979) after he completed a comparative analysis of 18 therapy systems and a critical review of 300 therapy outcome studies. From the analysis and review Prochaska found that some common processes were involved in change.

The first stage of the TTM is precontemplation. This initial stage is defined as a time when someone is not seriously thinking about changing her behavior during the next six months. The second stage, contemplation, is when someone is

Table 6.2
Stages of the transtheoretical model

Stages	Timeframe
Precontemplation	Not thinking about change in the next 6 months
Contemplation	Seriously thinking about change in the next 6 months
Action	Six-month period following overt modification
Maintenance	Six-month period after overt modification until termination
Relapse	Reverting back to old behavior
Termination	Zero temptation and ability to resist relapse

seriously thinking about a behavior change during the next six months. The third stage is called action—the six-month period following an overt modification of a behavior. If all goes well, the person will progress to the next stage, maintenance, defined as the period after action until the unwanted behavior is finally terminated. However, for whatever reason, some people are not successful in the maintenance stage and relapse to their old behavior. When this occurs, most do not give up but rather go back to the contemplation stage and consider other action. Termination, the final stage of the model, takes place when the person is no longer tempted by the unwanted behavior and feels confident in the ability to resist relapse in all situations. The spiral representation of the model in Figure 6.7 suggests that most people learn from their relapse episodes instead of going in circles and making no progress (Prochaska, 1989, August).

Figure 6.7
Diagram of the transtheoretical model (From "What Causes People to Change from Unhealthy to Health-Enhancing Behavior?" by J. O. Prochaska, 1989, August, paper presented at the American Cancer Society's Human Behavior and Cancer Risk Reduction Conference, Bloomington, IN. Reprinted by permission.)

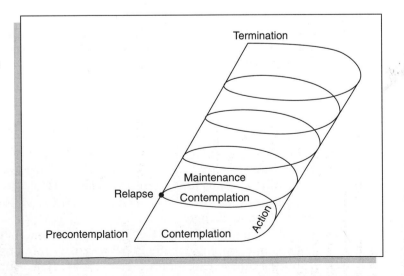

Table 6.3
Major components of the theories and models that underlie health promotion interventions

Stimulus Response Theory	Social Cognitive Theory	Theory of Reasoned Action	Theory of Planned Behavior	Problem Behavior Theory	Theory of Freeing	Health Belief Model	Transtheoretical Model
Operant behavior	Reinforcement 1. Direct 2. Vicariously 3. Self-management	Attitude toward behavior	Attitude toward behavior	Personality system	Free	Perceived susceptibility	Pre-contemplation
Consequences	Behavioral capability	Subjective norm	Subjective norm	Perceived environment system	Oppressed	Perceived seriousness	Contemplation
Positive reinforcement	Expectations	Intentions	Perceived behavioral control	Behavior system	Critical consciousness	Perceived benefits	Action
Negative reinforcement	Expectancies	Behavior	Intentions	Antecedent variables	Education	Perceived barriers	Maintenance
Positive punishment	Self-control		Behavior	Background variables		Motivation	Relapse
Negative punishment	Self-efficacy						Termination
	Emotional coping response						
	Reciprocal determinism						

Since its development, the model has been useful in several different ways. The first is that it makes program planners aware that not everyone is ready for change "right now," even though there is a program that can help people modify their behavior. People proceed through behavior change at different paces. Second, if a person is not ready for action right now, then other programs can be developed to help her become ready for action. Third, the model has been very useful in helping to identify individuals who are truly ready for change and in predicting who may be successful in trying to change a health behavior. This third aspect fits in nicely with the effort to market a program and is discussed further in Chapter 10.

 ## SUMMARY

This chapter presented an overview of several theories and two models that underlie the interventions used in many of today's health promotion programs. These theories and models are important components for planning and evaluating health promotion programs because they provide planners with ideas that have been tried and tested. They provide the framework on which to build. The theories and models reviewed include: stimulus response theory, social cognitive theory, theory of reasoned action, theory of planned behavior, problem-behavior theory, theory of freeing, health belief model, and transtheoretical model (see Table 6.3 (p. 83) for a summary of the major components).

QUESTIONS

1. Define *theory*, using your own words.
2. Why is it important to use theories when planning and evaluating health promotion programs?
3. What is the underlying concept for each of the following theories?
   a. Stimulus response theory
   b. Social cognitive theory
   c. Theory of reasoned action
   d. Theory of planned behavior
   e. Theory of freeing
   f. Problem-behavior theory
4. What are the major components of the health belief model? Explain each.
5. What are the stages of the transtheoretical model? Why is it important to understand this model?

⬜ ACTIVITIES

Write a paragraph on each of the following:

1. Using the stimulus response theory, explain why a person might smoke.
2. Using the social cognitive theory, explain how you could help people change their diets.
3. Explain how the SCT construct of behavioral capability applies to managing stress.
4. Explain the differences between and the relationship of the SCT constructs of expectations and expectancies.
5. Explain what would have to take place for a person to be self-efficacious with regard to being able to take her insulin.
6. According to the theory of reasoned action, what would increase intent to exercise?
7. Use the theory of planned behavior to explain how a smoker stops smoking.
8. Using the theory of freeing, describe an ideal teacher.
9. Apply the health belief model to getting a person to take a "flu shot."
10. Apply the transtheoretical model to getting a person to try to stop smoking.

7

Interventions

After reading this chapter and answering the questions at the end, you should be able to:

❑   Define the word *intervention* and apply it to a health promotion setting.

❑   Provide a rationale for selecting an intervention strategy.

❑   Explain the advantages of using a combination of several intervention activities rather than a single intervention activity.

❑   Explain the difference between micro and macro interventions.

❑   List and explain the different categories of intervention activities.

❑   List some of the documents that provide guidelines or criteria for developing health promotion programs and interventions.

❑   Discuss the ethical concerns related to intervention development.

❑   Identify the major components of a micro health promotion intervention.

❑   Explain how the term *relapse* applies to health promotion interventions.

KEY TERMS

codes of practice

ethics

field test

incentives

intervention

intervention activity

locus of control

macro intervention

mandated activities

micro intervention

penetration rate

recidivism

relapse

relapse prevention

risk appraisal

risk reduction

self-efficacious

treatment

Once goals and objectives have been developed, program planners need to decide on the most appropriate means of reaching, or attaining, the goals and objectives. The planners must identify an activity or set of activities that would permit the most *effective* (leads to desired outcome) and *efficient* (uses resources in a responsible manner) achievement of the outcomes stated in the goals and objectives. These planned activities make up the **intervention**, or what some refer to as **treatment**. The intervention is the activity or experience to which those in the target population will be exposed or in which they will take part. In the strictest sense, *intervention* means "to occur, fall, or come between points of time or events" (Woolf, 1979, p. 600). When applied to the planning of health promotion programs, it is usually thought of as something that occurs between the beginning and the end of a program or between pre- and post-program measurements. For example, let's say that we want the employees of Company S to increase their use of safety belts while riding in company-owned vehicles. We can measure their safety belt use before doing anything, by observing them driving out of the motor pool; this would be a preprogram measure. Then we can intervene in a variety of ways. For example, we could provide an incentive by stating that all employees seen wearing their safety belt would receive a ten-dollar bonus in their next paycheck. Or we could put a pamphlet on the importance of wearing safety belts in each employee's pay envelope. We could institute a company policy requiring all employees to wear safety belts while driving company-owned vehicles. Each of these activities for getting employees to increase their use of safety belts would be considered part of an intervention. After the intervention we would complete a postprogram measurement of safety belt use to determine the success of the program.

The term *intervention* is used to describe all the activities that occur between the two measurement points. Thus an intervention may be a single activity, or it may be a combination of two or more activities. In the case of the example just given, we could use an incentive by itself and call it an intervention, or we could use an incentive, pamphlets, and a company policy all at the same time to increase safety belt use and refer to the combination as an intervention.

With regard to the number of activities that should be included in an intervention, research (Erfurt, Foote, Heirich & Gregg, 1990; Shea & Basch, 1990) shows that interventions that include several activities are more likely to have an effect on the target population than are those that consist of only a single activity. In other words, "dosage" is important in health promotion. Few people change their behavior based on a single exposure (or dose); instead, multiple exposures (doses) are generally needed to change most behaviors. It stands to reason that "hitting" the target population from several angles or through multiple channels should increase the chances of making an impact. Although research has shown that several activities are better than one, it has not identified an exact number of activities or a specific combination of activities that yields the best results. It is still a best-guess situation. It is possible, however, to determine the effectiveness of an **intervention activity** or activities by measuring the number of people who comply with the health message of the intervention. The specifics of how to measure the effectiveness of an intervention are discussed in detail beginning in Chapter 12.

MACRO VERSUS MICRO INTERVENTIONS

Interventions can be classified into two major categories—macro and micro. **Macro interventions** are usually planned and implemented for a group of people (or a community or society) and are not aimed at a specific individual. Mandates to use safety belts are a good example. These interventions may take the form of a company's chief executive officer creating a policy that requires employees to wear a safety belt while driving a company-owned vehicle, or they may come in the form of a state law concerning safety belt use. In both cases, these interventions affect large groups of people: all those who work for the company that establishes such a policy, and all those who drive or ride in motor vehicles in the state that has such a law. No single person is identified as the recipient of the intervention; rather, the intervention is aimed at a group of people. Health messages sent as public service announcements in the mass media (television, radio, or newspapers) are another example of macro interventions.

Micro interventions, on the other hand, are aimed at individuals, even though those individuals may meet in a group. For example, a smoking cessation program for a group of 10 employees is considered a micro intervention. Individually prescribed diet and exercise regimens for those in a weight loss program would be considered micro interventions.

Usually it is thought that macro interventions affect a relatively larger number of people than micro interventions, but that is not always the case. For example, a small business with, say, 30 employees may be exposed to a macro intervention in the form of a safety belt policy, while there may be 30 people enrolled in a micro intervention program for smoking cessation. The real distinction between macro and micro interventions is whether the intervention is aimed at specific individuals or at groups. The old concept of public or community health interventions (macro) versus personal health interventions (micro) may be one way to keep the distinction clear.

To date, much of the work of health promotion planners has dealt with micro interventions. O'Rourke and Macrina (1989) believe that continued emphasis on the micro interventions will limit the approaches that can be taken in improving the level of health of American society. They have suggested that health promotion planners redirect their efforts to work toward more public policies that combine micro and macro interventions.

SELECTING APPROPRIATE INTERVENTION ACTIVITIES

Selection of intervention activities for a health promotion program should be based upon a sound rationale as opposed to chance; an activity should not be selected just because the planners think it "sounds good," or because they have a "feeling" that it will work. As mentioned earlier, planners should choose an intervention that will be both effective and efficient. Although no prescription for an appropriate intervention has been developed, experience has indicated that the results of some interventions are more predictable than others. We present here a list of questions that planners should consider before selecting interventions. Because of the limited opportunities and resources available for health promotion, planners rarely have the opportunity to experiment; therefore, they must be sure they are using the best available interventions.

Are the activities based upon an appropriate theory?

Interventions have a much greater chance of reaching the desired outcome if they are planned using sound learning and educational theories that have proved their worth through experience and social science research. Interventions should not be without a solid basis in theory. Figure 7.1 shows how theories and models relate to intervention activities.

Are the necessary resources available to implement the intervention selected?

Obviously, some intervention activities require more money, time, personnel, or space to implement than others.

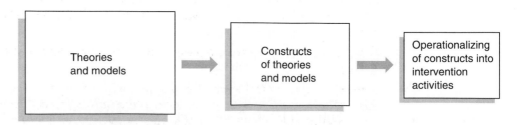

Figure 7.1
Relationship of theories and models to intervention activities

Would it be better to use an intervention that consists of a single activity, or one that is made up of multiple activities?

A single-activity intervention would most likely be easier and less expensive to implement and easier to evaluate. There are, however, some real advantages to using several activities. These advantages include: (1) "hitting" the target population with a message in a variety of ways; (2) appealing to the variety of learning styles within any target population; (3) keeping the health message constantly before the target population; (4) hoping that at least one activity appeals enough to the target population to help bring about the expected outcome; and (5) appealing to the various senses (such as sight, hearing, or touch) of each individual in the target population. Probably the biggest drawback to using multiple activities is the difficulty of separating the effects of one activity from the effects of others in evaluating the impact of the total program and of individual components (Ad Hoc Work Group, 1987).

Is the intervention appropriate for the demographics (age, gender, or socioeconomic status), knowledge, skills, and behavior of the target population?

Experience has shown that not all target populations react the same way to a standard intervention.

Are the activities developmentally appropriate for the target population?

For example, when working with a group of kindergarteners, it is not realistic to expect them to sit quietly for an hour while a lesson (the intervention) is presented, but adults should be able to do so.

What types of intervention activities are known to be most effective (that is, have been successfully used in previous programs) in dealing with the the program focus?

For example, by checking the literature, a planner could find out what interventions have been documented to best help people in managing their stress.

Do the intervention activities fit the purpose of the program?

If the single purpose of a program is to increase the awareness of the target population, the intervention would be much different than if the purpose is to change behavior.

Are the proposed intervention activities appropriate for the number of people?

Some strategies work better with groups (small or large), while others are more effective with single individuals. If the target population happens to be a handful of employees trying to stop smoking, the intervention would be much different than if one were trying to persuade a community of 50,000 people to get flu shots.

TYPES OF INTERVENTION ACTIVITIES

As mentioned earlier, there are many different types of activities that planners can use as part of an intervention. We present here several categories covering the more common activities, but in actuality the variety of activities is limited only by the planner's imagination. We have categorized activities into the following groups: (1) traditional educational activities or methods; (2) activities based upon behavior modification; (3) environmental change activities; (4) regulatory activities; (5) community participation activities to influence public policy; (6) activities affecting organizational culture; (7) communication activities; (8) economic and other incentives; and (9) social intervention activities.

Traditional Educational Activities

Traditional educational activities are those usually associated with formal education in courses, seminars, and workshops. This includes educational methods such as lecture, discussion, and group work, as well as audiovisual materials, laboratory exercises, and written materials (books and periodicals). This class of

Table 7.1
Commonly used educational methods

A. Audiovisual materials and equipment
   1.   Audio tapes, records, and compact disks
   2.   Bulletin, chalk, cloth, flannel, magnetic, and peg boards
   3.   Charts, pictures, and posters
   4.   Computers
   5.   Films and filmstrips
   6.   Instructional television
   7.   Opaque projector
   8.   Slides and slide projectors
   9.   Transparencies and overhead projector
   10. Video disks and tapes
B. Printed educational materials
   1.   Instructor-made handouts and worksheets
   2.   Pamphlets
   3.   Study guides (commercial and instructor-made)
   4.   Text and reference books
   5.   Workbooks
C. Teaching strategies and techniques for the classroom
   1.   Brainstorming
   2.   Case studies
   3.   Debates
   4.   Demonstrations and experiments

activities seems to be most useful in programs aimed at the first four levels of objectives (awareness, attitudes, knowledge, and skill development) noted in Chapter 5. Table 7.1 provides a more complete listing of educational methods.

Behavior Modification Activities

This group of activities, most often used in micro interventions, includes techniques intended to help those in the target population experience a change in behavior. Behavior modification is usually thought of as a systematic procedure for changing a specific behavior. The process is based on the stimulus response theory. As applied to health behavior, emphasis is placed on a specific behavior that one might want either to increase (such as exercise or stress management techniques) or to decrease (such as smoking or consumption of fats). Particular attention is then given to changing the events that are antecedent or subsequent to the behavior that is to be modified.

In changing a health behavior, the behavior modification activity often begins by having those in the target population keep records (diaries, logs, or journals) for a specific period of time (24–48 hours, 1 week, or 1 month) concerning the behavior (such as eating, smoking, or exercise) they want to alter. Using

5. Discovery or guided discovery
6. Discussion
7. Group discussion
8. Guest speakers
9. Lecture
10. Lecture/discussion
11. Newspaper and magazine articles
12. Panel discussions
13. Peer group teaching
14. Poems, songs, and stories
15. Problem solving
16. Puppets
17. Questioning
18. Role playing and plays
19. Simulation, games, and puzzles
20. Tutoring
21. Values clarification activities
D. Teaching strategies and techniques for outside of the classroom
    1. Community resources
    2. Field trips
    3. Health fairs
    4. Health museums

the information recorded, one can plan an activity to modify that behavior. For example, facilitators of smoking cessation programs often will ask participants to keep a record of all the cigarettes they smoke from one class session to the next (see Figure 7.2 for an example of such a record). After keeping the record, partici-

Name _____

Date _____

Number of cigarettes during the day	Time of day	Need rating*	Place or activity	With whom	Mood or reason
1.	_____	1 2 3	_____	_____	_____
2.	_____	1 2 3	_____	_____	_____
3.	_____	1 2 3	_____	_____	_____
4.	_____	1 2 3	_____	_____	_____
5.	_____	1 2 3	_____	_____	_____
6.	_____	1 2 3	_____	_____	_____
7.	_____	1 2 3	_____	_____	_____
8.	_____	1 2 3	_____	_____	_____
9.	_____	1 2 3	_____	_____	_____
10.	_____	1 2 3	_____	_____	_____
11.	_____	1 2 3	_____	_____	_____
12.	_____	1 2 3	_____	_____	_____
13.	_____	1 2 3	_____	_____	_____
14.	_____	1 2 3	_____	_____	_____
15.	_____	1 2 3	_____	_____	_____
16.	_____	1 2 3	_____	_____	_____
17.	_____	1 2 3	_____	_____	_____
18.	_____	1 2 3	_____	_____	_____
19.	_____	1 2 3	_____	_____	_____
20.	_____	1 2 3	_____	_____	_____
21.	_____	1 2 3	_____	_____	_____
22.	_____	1 2 3	_____	_____	_____
23.	_____	1 2 3	_____	_____	_____
24.	_____	1 2 3	_____	_____	_____
25.	_____	1 2 3	_____	_____	_____
26.	_____	1 2 3	_____	_____	_____
27.	_____	1 2 3	_____	_____	_____
28.	_____	1 2 3	_____	_____	_____
29.	_____	1 2 3	_____	_____	_____
30.	_____	1 2 3	_____	_____	_____

*Need rating: How important is the cigarette to you at this time?
1 = Most important, I would miss it very much.
2 = Average
3 = Least important, I would not miss it.

Figure 7.2
Twenty-four-hour cigarette count

pants are asked to analyze it to see what kind of smoking habit they have. They may be asked questions such as these: "What three cigarettes seem to be the most important of the day to you?" "In what three places or activities do you find yourself smoking the most?" "With whom do you find yourself smoking most often?" "Is there a primary reason or mood for your smoking?" "When during the day do you find yourself smoking the most and the least?" Once the participant has answered these questions, appropriate interventions can be designed to deal with the problem behavior. For example, if a participant says he only smokes when he is by himself, then activities would be planned so that he does not spend a lot of time alone. If another participant seemed to do most of his smoking while drinking coffee, an activity would be developed to provide some type of substitute. If a person seemed to smoke the most while sitting at the table after meals, activities could be planned to get the person away from the dinner table and doing something that would occupy his hands.

Environmental Change Activities

Another group of activities that have proven to be useful in reaching desired outcomes falls into the category of environmental change. These activities are more often used in macro interventions because they usually affect a group of people. They are characterized by changes in those things "around" individuals that may influence their awareness, knowledge, attitudes, skills, or behavior. Some of these activities provide a "forced choice" situation, as when the selection of foods and beverages in vending machines or cafeterias is changed to include only "healthy" foods. If people want to eat foods from these sources, they are forced to eat certain types of foods. Other activities in this category may provide those in the target population with health messages and environmental cues for certain types of behavior. Examples would be the posting of no-smoking signs, elimination of ash trays, provision of lockers and showers, use of role modeling by others, playing of soft music in a work area, and point-of-purchase education, such as a sign on a vending machine or food labeling on the food lines in the cafeteria.

Regulatory Activities

This group of activities includes laws, policies, position statements, regulations, and rules. These could be classified as **mandated activities** or regulated activities because they are ones that are required by an administrator, board, or legislative body. These activities are commonly part of macro interventions. Examples include state laws requiring the use of safety belts and motorcycle helmets or raising the taxes on cigarettes, company policy stating that there will be no smoking in corporate offices and company-owned vehicles, a board of education adopting a position statement that it will provide only well-balanced meals in its cafeterias.

This type of intervention activity may be controversial. It has been criticized by some because it mandates a particular response from an individual. It takes away individual freedoms and sometimes plays on a person's pride, "pocketbook," and psyche. This type of activity must be sold on the concept of "common good." That is, the justification for this type of societal action is to protect the public's health. Regulatory activities exist for the protection of the community and of individual rights. In other words, "officials are willing to intercede into the private activities and lives of people in order to protect the larger population. When such intervention occurs it is usually very narrow and very specifically defined. There also tend to be sanctions attached if people do not comply. For example, in the case of inoculations, if a mother and father did not have their child inoculated that child cannot attend school. If parents do not send their child to school they are in violation of the law, and there are criminal and civil penalties that are involved" (Rich & Sugrue, 1989, p. 33).

Some would say that regulatory activities do not allow for the "voluntary adaptations of behavior conducive to health" that are suggested by Green and colleagues (1980, p. 7) in their definition of health education. But, at the same time, this kind of activity can get people to change their behavior when other strategies have failed. For example, before the passage of safety belt laws, most states were reporting about a 14% use rate by drivers of automobiles and were trying to attack the problem through traditional educational activities using the mass media. Now that safety belt laws are in effect in about half of the states, usage rates in those states are closer to 50%; in some states where there is strict enforcement, usage rates approach 80%. Another example is the work of Sorensen, Rigotti, Rosen, Pinney, and Prible (1991), which showed a 21% reduction in the number of employees who smoked in a company that put a nonsmoking policy in effect. Both of these examples show that regulatory activities are necessary to reinforce and support prevention messages.

Since regulatory activities are mandatory, it is particularly important to use good judgment and show respect for others when implementing such activities. In some instances, program planners will be faced with ethical decisions. If a program will make use of regulatory intervention activities, the planner should remember that, as in any political process, there is likely to be both pro and con feeling toward the "mandatory" action. Thus when developing and implementing any mandatory action, planners should bear in mind the following points:

1.   Have top-level support of the mandated action (Emont & Cummings, 1989).

2.   Have a representative group (committee) from the target population help formulate the "mandatory" action.

3.   Make sure expert advice on the subject of the mandated action is available to the group developing it.

4.   Seek a legal opinion if necessary.

5.   Examine the work of others and review the issues they faced when implementing "mandatory" actions.

6.   Be sure that regulatory activities are based on sound principles.

7.   Seek input and debate/discussion concerning the mandated action from the target population while it is being formulated.

8. Consider implementing the new regulation a little bit at a time. For example, if a no-smoking policy is going to be implemented, the planner may want to begin by restricting smoking in certain areas before banning it altogether. This not only helps people change gradually, but also expresses concern for them.

9. Ensure that, once formulated, the "mandatory" actions

    a. are actively communicated to those in the target population.

    b. are reviewed on a regular basis for the purposes of evaluating and revising if necessary.

    c. apply to all in the target population and not just to select groups.

    d. are consistently enforced.

    e. are enforced as a shared responsibility of all in the institution.

To help gain a sense of the difficulty of dealing with regulatory activities, let's examine the options available to a group of department heads trying to decide whether or not they should continue to allow the public to smoke in the lobby of the building and employees to smoke in their individual, self-contained offices. Several options are available to this administrative group:

1. Decide to have no explicit policy.
2. Make no changes, and continue with the status quo.
3. Eliminate only public smoking in the building.
4. Designate a different area or room within the building for public smoking.
5. Allow smoking only in individual offices.
6. Designate the entire building as a "smoke free building."
7. Request that all employees hired in the future be nonsmokers.
8. A combination of items 1–7.

Each of these options poses special concerns for administrative groups. Policies are seldom easy to develop, but looking at others that have already been developed helps in the creation of a new policy. For this reason, we provide several examples in the appendices to this book. Appendix C presents a model for developing an alcohol policy on a college campus (Sherwood, 1987). The steps outlined in this model could be useful in developing and implementing health-related mandates in other settings. Appendix D presents the safety belt policy of the Indiana Bell Telephone Company. This company policy was in effect before former transportation secretary Elizabeth Dole's push to implement the Occupational Safety and Health Administration (OSHA) standard of safety belt use for employees of companies that are regulated by such standards. Appendix E presents a "Model Ordinance Eliminating Smoking in Workplaces and Enclosed Public Places" developed by Americans for Nonsmokers' Rights. An additional source for planners interested in developing policies regulating smoking in the workplace is a publication of the U.S. Department of Health and Human Services (USDHHS, 1985).

Community Participation Activities to Influence Public Policy

Not to be confused with regulatory activities, community participation activities are used to influence public policy. Community participation is a process in which the people of the community become involved in the institutions and decisions that will have an impact on their lives. It has the potential for creating more support, keeping people informed, influencing decisions, activating nonparticipants, improving service, and making people, plans, and programs more responsive (Checkoway, 1989). But community participation is not without costs: in most situations it requires time and effort, as well as persistence. Yet it can have a big impact on public policy issues involving health. Checkoway (1989) described several different types of community participation that may be useful in shaping health policy. These include: mass mobilization, social action, community planning, community services development, community education, and community advocacy. These different types of community participation are not mutually exclusive and thus can overlap each other. Mass mobilization brings people together in efforts to create or oppose change, such as a rally. Social action is used to build a powerful group at the community level, such as a group of "Citizens Against Poverty." Community planning means getting those within a community involved in planning the programs that they will "consume"—that is, helping to build a sense of ownership. Community service development includes efforts that emphasize self-sufficiency and community control, such as individual communities working to help the hungry and homeless. Community education includes both formal and informal means of increasing awareness and knowledge on specific issues. This could occur at adult education classes or public forums. Community advocacy is carried out by people seeking to influence decision makers (or those who enforce decisions) regarding legislation and policy. Lobbying and letter-writing campaigns are good examples of advocacy programs. When trying to influence decision makers, it is important to do the following:

1. Gather and use data wisely.
2. Identify committed leadership.
3. Gain grassroots support.
4. Look for other related issues that could further the effort.
5. Gain bipartisan support.
6. Work with appropriate lobbyists.
7. Spend resources carefully.

An effort to solicit support through a letter-writing campaign is presented in Appendix F. The letter reproduced in this appendix was written in August 1990 by the then president of the American Public Health Association (APHA) to solicit support from the membership for a congressional resolution on "Health Care For All." The mechanics of organizing community participation are discussed in Chapter 8.

Activities Affecting Organizational Culture

Closely aligned with environmental change activities is the category of activities that affect organizational culture. Culture is usually associated with norms and traditions that are generated by and linked to a "community" of people. Organizations, which are made up of people, also can have their own culture. The culture of an organization can be thought of as its personality. The culture expresses what is and what is not considered important. The nature of the culture depends on the type of organization—corporation, school, or nonprofit group.

Many people think that it takes a long time to establish norms and traditions, and it often does. Still, change can occur very quickly if the decision makers in an organization support it. For example, if organizational decision makers believe exercise is important, they may provide employees with an extra 20 minutes at lunchtime for exercise. Similarly, it is surprising to see how many young executives will use a corporation's exercise facility because the chief executive officer does. Other examples of activities that affect organizational culture might include changing the types of foods found in vending machines, closing the "junk food" machines during lunch periods at school, and offering discounts on the healthy foods found in the company cafeteria. Because these activities have the potential to affect a large group of people, they are usually thought of as macro interventions.

Communication Activities

Communication activities play an important part in most health promotion interventions. Among the best examples of the importance of communication activities are those activities associated with attempts by government agencies to communicate environmental health risks to the public (Chess, Salomone & Sandman, 1991; Covello & Allen, 1988; Covello, McCallum & Pavlova, 1989). However, the usefulness of communication activities goes well beyond their use in communicating environmental health risks. With regard to other health promotion interventions, communication activities have been shown to (1) increase awareness; (2) increase knowledge; (3) change attitudes (for example, about blood pressure, cancer screenings, and ills of smoking); (4) reinforce attitudes (for example, about smoking in public places); (5) maintain interest (for example, for those contemplating a behavior change); (6) provide cues for action; and (7) demonstrate simple skills (as in self-screening) (Bellicha & McGrath, 1990; Erickson, McKenna & Romano, 1990). Because of the techniques used, communication activities probably have the highest **penetration rate** (number in the target population exposed or reached) of any of the intervention activities. Thus they are most often used in macro interventions. They are also much more cost effective and less threatening than many other types of intervention activities.

Probably the most visible forms of communication activities are those in the mass media, which include: daily newspapers with national or local circulation; local weekly newspapers; local, public, and network television, including cable television; public and commercial radio stations; and magazines with either a broad readership or a narrow focus. There are many ways to convey a message using the mass media. These include news coverage, public affairs coverage, talk shows, public service roundtables, entertainment, public service announcements (PSAs) (see Appendix G for examples of PSAs used by the Indiana Board of Health), paid advertisements, editorials, letters to the editor, comic strips, and columnists' commentaries (Arkin, 1990). But communication activities are not limited to mass media; they can take many other forms. Information can be presented on billboards, in booklets, on bulletin boards, in church bulletins, in fliers, through direct mail (such as the mailing on the subject of AIDS sent by the Public Health Service to every U.S. household in 1988), on product labels (for alcohol, foods, and cigarettes), in newsletters, in pamphlets, on posters, and through self-help materials in print or on audio and video. The cost of communication activities can range from almost nothing (as when elementary school children make posters for a health awareness campaign in a community) to very expensive (a prime-time television commercial). No matter what the cost, for communication activities to be effective, they need to be carefully planned.

Several different authors have suggested procedures for effectively designing communication activities. Three such procedures are presented here. One of the most often used procedures for developing communication activities for health educators was developed by McGuire (1981). McGuire set out a seven-step approach for designing a public health communications campaign. The first step involves analyzing the situation to determine if the health problem of concern is sufficiently severe, if corrective behaviors for the problem are available, and if such behaviors can be effectively promoted through communication activities. The second step determines whether the communication activity is cost beneficial compared to other means of dealing with the problem. The third step examines the sociocultural factors of the target population to determine which could facilitate or impede the campaign's effectiveness. In the fourth step, planners seek to find out the psychological matrix of thoughts, feelings, and behaviors that instigate and sustain undesirable health behavior. For example, do those in the target population not eat properly because they do not know any better, cannot afford it, or do not care? The fifth step consists of analyzing the data collected in the first four steps to pick out the most promising target groups and techniques for the communication activities. The sixth step includes the construction of the persuasive communication by choosing the source, message, channel, receiver, and destination variables that have the greatest promise for changing the undesirable behavior. The seventh and last step, as with many planning procedures, is to evaluate the effectiveness of the campaign by monitoring each of the previous six steps and examining the end results.

The National Cancer Institute compiled a book (USDHHS, 1989) that is most useful for developing communication activities in both mass media and printed materials (other than newspapers). The book is organized around six stages in health communication. Figure 7.3 graphically represents these stages. The first stage is planning and strategy selection. This includes studying the health problem and the target population, deciding what objectives are to be accomplished, and deciding what the target population should be told. Stage 2 deals with selecting the appropriate communication channels (worksite, mass media, face-to-face) to be used and deciding which format (booklets, videotapes, newsletters) will best suit the channels and messages. Stage 3 consists of developing the materials and pretesting them with the target population. Feedback from the target population is most important at this stage. The fourth stage is the implementation of the activity. During this stage, the effect of the activity is tracked to determine if any alterations are needed. The fifth stage is evaluation, which should be based on the objectives identified in stage 1. The sixth stage, which loops right back to stage 1, incorporates feedback gained in the other stages to prepare for a new cycle of the communication. This method answers many key questions: What worked and did not work? How can we improve it the next time? Knowing the answers to these questions will lead to better future interventions.

Adcock, Nagy, and Adcock (1990) presented very useful information on how to better use the mass media to promote health education. They outline a step-by-step approach that includes, first, planning a press conference by selecting a site, day, and time; identifying a "newspeg" (a special event that heightens interest in the news release); and contacting the media. The second step is writing a press release; the third is conducting the press conference.

Economic and Other Incentives

The use of **incentives** to influence health outcomes is a common type of activity. This activity is based upon the stimulus response theory, which holds that peo-

Figure 7.3

Stages in health communication

Source: From *Making Health Communication Programs Work: A Planner's Guide* (p. 5) by U.S. Department of Health and Human Services (USDHHS), 1989, Washington, DC: Government Printing Office. NIH Publication No. 89-1493.

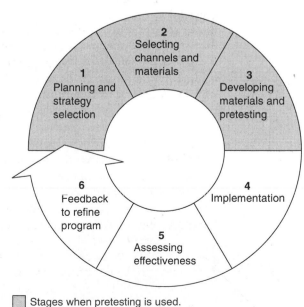

☐ Stages when pretesting is used.

ple are more likely to act in a certain manner if they are reinforced to do so. An incentive can increase the perceived value of an activity (Patton, Corry, Gettman & Graf, 1986). The key to motivating someone with an incentive is to know what will incite an individual to action. Thus, for this type of activity to work, the planner needs to match the incentives with the needs, wants, or desires of the target population. However, this is not easy, for what is an incentive for one person may be a deterrent for another, and vice versa. It has been suggested that incentives should even be tailored to the socioeconomic characteristics of the participants (Chenoweth, 1987) and, for that matter, the individual characteristics of each person.

For the planners, the task becomes one of matching the needs of the program participant or potential program participant with available incentives. Two approaches have been used to accomplish this. The first is to include questions about incentives as part of any needs assessment conducted in program planning. For example, a workforce needs survey might include questions on incentives, such as "What incentives would entice you to participate in the exercise program?" or "What would it take to get you to participate in this program?" or "What would it take to keep you involved in a health promotion program?" or "Would you continue to participate in an exercise program if you knew you were going to be given a nice tee shirt after logging 100 miles running or walking, or participating for 50 days in an aerobic dance or swimming program?" The responses to these questions should provide some indication of the type of incentives that would be most useful for this target population. The second is the shotgun approach, based upon previous experience or the experience reported by others. The shotgun approach offers a variety of incentives to meet the needs of a large percentage of the program's target population. However, we recommend the former approach as being more likely to meet the targeted needs and wants.

Based upon the idea that incentives should meet the individual needs of the target population, the number of different types of incentives is almost endless. Feldman (1983) has suggested two major categories of incentives or reinforcers. The first group includes incentives that would be considered social reinforcers, while the second group includes incentives that are considered material reinforcers, or what we refer to as economic incentives. A listing of such reinforcers is presented in Chapter 10.

As a final comment on incentives, planners should remember that incentives can be used to keep the target population from doing something as well for getting them to do something. For example, Penner (1989) reports on the use of a surcharge for health insurance to influence the behavior of those who continue to use tobacco products.

Social Intervention Activities

The importance of social support to behavior change and its relationship to health have been noted by several researchers (Becker & Green, 1975; Berkman & Syme, 1979; Colletti & Brownell, 1982; Horman, 1989; Kaplan & Cassell, 1977; Cummings, Becker & Maile, 1980). Many people find it much easier to change a behavior if those around them provide support or are willing to be partners in the behavior change process. One of the major reasons why worksite health promotion programs have been so well received is because of the built-in social support from coworkers (Behrens, 1983).

Reference has already been made to how social support could work as an incentive. That would be one form of a social activity. Other social interventions could include support groups, social activities, and social networks. These intervention activities have been used both in micro and macro interventions with much success.

Support Groups

The importance of support groups as part of comprehensive interventions has been well established. One need only look to the 12-step programs, such as Alcoholics Anonymous, Overeaters Anonymous, Gamblers Anonymous, and also commercial programs (such as Weight Watchers and Optifast) to realize the importance of people coming together to share their experiences and support one another's efforts. A support group need not be large; it might be as small as just two people. Sometimes this group of two is thought of as a buddy system, in which two individuals support each other, whether this means helping each other to stay on a special diet or meeting each other at 6 a.m. for exercise.

Special elements that can be added to the support group or buddy system are the use of competition or a contract. Competition can take place between individual group members over such things as who can lose the most weight, who can walk/run the most miles, or who can go the longest without a cigarette. Competition could also be based upon teams within the target population (such as two different companies, two schools, or departments within an organization) using similar criteria but now based on group total figures (pounds, miles, or cigarettes).

Contracts could be used by having one member of the target population enter into an agreement with another member or with another person (such as the program facilitator, a friend, or spouse) over a change in some health behavior. The major component of a contract is the contingency. The contingency is a statement of what will happen if a contract is met or not met. For example, if a person meets the terms of his contract by losing 10 pounds in 5 weeks, he can then expect to receive something specified (an intangible, such as praise, or a material object) from the person who agreed to the contract. If the terms are not met, then the person for whom the contract was written must forfeit something specified (perhaps time volunteered to a community service or a material object of his own).

Social Activities

Social activities can be an an important type of social intervention. Bringing people together who may be confronting similar problems for the purpose of purely social interaction not related to the problem can indirectly help them deal with the problem. Examples of such activities might be single parents having a cookout or a group of senior citizens attending a play. Although these activities do not deal directly with their common problems, they do help fill voids in people's lives and thus indirectly help with the problem.

Social Networks

Social networks are another type of social intervention. Networks are matrices linked by relationships or "ties." The nature of a tie can be quite varied, consisting of almost anything that creates a special feeling: need, concern, loyalty, frustration, power, affection, or obligation, to name just a few. When people are "networking" they are said to be looking for relationships that would be useful in helping them with their concerns, such as problem solving, program development, resource identification, and others. As part of a health promotion intervention, social networking may take the form of having program participants trade telephone numbers for the purpose of calling each other when they are trying to resist smoking a cigarette or trying to locate a needed resource to solve a problem.

DESIGNING HEALTH PROMOTION INTERVENTIONS

Once program planners have completed a needs assessment, written program goals and objectives, and considered different types of intervention activities, they are in a position to begin designing an appropriate intervention.

Criteria and Guidelines for Developing a Health Promotion Intervention

There is no one best way of intervening to accomplish a specific program goal that can be generalized to all target populations. Each target population has its own needs and wants that must be addressed. Nevertheless, successful and responsible health promotion programs generally adhere to some common set of guidelines, standards, or criteria around which their interventions are planned (Ad Hoc Work Group, 1987). Such guidelines help to standardize and ensure the quality of the program, give credibility to a program, help with program accountability, provide a legal defense if a liability situation might arise, and identify ethical concerns that need to be addressed as a part of planning, implementing, and evaluating programs.

In 1987, the American Public Health Association (APHA) in collaboration with the Center for Health Promotion and Education of the Centers for Disease Control (CDC) developed a set of criteria to serve as guidelines for establishing the feasibility and/or the appropriateness of health education and promotion programs in a variety of settings (industrial, hospital, worksite, voluntary and official agencies) before making a decision to implement them. The criteria were not developed to assure successful programs, but rather to suggest issues that need to be considered in the decision-making process leading to the allocation of resources or the setting of program priorities (Ad Hoc Work Group, 1987, pp. 89–92). The five criteria suggested by the Work Group are:

1.   A health promotion program should address one or more risk factors which are carefully defined, measurable, modifiable, and prevalent among the members of a chosen target group, factors which constitute a threat to the health status and the quality of life of target group members.

2.   A health promotion program should reflect a consideration of the special characteristics, needs, and preferences of its target group(s).

3.   Health promotion programs should include interventions which will clearly and effectively reduce a target risk factor and are appropriate for a particular setting.

4.   A health promotion program should identify and implement interventions which make optimum use of the available resources.

5.   From the outset, a health promotion program should be organized, planned, and implemented in such a way that its operation and effects can be evaluated.

In addition to the criteria set forth by APHA and CDC, other agencies and organizations have suggested criteria and guidelines. The Society of Prospective Medicine has developed some definitions of commonly used terms in health education and promotion and a set of "Guidelines for Health Risk Appraisal/Reduction Systems." This organization refers to the individual guidelines as essentials. The essentials are the basic attributes that need to be present in any **risk appraisal/risk reduction** program, no matter who provides it, where it is offered, or how long it runs. The seven essentials offered by the society (Task Force, 1981) state that every program should:

1.   Have a written statement of objectives of the program and limitations.

2.   Have evidence of a scientific base for the risk appraisal instrument.

3.   Show that appropriate risk reduction resources are available to participants.

4.   Be able to demonstrate the staff's capability to organize and conduct risk appraisal/reduction programs in accordance with stated objectives.

5.   Ensure that participants receive the results of their appraisals in a form they can comprehend, including recommendations to consult an appropriate health provider when needed.

6.   Have mechanisms to protect the confidentiality of the data on individual participants.

7.   Have evidence of efforts to evaluate the program periodically in relation to objectives.

Some organizations and professionals have set guidelines, criteria, or **codes of practice** for specific types of health promotion programs. Examples are the criteria set forth by the American College of Sports Medicine (1980) for exercise programs, the guidelines established by the American College of Obstetricians and Gynecologists for exercise during pregnancy, and the "Code of Practice for Smoking Cessation Programs" (see Appendix H for a copy of this code) agreed upon by the American Cancer Society, the American Health Foundation, the American Heart Association, the American Lung Association, the Five-Day Plan to Stop Smoking, and SmokEnders. Another example is the guidelines for conducting smoking cessation programs put forth by Bartlett, Windsor, Lowe, and Nelson (1986).

Obviously, the guidelines and criteria listed here are not all that are available. Prudent planners should seek out, through inquiry and networking, other criteria and guidelines that apply to programs they are planning.

Ethics and Health Promotion Interventions

It is not unusual for program planners to be faced with decisions about **ethics** when designing interventions. Is it ethical to require people to wear safety belts and fine them if they do not? To try to persuade people to do something they do not want to do? To try out a new smoking cessation treatment on a group without their knowledge? To withhold treatment from people because they cannot afford it? To help people lose weight in any way possible as long as they succeed in losing it? To use a sensationalist or fear-arousing method in teaching? To largely ignore the content recommendations of parents when teaching school health classes? To grade students on health behaviors or behavior change? These are just a few of the ethical questions that program planners may have to address.

As program planners begin to develop interventions, the following moral and ethical concerns need to be addressed (Shirreffs, Odom, McLeroy, Cryer & Fors, 1990):

1. Respect the goals and values of those in the target population.
2. Be aware of the degrees of autonomy related to health behavior.
    a. Facilitation—assist in achieving objectives set by a target group (for example, putting safety belts in cars).
    b. Persuasion—argue and reason with others (for example, telling others about the importance of safety belts).
    c. Manipulation—modifying environment or psychic disposition (for example, automatic safety belts or passive restraints).
    d. Coercion—threat of deprivation (for example, a safety belt law and fine).
3. Follow the necessary steps to provide informed consent to those in the target population.
    a. Explanation of nature and purposes of procedures.
    b. Explanation of discomfort or risks.
    c. Explanation of expected benefits.
    d. Disclosure of alternate procedures.
    e. Offer to answer questions.
    f. Indication that the person is free to discontinue participation.

4.   Be just and fair.

5.   Protect the confidentiality and privacy of those in the target population.

6.   Do not cause harm (nonmaleficence). Do not omit something you should include (omission) and do not do something you should not (commission).

7.   Work to bring about or do good (beneficence).

A Model for Designing Interventions

What should be included in a health promotion intervention? This question is constantly asked by those who are responsible for planning programs. The criteria and guidelines listed earlier in this chapter and the theories presented in Chapter 6 provide a partial answer to this question, but more guidance is needed to help planners in the development of well-conceived interventions. For this reason we felt it was important to present a model that would be useful in planning a comprehensive intervention. By this we mean an intervention that could address several of the eight objective levels presented in Chapter 5 and would include several different intervention activities. Although the major focus of this model is to change health behavior, it also addresses the levels of awareness, knowledge, skill development, and health service; if behavior change takes place then, at least in theory, the risk will be reduced and health status will improve. We have chosen to develop a model aimed at behavior change because, in reality, much of what is done in the name of health promotion is aimed at health behavior change.

The model (Figure 7.4) includes eight components and brings together the theories, models, and ideas of several different authors (Cummings, Becker &

Figure 7.4
Model for building a comprehensive intervention

Maile, 1980; Dennison, 1984; Green et al., 1980; Marlatt, 1985; McKenzie, 1988; McKenzie & Dunn, 1984). Although it may not be feasible for program planners to use all steps in the model, because of limitations specific to their situation, the model does provide planners with a "skeleton" on which to build a comprehensive intervention. However, whether program planners use this model or another, they should devote much thought to the health problem or concern, the desired program outcome(s), at what points to intervene, and the most effective intervention activities for the problem. The following sections describe the components of our model.

First Component: Education and Awareness Building

This component of the model is included to provide the target population with the awareness and the necessary background to understand the scope of the health concern or problem the program is intended to address (Cummings et al., 1980; McKenzie & Dunn, 1984). For instance, if a program is aimed at changing the behavior of people in order to lower their serum cholesterol levels, after experiencing this component of the intervention those in the target population should know (1) what cholesterol is; (2) why it is a health concern; (3) what contributes to the level found in one's blood; and (4) what are acceptable cholesterol readings. Answering these questions could be the basis of a semester-long college course, but the purpose of this component is not to provide in-depth information on the health concern or problem; rather, it should provide an overview. After experiencing this component, the participants should have a general understanding of the health concern or problem and should not be mystified by medical jargon and statistics. This component could be accomplished through an introductory session of a program, through a pamphlet distributed to all those in the target population, or through a series of public service announcements on television or radio.

Second Component: Personal Assessment

Once the program participants have an overall understanding of the health concern or problem, they need to see how the problem relates to their own life or situation. Therefore, we suggest that planners allow the participants either to assess themselves or, if that is not possible, to be assessed by someone else to find out how they compare to norms or averages with regard to the health concern or problem. This component will help make the program more relevant to the individual participants, thus increasing their interest and motivation. Typical assessments could include: (1) a health risk appraisal (HRA); (2) disease-specific risk appraisals like Risko or Cancer Risks (see Table 4.1 in Chapter 4 for a listing of commonly used, problem-specific, paper-and-pencil HRA instruments); (3) a **field test**, such as Cooper's 12-minute or 1.5-mile run (Cooper, 1982) or a treadmill test for physical fitness; (4) a health screening (blood pressure, body composition, or cholesterol); (5) a paper-and-pencil assessment for stress, stress management, or personality type; or (6) a record of consumption patterns for tobacco, alcohol, or food, as is commonly done with the 24- and 48-hour diaries.

The personal assessment is completed primarily for the benefit of the program participants, even though it can also provide valuable information for the program facilitators. There is, however, another assessment that can be very helpful for the program planners at this point of the intervention: one that is used to determine participants' attitude toward health in general and toward the specific health concern or problem being addressed in the program (Cummings et al., 1980). What value do the program participants put on health? Are the program participants **self-efficacious** (the internal state that individuals experience as "competent" to perform certain desired tasks or behaviors) with regard to skills or behavior necessary to deal with the concern or problem? What type of health **locus of control** (a psychosocial variable that measures people's feelings of whether they are in control of their behavior) do the program participants have? Are the participants ready for change? Answers to these questions could go a long way in helping program planners in selecting and designing appropriate program interventions. There are several instruments available to help collect this type of data. They include the Value Survey (K. A. Wallston, personal communication, 1984), Multi-dimensional Health Locus of Control (MHLC) Scales (Wallston, Wallston & DeVellis, 1978), Terminal Values (Rokeach, 1969), Stages of Change (McConnaughy, Prochaska & Velicer, 1983), and the Rotter Internal-External Locus of Control Scale (Rotter, 1966). Other valuable assessment scales may be found in a set of books from IOX Assessment Associates (1988) that should be useful with this component of the model.

The first two components of this model should provide both the program participants and the program planners with a good understanding of the predisposing factors (see Chapter 2 for a definition of this term) to which Green and colleagues (1980) have referred.

Third Component: Goal Setting

Once those in the target population have an understanding of the health concern or problem and know what their own status is in relationship to it, they are ready to set goals for themselves. These goals are not to be confused with the program goals discussed in Chapter 5. The goals we are referring to now are individual or personal goals for the participants. Individual goal setting should help to maintain participants' interest, individualize the program as much as possible, and motivate the participants to continue their participation in the program. In the goal-setting process, program planners need to make sure that the participants set realistic goals for themselves. An unrealistic goal can be just as detrimental to a participant as a realistic goal can be motivating. In addition to being realistic, program goals should be based upon the best available information and research on the health concern or problem.

To guide health planners in understanding the difference between appropriate (realistic and soundly based) and inappropriate (unrealistic goals or goals that are not based on sound information) goals, we present several examples of each. After each inappropriate goal the reason why it is inappropriate is stated in parentheses.

Inappropriate goals for program participants

1.   I plan to lose 30 pounds during this four-week weight loss program. (Research has shown that a healthy weight loss rate is 1–2 pounds per week.)

2.   I will lose 10 pounds using the grapefruit diet. (Weight loss should incorporate sound eating habits and exercise.)

3.   I want to lose 10 pounds during my participation in the program. (Why 10 pounds? Is this figure based upon a body composition test or weighing oneself, or is it based on the feeling that "I look better when I am ten pounds lighter"?)

4.   As an alcoholic, I plan to reduce my alcohol intake to zero, then just drink socially. (Recovering alcoholics cannot drink socially.)

5.   After the first six weeks of my aerobics exercise program, I want to be in good enough shape to run a marathon. (Training for a long endurance race takes much longer than six weeks, especially for the beginning exerciser.)

Appropriate participant goals

1.   Based upon my body composition test, I will lose 10 pounds. This will put my percentage of body fat at 15% (for males; 22% for females).

2.   One year after the last class of the smoking cessation program, I will no longer be smoking.

3.   I will burn 400 calories more per day than I am doing now.

4.   At the end of this program, I will be able to conduct a breast self-examination (or a testicular self-examination) and explain it to someone else.

5.   I will incorporate one stress management technique into my daily schedule.

Fourth Component: Knowledge and Skill Building

Upon completion of any health promotion program, those in the target population should possess the necessary knowledge and skills to behave in a healthy manner with regard to the health concern of interest. If people want to eat in a healthy manner, they must first know what the "healthy manner" is and, second, have the necessary skills to prepare or choose the appropriate foods to eat. If people want to begin an aerobic exercise program, they need to know how to exercise and to have the skills to do so properly. This component of the model would be included in what Green and colleagues (1980) have referred to as enabling factors (see Chapter 2 for a definition of this term).

This is the component of the model in which those in the target population learn most of the information about the concern or problem, and also learn the skills necessary to deal with it. The actual time needed to incorporate this component may be just a one-hour session, as with a breast self-examination or a testicular self-examination program; it may take 4–12 hours, as for a course in cardiopulmonary resuscitation (CPR); or it may take weeks, as with weight loss, exercise, or nutrition programs.

Fifth Component: Opportunity to Practice the Behavior

This component of the model has three major aspects. The first is to make sure that the planned intervention includes activities for removing barriers that stand between those in the target population and healthier behavior. Planners should consider barriers such as limited access, availability, and resources, and prohibitive policies and laws.

The second aspect of this component is to allow those in the target group an opportunity to put into practice the new knowledge and skills learned in the fourth component. Too many health promotion programs provide people with the knowledge and skills to behave in a healthy manner, but never give them an opportunity to practice the activity. If people are going to stop smoking, they need to practice those skills to stop. If people want to become involved in a program of regular exercise, they need to experience it, not just read or be told about exercising (Dennison, 1984).

Most, but not all, interventions can be planned to incorporate this "get them involved" step, in which program participants can experience the new behavior. In preparing the program participants for situations in which they cannot actually experience the new behavior, a lifelike experience may be the next best thing. An example of this may be the social pressure people experience when trying to break a habit, like smoking. There always seems to be someone around who tries to pressure the person to have "just one." In this case, a lifelike experience could include a role-playing activity; other possibilities would be responding to a case study or analyzing a critical incident. All of these "next best" experiences allow people to think about and react to a situation before they experience it in real life.

The third important aspect of this component is letting the program participants see others practicing healthy behaviors. People not only learn vicariously (by seeing others doing the behavior), but also they can become self-efficacious (an internal feeling that they indeed can do the behavior) from watching others. Allowing new participants in a weight loss program to interact with those who have been through it previously, letting new exercise participants watch an exercise class in session, or making sure employees see the executives wearing their safety belts while driving company-owned cars are all very important.

Sixth Component: Relapse Prevention Skills

It has been said that getting people to change behavior is hard, but having them maintain the behavior is much harder. This is nicely illustrated by the old saying, "giving up smoking is easy, I've done it a hundred times." At one time, it was enough for health promotion program planners just to get people to change their behavior, now they need to do more. Because of the difficulty of maintaining a new behavior, program planners need to give special attention to helping those in the target population from slipping back to their previous behaviors.

Although much of the early research dealing with this concept of slipping back was conducted using addictive behaviors, such as substance abuse and gambling, the concept applies to all behavior change, including preventive health behaviors. Marlatt (1982) indicates that a high percentage of individuals who enter programs for health behavior change **relapse** to their former behaviors within one year. More specifically, researchers have warned program planners of **recidivism** problems with participants in exercise (Dishman, Sallis & Orenstein, 1985; Horne, 1975), weight loss (Stunkard & Braunwell, 1980), and smoking cessation (Leventhal & Cleary, 1980) programs. Therefore, planners need to make sure that program interventions include the skills necessary for dealing with those difficult times during behavior change.

Marlatt (1982) has referred to the process of trying to prevent slipping back as **relapse prevention**. Relapse prevention, which is based on social cognitive theory, "is a self-control program designed to teach individuals who are trying to change their behavior how to anticipate and cope with the problem of relapse" (Marlatt, 1982, p. 329). Relapse is triggered by high risk situations. "A high risk situation is defined broadly as any situation which poses a threat to the individual's sense of control and increases the risk of potential relapse" (Marlatt, 1982, p. 338). Cummings, Gordon, and Marlatt (1980), in a study of clients with a variety of problem behaviors (drinking, smoking, heroin addiction, gambling, and overeating), found high risk situations to fall into two major categories—intrapersonal and interpersonal determinants. They found that 56% of the relapse situations were caused by intrapersonal determinants, such as negative emotional states (35%), negative physical states (3%), positive emotional states (4%), testing personal control (5%), and urges and temptations (9%). The 44% of the situations represented by interpersonal determinants included interpersonal

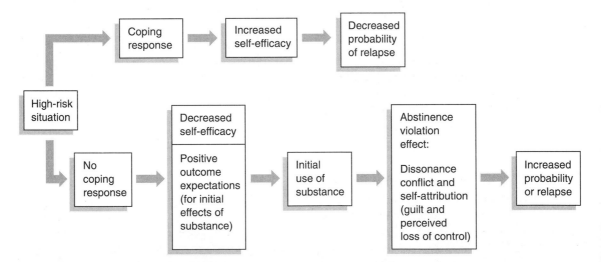

Figure 7.5
Cognitive-behavioral model of the relapse process
Source: From "Relapse Prevention: Theoretical Rationale and Overview of the Model" by G. A. Marlatt, in G. A. Marlatt and J. R. Gordon (Eds.), *Relapse Prevention* (p. 38), 1985, New York: Guilford Press. Reprinted by permission of Guilford Press.

conflicts (16%), social pressure (20%), and positive emotional states (8%). These determinants can be referred to as the covert antecedents of relapse. That is to say, these high risk situations do not just happen; instead, they are created by what Marlatt (1982) calls lifestyle imbalances.

People who have the coping skills to deal with a high risk situation have a much greater chance of preventing relapse than those who do not. Figure 7.5 illustrates the possible paths one may take in a high risk situation (Marlatt, 1982).

Marlatt has developed both global (Figure 7.6) and specific (Figure 7.7) self-control strategies for relapse intervention. Specific intervention procedures are designed to help participants anticipate and cope with the relapse episode itself, while the global intervention procedures are designed to modify the early antecedents of relapse, including restructuring of the participant's general style of life. A complete application of the relapse prevention model would include both specific and global interventions (Marlatt, 1982).

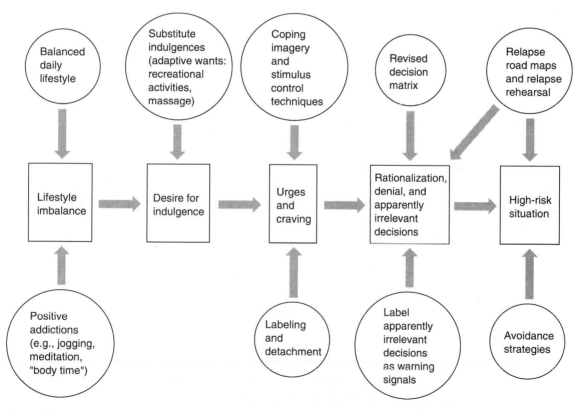

Figure 7.6
Relapse prevention: global self-control strategies

Source: From "Relapse Prevention: Theoretical Rationale and Overview of the Model" by G. A. Marlatt, in G. A. Marlatt and J. R. Gordon (Eds.), *Relapse Prevention* (p. 61), 1985, New York: Guilford Press. Reprinted by permission of Guilford Press.

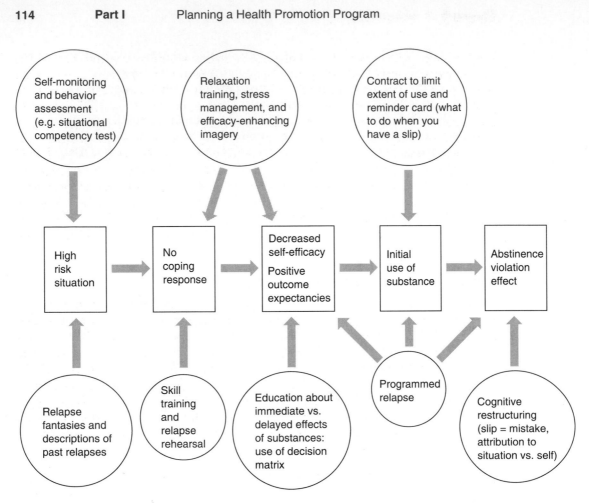

Figure 7.7
Relapse prevention: specific intervention strategies
Source: From "Relapse Prevention: Theoretical Rationale and Overview of the Model" by G. A. Marlatt, in G. A. Marlatt and J. R. Gordon (Eds.), *Relapse Prevention* (p. 54), 1985, New York: Guilford Press. Reprinted by permission of Guilford Press.

Seventh Component: Monitoring Progress of the Target Population

After those in the target population have had the opportunity to experience their new behavior, either actually or through a lifelike situation, they need to reflect on, critique, and monitor their progress. This monitoring process will provide the participants and planners with feedback that can be used to: (1) reinforce what is being done; (2) check learning; (3) help prevent relapse; and (4) identify areas that should be corrected and not reinforced.

The monitoring process can be completed by anyone involved in the program; it may take many different forms depending on the program goals and objectives. It can be completed by the participants themselves, by other participants, by the facilitators of the program, or by a combination of these individuals. Commonly used techniques for participants to self-monitor their progress are keeping logs of their activity or behavior (weight loss, miles walked, percentage of a particular group adhering to a specific behavior) or charting or graphing their progress. Other participants could be involved in the monitoring process by providing verbal feedback on the behavior of their peers after a role-playing situation, by giving their opinion on progress made to date, or by reviewing a videotape of a role-playing situation, critical incident, or even a real situation. This responsibility has traditionally been approached by having program facilitators monitor the target population's progress. Techniques have included various forms of testing, verbal feedback, written critiques of work, and use of checklists.

No matter what technique is used, it is most important that progress be monitored and feedback provided. This component, which leads into the eighth component, is encompassed in what Green and colleagues (1980) refer to as reinforcing factors (see Chapter 2 for a definition of this term).

Eighth Component: Redefining Participant Goals

After the program participants have had the opportunity either to monitor their own progress or to have it monitored by another, they need to compare their progress to the goal(s) they set in the third component of the model. If their goals are still realistic, given the progress made to date, they should continue. If not, they should rework the goals with the program facilitator to make them realistic. This would mean repeating the activity described in component 3 concerning goal setting and then working through the remaining components as they apply to the new goal(s). This component could be completed in a group setting with discussion, in one-on-one sessions between participant and facilitator, or by the participants themselves.

☐ SUMMARY

Interventions are activities used by program planners to bring about the outcomes identified in the program objectives. These activities are also sometimes referred to as "treatments." Although many times an intervention is made up of a single activity, it is more common for planners to use a variety of activities to make up an intervention for a program. In this chapter, intervention activities were categorized into the following groups: (1) traditional educational activities or methods; (2) activities based upon behavior modification; (3) environmental change activities; (4) regulatory activities; (5) community participation activities to influence public policy; (6) activities affecting the organizational culture; (7) communication activities; (8) economic and other incentives; and (9) social intervention activities.

Additionally, this chapter identified the need for program planners to be aware of recommended standards/criteria/guidelines when planning program interventions. Some examples were reviewed of general, as well as program-specific, guidelines that have been set forth by both professional organizations and individual professionals. Finally, this chapter presented an eight-component model that planners can use in developing health education interventions.

❑ QUESTIONS

1. What is an intervention?

2. What are the advantages of using a multiactivity intervention over one that includes a single activity? Are there any disadvantages?

3. What are the major categories of interventions? Explain each.

4. Why should program planners be concerned with program guidelines that have been developed by professional organizations?

5. Name and briefly describe the major categories of ethical concerns related to intervention development.

6. What are some of the documents and sponsoring groups that have suggested standards, criteria, or guidelines for program development?

7. Name and briefly explain the eight components of the model set forth in this chapter.

8. What is meant by *relapse, relapse prevention,* and *recidivism?*

❑ ACTIVITIES

1. Using one of the *behavior* objectives you created in activity 1 of Chapter 5, design and describe a multiactivity intervention to accomplish the objective. Try to develop an intervention for each component of the model presented in this chapter. Explain in detail each of the activities you select and why you are using it, and identify on which theoretical construct the activity is based (you may want to refer to Chapter 6). You may find it helpful to use the following chart.

   Objective

Activity	Rationale	Theoretical Construct

   1.

   2.

   3.

   4.

   5.

   6.

7.

8.

2.   Create a multiactivity intervention for a program that has as its goal "to get third-grade students to wear helmets while riding their bicycles."

3.   Create a multiactivity intervention for a program that has as its goal "to eliminate smoking of all employees of company X."

4.   Create a multiactivity intervention for a program that has as its goal "the rehydration of young children in the small village of Y in the Third World country of Q."

5.   Write a one-paragraph statement outlining the ethical stand your organization will take with regard to program development.

6.   Develop a three-fold pamphlet that can be used as an informational piece for a program you are planning.

7.   With other students in your class, write a PSA script for a program you are planning. Then rehearse the script and have it videotaped.

8.   Write a two-page, double-spaced news release that describes a program you are planning.

9.   Write a letter to your state or federal senators or representatives requesting their support of a piece of health-related legislation that is currently being considered.

10.   Describe a set of relapse prevention skills necessary for a person who is losing weight through a diet and exercise program.

Part II

Implementing a Health Promotion Program

8
Community Organization

After reading this chapter and answering the questions at the end, you should be able to:

❑ Define *community, community organization, community development,* and *coalitions.*

❑ Outline a process for organizing a community.

❑ Provide an overview of PATCH.

KEY TERMS

active participants

bottom-up

citizen initiated

citizen participation

coalitions

community

community organization

gatekeepers

grass-roots participation

locality development

network

networking

occasional participants

ownership

PATCH

social action

social planning

stakeholders

supporting participants

top down

H ealth educators most often implement health promotion programs with small communities of people. By **community**, we mean a group of people (social unit) who have some common characteristic. This common element might be a geographic area (neighborhood, village, town, city, county, district, state, or region), a work group (employees of a business, workers in an industry, or students or staff in a school district), a shared interest or function (welfare, agriculture, education, or religion), a social concern (issues and causes), an ethnic background, or any other commonality. Thus it is not uncommon for health educators to implement a smoking cessation program in a corporate setting, organize a support group for families affected by a chronic disease, or present a drug education program for school-age children. However, health educators sometimes work with large communities, a task that involves organizing the people in a community to work together to implement a solution to a communitywide problem, concern, or issue. This chapter addresses the fundamental elements of organizing large communities for action.

COMMUNITY ORGANIZATION AND ITS ASSUMPTIONS

When one begins to read the literature regarding community organization, it becomes apparent that not everyone defines community organization in the same way. As a matter of fact, several terms are used that have similar or overlapping definitions. Terms such as **citizen participation**, *community participation*, **grass-roots participation**, *macro practice*, and *community development* seem to be intertwined in the literature (Archer, Kelly & Bisch, 1984; Brager, Specht & Torczyner, 1987; Checkoway, 1989; Checkoway & Van Til, 1978; Connor, 1968; Kickbusch, 1989; Perlman, 1978; Perlman & Gurin, 1972; Rifkin, 1986; Ross, 1967;

Rothman & Tropman, 1987). The term *community development* is often mixed with *community organization*; their definitions are very similar. Probably the most accepted definition of *community development* is found in a United Nations (1955, p. 6) publication, where the term is defined as "a process designed to create conditions of economic and social progress for the whole community with its active participation and the fullest possible reliance on the community's initiative."

The term **community organization** comes from the social work literature and refers to various methods of intervention to deal with social problems. "Most problems or goals requiring a community organization effort are by definition larger than any one organization can be expected to handle, and stakes in the community issue often affect many different interest groups" (Green, 1990, pp. 175–76). *Community organization* has been defined as "the method of intervention whereby individuals, groups, and organizations engage in planned action to influence social problems. It is concerned with the enrichment, development, and/or change of social institutions" (Brager et al., 1987, p. 55). It is not a science but an art of building consensus within a democratic process (Ross, 1967).

Even though formal community organization has taken place for a long time, the needs and efforts to organize communities now seem to be greater than in years past. In the early history of the United States a sense of community was inherent in everyday life (Green, 1989, March). It was natural for communities to pool their resources to deal with shared problems. As time has passed, technology has improved greatly, resources have become more centralized, and American society has become more mobile. As a result of these changes, communities have become more dependent on those outside the community and have fewer reasons to interact with neighboring communities. "From self-sufficient farming communities of colonial America to the single-industry towns of the westward expansion and the industrial revolution to the Silicon Valleys of today's information and service era, communities have become increasingly dependent on other communities and on higher levels of organization and government to facilitate, coordinate, and regulate their interdependence (Green, 1990, p. 165).

Although community organization may not be as "natural" as it once was, communities can still organize to analyze and solve problems through collective action (Table 8.1). In working toward this end, those who try to organize communities must make several assumptions. Ross (1967, pp. 86–92) has stated these as follows:

1. "Communities of people can develop capacity to deal with their own problems."
2. "People want to change and can change."
3. "People should participate in making, adjusting, or controlling the major changes taking place in their communities."

Table 8.1
Terms associated with community organization

Citizen participation—the bottom-up, grass-roots mobilization of citizens for the purpose of undertaking activities to improve the condition of something in the community.

Community development—"a process designed to create conditions of economic and social progress for the whole community with its active participation and the fullest possible reliance on the community's initiative" (United Nations, 1955, p. 6).

Community organization—"the method of intervention whereby individuals, groups, and organizations engage in planned action to influence social problems. It is concerned with the enrichment, development, and/or change of social institutions" (Brager et al., 1987, p. 55).

Community participation—"a process of involving people in the institutions or decisions that affect their lives" (Checkoway, 1989, p. 18).

Grass-roots participation—"bottom-up efforts of people taking collective actions on their own behalf, and they involve the use of a sophisticated blend of confrontation and cooperation in order to achieve their ends" (Perlman, 1978, p. 65).

Macro practice—the methods of professional change that deal with issues beyond the individual, family, and small group level.

4.   "Changes in community living that are self-imposed or self-developed have a meaning and permanence that imposed changes do not have."

5.   "A `holistic approach' can deal successfully with problems with which a `fragmented approach' cannot cope."

6.   "Democracy requires cooperative participation and action in the affairs of the community, and that the people must learn the skills which make this possible."

7.   "Frequently communities of people need help in organizing to deal with their needs, just as many individuals require help in coping with their individual problems."

THE PROCESS OF COMMUNITY ORGANIZATION

There is no one specific method for organizing a community. In fact, Rothman and Tropman (1987, pp. 4–5) have stated, "We should speak of community organization methods rather than the community organization method." Over the years, several different community organization methods have been used, including revolutionary techniques (Alinsky, 1971). However, in recent years three models of community organization have been developed (Rothman & Tropman, 1987). They are locality development, social planning, and social action. **Locality development** is most like community development and seeks community change through broad self-help participation from the local community. The Peace Corps is a good example. **Social planning** emphasizes a technical process of problem solving that includes various levels of participation, ranging from a little to a lot, and involves outside planners. The United Way is an example of social planning. **Social action** deals with organizing a disadvantaged segment of the population. It aims at making change in institutions and communities and often seeks a redistribution of resources and power. Although this model is no longer used as often as it once was, it was most useful during the civil rights and homosexual rights movements.

At the risk of violating Rothman and Tropman's (1987) maxim that there are various ways of organizing a community based upon existing resources and problems, and since our purpose in this chapter is to provide an overview of community organization, we present a very general or generic approach to organizing a community (see Figure 8.1). It does not include everything planners need to know about community organization, but it does present the basic elements. Our model relies heavily on social planning but also includes some specific elements from locality development and social action. For further information about community organization, readers should refer to any of several books listed in the References that are devoted entirely to the subject. Also, there are several works that deal specifically with the application of community organization to health promotion activities (Blackburn, 1983; Kumpfer, Turner & Alvarado, 1991; Maccoby & Solomon, 1981; McAlister, Puska, Salonen, Tuomilehot & Koskelia, 1982, and Pentz, Johnson, Dwyer, MacKinnon, Hansen & Flay, 1989).

Recognizing the Problem

The process of community organization begins when an individual, group, or organization recognizes that a problem (or concern or issue) exists in the community and that something needs to be done about it. For the purposes of our discussion, we will assume that the problem is a health problem, but the community organization process could be used with any type of problem found in a community. Problems can be as specific as trying to get a certain piece of legislation passed to something as general as advocating for a drug-free community.

The recognition of a health problem can occur from inside or outside the community. A concerned citizen or a church leader from within the community may point out the problem, or it may first be identified by someone outside the community, such as an employee of a local or state health department, a state legislator, or someone from a local voluntary health agency. Internal recognition of the problem is referred to as **citizen initiated** and includes **bottom-up**, or grass-roots, groups. When recognition occurs from outside, it is thought of as mandated from the **top down**, and efforts are then made to gain citizen involvement (Perlman, 1978).

Making Entry into the Community

Recognition of a problem does not mean that people should immediately set about correcting it. Instead, they should follow a set of steps to deal with the problem: making proper "entry" into the community is the first step. Braithwaite, Murphy, Lythcott, and Blumenthal (1989) have stressed the importance of tactfully negotiating entry into a community with the individuals who

Figure 8.1
Summary of the steps of
community organization

Recognizing the problem

Making entry into the community

Organizing the people

Identifying the specific problem to handle

Determining the priorities and setting goals

Selecting a solution to the problem

Implementing the plan

Evaluating the outcomes of the plan of action

Maintaining the outcomes in the community

Looping back

control, both formally and informally, the "political climate" of the community. These individuals are referred to as **gatekeepers**, or community opinion leaders. They may include people such as business leaders, education leaders, heads of law enforcement agencies, leaders of community activist groups, parent and teacher groups, clergy, politicians, and others. Their support is absolutely essential to the success of any attempt to organize a community.

To make entry, community organizers must first be familiar with the community they want to help. They must know: (1) with whom the power lies; (2) what type of political interactions take place within the community; and (3) whether the problem has been recognized before and, if so, how it was addressed. In other words, community organizers must have a thorough knowledge of the community and the people living there before they try to enter the informal boundaries of the community (Braithwaite et al., 1989). Having a thorough understanding of the community and tactfully approaching its gatekeepers will help community organizers to develop credibility and trust with those in the community. It is not easy to bring a problem to the attention of those in the community. Few people are glad to know they have a problem, and fewer still like for others to tell them they have a problem. Move with caution, and do not be too aggressive!

A specific strategy for "making entry into the community" would be to work with an established organization/institution that is well received in the community. Green (1990) has suggested that the academic health center might be the ideal convener to address health services, health protection, or health promotion issues. "It has the deep roots in the community, it is not typically beholden to an out-of-state master, it can cut deals with local organizations, and it can draw upon resources to leverage commitments and resources from other organizations" (Green, 1990, p. 175).

Organizing the People

Once entry into a community has been gained, work must begin to organize those in the community. It is best to begin with those individuals who are already interested in solving the problem. This is not the time either to try to convert people to the cause or to make sure all the key players of the community are involved. It is best to begin with a core group of people who want to see change occur. Make sure this group includes people who are affected by the problem. For example, if you are dealing with a teenage drug problem, include teens in the core group. If you are trying to help low-income individuals who need housing, make sure they are involved. More often than not, this core group will be small and will consist of people who are committed to the resolution of the problem regardless of the time frame. Brager and colleagues (1987) have referred to this core group as executive participants. From among the core group, a leader or coordinator must be identified. If at all possible, the leader should be someone with leadership skills and a good knowledge of the problem. One of the early tasks of the leader will be to help build group cohesion.

With the core group in place, the next step is to expand the group to build support for dealing with the problem—that is, to broaden the constituency. Brager and colleagues (1987) have noted that other group participants will include active, occasional, and supporting participants. The **active participants** (who may also be executive participants) take part in most group activities and are not afraid to do the work that needs to be done. The **occasional participants** become involved on an irregular basis and usually only when major decisions are made. The **supporting participants** are seldom involved but help swell the ranks and may contribute in nonactive ways or through financial contributions. When expanding the group, look for others who may be interested in helping, and ask current group members for names of people who might be interested. Look for people who may already be dealing with the problem through their present work or who have the resources to contribute. This search should include existing social groups, such as voluntary health agencies, agricultural extension services, church groups, hospitals, health care providers, political officeholders, policy makers, police, educators, lay citizens, or special interest groups.

Getting people involved in community organization efforts is not an easy task. Organizers must ask people to give of their time and energy to help. Both time and energy are precious to most people, so organizers should make it as easy as possible for people to become involved. To this end, they may even provide rewards and perquisites, or "perks." One way to do this is to allow people in the larger group to work in their areas of strength (for example, having educators work with other educators, or police with other police) and to provide the training needed so people can feel compatible carrying out their assigned tasks. For example, one should not ask people to solicit contributions by telephone if they have not been trained to do so.

These expanded community groups are sometimes referred to as associations, task forces, or **coalitions**. These types of groups build a constituency in support of the problem; there is power in numbers, and pooled resources can maximize the energy of those involved. Of these types of community groups, the coalition is probably considered the most formal. A coalition can be defined as a temporary union of two or more individuals and/or organizations to achieve a common purpose (often, to compensate for deficits in power, resources and expertise). The underlying concept behind coalitions is collaboration, for several individuals, groups, or organizations with their collective resources have a better chance of solving the problem than any single entity.

Table 8.2 provides a modified list of guidelines (Lindsay & Edwards, 1988) for keeping a coalition dynamic, viable, and effective.

Identifying the Specific Problem to Tackle

With the expanded community group in place, the first task is to isolate the specific problems to be addressed. For example, consider a community in which community organizers initially saw the problem to be drug abuse by teens. What

Table 8.2
Guidelines for effective coalitions

1. Be sensitive to turf issues.
2. Make sure the coalition is genuine.
3. Clarify the exact purpose of the coalition.
4. Limit the number of agencies involved in the coalition.
5. Allow enough time for decisions to be made.
6. Communicate with other coalitions from other geographic areas dealing with the same problem.
7. Make sure the visibility and recognition of the agencies involved in the coalition are increased as a result of their participation.
8. Secure a financial commitment from agencies involved in the coalition.
9. Have infrequent but worthwhile meetings.
10. Make sure someone is accountable for the work of the coalition.
11. Be sure to distribute the workload of the coalition among participating agencies.

Source: From "Creating Effective Health Coalitions" by G. B. Lindsay and G. Edwards, 1988, *Health Education, 19*(4), pp. 35–36.

are the underlying problems that lead to teenage drug abuse? Answering this question will help to guide the group in its work.

An appropriately conducted needs assessment can help to identify these underlying problems. The needs assessment should be thorough enough to provide the expanded group with the knowledge needed to begin tackling the problem. This assessment is also useful in setting priorities and providing a baseline for further evaluation. An important follow-up to the needs assessment is an assessment of the "culture" of the community. This should identify the values of the community—what is seen as important. It should also identify the skills and limitations of the community, and the formal and informal political influences in the community.

A good way to approach this step in the community organization process is through **networking**. A **network** is thought of as a system of elements (professional counterparts) who work collaboratively as consultants and consultees. For example, if community organizers are interested in determining what resources there are in a community to deal with drug abuse, they may network with education leaders, church leaders, law enforcement agencies, hospitals, mental health centers, treatment centers, and the local health department. As a part of assessing the culture of the community, organizers need to identify the power base within the community and figure out what it takes to get the power base to act. The political reality of community organization is that no matter how hard organizers may work, the power base may prevent a resolution of the problem or issue. Community problems are complex, and the reality is that someone usually benefits if a problem remains unsolved (Archer & Fleshman, 1985). Do not be naive concerning a community's power base and political influences.

Determining Priorities and Setting Goals

Once the needs of the community have been assessed, the community group is ready to develop its goals. The goal-setting process includes two phases. The first phase consists of identifying the priorities of the group—what the group wants to accomplish. The priorities should be determined through consensus rather than through an individual or small group decision. The second phase consists of using the priority list to write the goals. To help ensure that the ideals of community organization take hold, the **stakeholders** (those in the community who have something to gain or lose from the community organization efforts) must be the ones to establish priorities and set goals. This may sound simple but in fact it may be the most difficult part of community organization. Getting the stakeholders to agree on priorities takes a skilled group facilitator because there is sure to be more than one point of view.

When working with coalitions and task forces, one is likely to find that determining priorities and setting goals causes turf struggles. Even though individuals or representatives of their organizations have come together to solve a problem, many people will still be concerned with finding specific solutions to the problems faced by their organization. For example, in the case of drug abuse in the community, consensus may indicate that the majority of people believe the problem lies in the educational system, but people who work in the treatment centers may believe the problem lies in the treatment of drug abuse. The facilitator will need special skills to keep these treatment center people involved after the priority-setting process does not identify their concern as a problem the group will attack. One means of dealing with this is to have subgoals, objectives that can be worked on by special interest subcommittees. Such an arrangement will allow the subcommittee to have a feeling of **ownership** in the process of solving the problem.

Selecting a Solution to the Problem

To achieve the goals that it has set, the group will need to identify alternative solutions and—again through consensus—choose a course of action. Most problems can be solved in any of several ways, however, each alternative has advantages and disadvantages. The group should examine the alternatives in terms of probable outcomes, acceptability to the community, probable long- and short-term effects on the community, and the cost of resources to solve the problem (Archer & Fleshman, 1985). Most of the interventions discussed in Chapter 7 are means by which the group can attack the problem.

Much of the work to identify the appropriate solution(s) can be accomplished through subcommittees. Subcommittees can complete specific tasks that will contribute to the larger plan of action. Their work should yield specific strategies that are culturally sensitive and appropriate to community needs. The plan of action is usually written in a proposal format and will be given final approval at a meeting of the full committee. It is important to take care in putting together this proposal; as many as possible of the ideas of the various subcommittees should be included. This will help to ensure approval of the entire plan. In the end, the real test of the course of action selected is whether it can provide whatever it is the people are seeking (Brager et al., 1987).

Final Steps in the Community Organization Process

The final four steps in a community organization process include implementing the plan, evaluating the outcomes of the plan of action, maintaining the outcomes in the community, and if necessary "looping" back to the appropriate point in the process to modify the steps and restructure the work plan. However, it may not be possible to succeed by handling the problem in a different way; some problems cannot be solved. Once the work of the group has been completed (that is, either the problem has been solved or it has been declared insoluble) the group can either disband or reorganize to take on another problem.

PLANNED APPROACH TO COMMUNITY HEALTH (PATCH)

What we have presented so far in this chapter is a general description of the process of organizing a community. However, there are some models for the community organization process that have been developed to guide community organizers. One model that has received considerable attention in the area of health promotion is the Planned Approach to Community Health, better known by its acronym, **PATCH**. PATCH was designed to help communities analyze their needs and then plan, implement, and evaluate health promotion programs to address these needs. The model is characterized as a bottom-up rather than a top-down approach; it begins at the grass-roots level with a small group of people within a community wanting to improve the overall health of those living in the community. It is a team approach in which the people of the community make the decisions (via a consensus process) and do the work, with technical assistance from the state and local health departments and the federal Centers for Disease Control. These team members not only facilitate the necessary work but also provide financial support for the project.

SUMMARY

Community organization refers to various methods of intervention whereby individuals, groups, and organizations engage in planned collective action to deal with social problems. The literature on community organization is not distinct; it is often intertwined with such terms as *citizen participation, community participation, grass-roots participation, macro practice,* and *community development.* The process of community organization has been used for many years in the area of social work, but its history in the area of health promotion is much more recent. Within this chapter a generic process for community organization was presented, which should be an adequate introduction to the process. Finally, a brief overview of the PATCH model was presented.

❑ QUESTIONS

1. What is meant by the term *community*?
2. Community organization originated out of what discipline?
3. What is the underlying concept of community organization?
4. What are some of the assumptions under which planners work when organizing a community?
5. What are the basic steps in the community organization process?
6. What is meant by the term *gatekeepers*?
7. What does the acronym PATCH stand for?

❑ ACTIVITIES

1. Assume that a core group of individuals have come together to deal with the problem of a high rate of teenage pregnancy in the community. Please identify (by job title/function) others whom you think should be invited to be part of the larger group. In addition, provide a one-sentence rationale for inviting each. Assume that this community is large enough to have most social service organizations.
2. Provide a list of at least 10 different community agencies that should be invited to make up an antismoking coalition in your home town. Provide a one-sentence rationale for including each.
3. Assume that you want to make entry into a community with which you are not familiar, in order to help to organize the community. Describe such a community, and then write a two-page paper to tell what steps you would take to gain entrance into the community.
4. If you wanted to find out more about your community's resources regarding exercise programs, with whom would you network? Provide a list of at least five contacts, and provide a one-sentence rationale for why you selected each.
5. Ask your professor if he or she is aware of any community organization efforts in a local community. If such a program exists, make an appointment along with three of your classmates to interview the community organization leader. Ask the leader to respond to the following questions:
    a. What is the problem being tackled?
    b. Who identified the initial problem?
    c. Who makes up the core group? How large is it?

d.   Did the group complete a needs assessment or community resource assessment?

e.   What type of intervention is being used?

f.   Will the problem be solved?

g.   What type of community organization model was used?

9

Identification and Allocation of Resources

After reading this chapter and answering the questions at the end, you should be able to:

❑   Define resources.

❑   List the common resources used in most health promotion programs.

❑   Identify the tasks to be carried out by program personnel.

❑   Explain the difference between internal and external resources.

❑   List the agencies/organizations that offer "canned" health promotion programs.

❑   Identify questions to ask vendors when they are selling their programs.

❑   List and explain common means of financing health promotion programs.

❑   Identify and explain the major components of a grant proposal.

KEY TERMS

canned program

curriculum

flex time

grant money

grantsmanship

hard money

in-house materials

ownership

peer education

proposal

request for proposals (RFP)

resources

soft money

speaker's bureau

vendors

voluntary health organizations

For a program to reach the identified goals and objectives, it must be supported with the appropriate **resources**. Resources include all the people and things needed to carry out the desired program. The quantity or amount of resources needed to plan, implement, and evaluate a program depends upon the scope and nature of the program. Most resources carry a "price tag," which planners must take into account. Thus, planners face the task of securing the financial resources necessary to carry out a program. However, several different resources are provided by organizations, mostly voluntary or governmental health organizations, that are free or inexpensive. This chapter identifies, describes, and suggests sources for obtaining the resources commonly needed in planning, implementing, and evaluating health promotion programs.

PERSONNEL

The key resource of any program is the individuals needed to carry out the program. Instead of trying to identify all the individuals necessary to ensure the program's success (because many times the same person is responsible for several different program components), planners should focus on the tasks that need to be completed by the program personnel. These tasks include planning, identifying resources, advertising, marketing, conducting the program, evaluating the program, making arrangements for space and program materials, handling clerical work, and keeping records (for program sign-up, collection of fees, attendance, and budgeting).

In some cases, the program participants themselves constitute a program resource. In the case of a worksite health promotion program, planners will need to find out whether the employees will participate on company time, on their own time before or after work hours, on a combination of company time and employee time, or on their own anytime during the work day as long as they put in their regular number of work hours. (This last option is known as **flex time**.) The current trend in worksite health promotion programs is to ask the employees to participate at least partially on their own time. The reasoning behind this trend is that this investment by the participant helps to promote a sense of program **ownership** ("I have put something into this program and therefore I am going to support it") and thus build loyalty among participants.

When identifying the personnel needed to conduct a program, planners have three basic options. One, referred to as internal resources, uses individuals from within the planning agency/organization or people from within the target population to supply the needed labor. For example, if a local health department was planning a health promotion program in a community, the employees of the health department might handle the planning, implementation, and evaluation of the program. If that same health department was planning a health promotion program for the faculty and staff of a school district, there would likely be many school employees (school nurse, health educator, physical education instructor, home economics teacher) who have the expertise (knowledge and skills) to carry out much of the program. If the department was planning a worksite program, there would probably be quite a few employees who would be qualified to conduct at least a portion of the program (for example, an employee who is certified to teach first aid or cardiopulmonary resuscitation).

Another internal resource that health promotion planners are using successfully in a variety of settings, especially in schools (from kindergarten to college), is **peer education**. The process is simple: individuals who have specific knowledge, skills, or understanding of a concept help to educate their peers. For example, college students may work with other college students to help educate them about the dangers of drinking and driving. The major advantages of peer education are its low cost and the credibility of the instructor. Children, for example, are greatly influenced by their peers.

A second source of personnel for a program is to bring in individuals from outside the planning agency/organization or the target population to conduct part or all of the program. Such individuals are considered external resources. There are now many companies that offer or sell programs, services, or consulting to groups wanting health promotion programs. These companies are referred to as **vendors**. Some vendors are for-profit groups, such as hospitals, consulting agencies, health promotion companies, or related businesses, while others are nonprofit organizations, such as voluntary health agencies, YMCAs, YWCAs, governmental health agencies, universities/colleges, extension services, or professional organizations. Because of the recent growth of interest in health promotion programs, the quality of vendors can vary greatly. Planners should screen vendors carefully before using their services. Harris, McKenzie, and Zuti (1986) provide a checklist for choosing an appropriate vendor (see Appendix I).

An often untapped source of personnel for health promotion programs is experts available through **speaker's bureaus**. Many voluntary health agencies and other health-related organizations maintain speaker's bureaus. The services of these experts are usually available at little or no cost to groups. Some examples of speaker's bureaus are local offices of **voluntary health organizations**, which have individuals available to speak on a variety of health-related topics, or hospitals willing to send their medical experts into the community to share their knowledge. The speaker's bureau is a win-win concept for both the group offering the service and the one receiving it. Groups that take advantage of a speaker's bureau gain access to expert information, but those delivering the information gain in terms of public relations and recognition.

There are advantages and disadvantages connected with using either internal or external personnel to conduct health promotion programs. Table 9.1 lists the pros and cons of each.

The third option for obtaining personnel to carry out a program is a combination of internal and external resources. This option is the one most commonly used because it allows the program planners to make use of the advantages of the first two options and avoid many of the disadvantages.

CURRICULA AND OTHER INSTRUCTIONAL RESOURCES

When it comes to selecting the **curriculum** and other instructional materials that will be used to present the content of the program, planners can proceed in three ways: (1) by developing their own materials (in-house) or having someone else

Table 9.1
Advantages and disadvantages of using internal and external personnel

Internal Program Personnel

Advantages
1. Reduce costs.
2. Internal arrangements can be made to free needed personnel.
3. More control over those involved.

Disadvantages
1. Limited by the interest of those on staff.
2. May have to train personnel or be limited by the expertise of those on staff.
3. Can spend more time developing the program than implementing it, thus reaching fewer people.

External Program Personnel

Advantages
1. Known expertise.
2. The responsibility for conducting the program becomes the work of another.
3. Can request product (program) guarantees.
4. External personnel sometimes more respected than internal personnel.

Disadvantages
1. Often more costly than using internal resources.
2. Subject to the limitations of any given vendor.
3. Sometimes less control over the program.

develop custom materials for them; (2) by purchasing or obtaining "canned" programs from outside vendors; or (3) by using a combination of in-house and canned materials. Each choice has both advantages and disadvantages.

Developing **in-house materials** or having someone else develop custom materials has the major advantage of allowing the developers to create materials that match very closely the needs of the target population. However, a serious drawback is the time, money, and effort necessary to develop a curriculum and other instructional materials. The exact amount of time necessary would obviously depend on the scope of the program and the expertise of those doing the work. No matter who does the work, however, the commitment of time and resources is sure to be considerable. In putting together an in-house program, planners should be aware of several different sources where they can obtain free or inexpensive materials to supplement the ones they develop. For example, most voluntary and official health agencies have up-to-date pamphlets on a variety of subjects that they are willing and eager to give away in quantity. Also, most communities have a public library with a film/video section that includes some health films/videos. If the public library does not carry health films/videos, almost all local and state health departments offer such a service. Planners who are unsure about what sources of information are available in their community can begin by checking the Yellow Pages of the local telephone directory. Table 9.2 provides a partial listing of organizations and the types of information available from each.

Purchasing or obtaining canned programs from vendors has become very popular in recent years because of the time and money needed to create programs. A **canned program** is one that has been developed by an outside group and includes all the components and materials necessary to implement a program. Because some vendors are for-profit groups while others are nonprofit organizations, the cost of these programs can range from nothing at all to thousands of dollars.

Most canned programs have five major components: (1) a participant's manual (printed material that is easy to follow and read and is handy for participants); (2) an instructor's manual (a much more comprehensive document than the participant's manual, which includes the program content, background information, and lesson and unit plans with ideas for presenting the material); (3) audiovisual materials that help present the program content (usually including films, video and audio tapes, overhead transparencies, charts, or posters); (4) training for the instructors (a concentrated experience that prepares individuals to become instructors); and (5) marketing (the "wrapping" that makes the program attractive to both the participants and the program planners who will purchase it to market to the participants). The advantages and disadvantages of these canned programs are just the opposite of those for materials developed in-house. No time is spent on development; however, the program may not exactly fit the needs or the demographics of the target population. For example, using the same canned smoking cessation program with middle-aged adults who realize the long-term hazards of cigarettes and with teenagers who are required to attend a smoking cessation program for disciplinary reasons may not be advis-

Table 9.2 (pp. 140 – 142)
Selected organization/agencies offering free or inexpensive health promotion materials

Organization/Agency	Topics covered	Address
American Cancer Society	Cancer, nutrition, smoking, smokeless tobacco, smoking cessation	Contact local affiliate
American Diabetes Assn.	Diabetes	Contact local affiliate
American Dietetic Assn.	Nutrition	ADA Sales Order Dept. Suite 1100 208 S. LaSalle St. Chicago, IL 60604-1003
American Heart Assn.	Cardiovascular disease, CPR, nutrition, smoking	Contact local affiliate
American Hospital Assn.	Variety of areas	AHA Center for Health Promotion 840 N. Lake Shore Dr. Chicago, IL 60611
American Lung Assn.	Lung diseases, smoking, smoking cessation	Contact local affiliate
American Red Cross	CPR, blood pressure, first aid, nutrition, safety, stress management	Contact local affiliate
Consumer Information Center	Variety of topics	Consumer Information Center Pueblo, CO 81009
Health Insurance Assn. of America	Worksite wellness	HIAA Public Relations Dept. 1001 Penn. Ave., NW Washington, D.C. 20004
Kidney Foundation	Kidney disease	Contact local affiliate
Local health department	All areas	Contact local department
Local public library	All areas	Contact local library
Local colleges and universities	Variety of areas	Check local telephone book
March of Dimes	Birth defects, pregnancy and worksite wellness	Contact local affiliate
National Cancer Institute	Cancer	NCI Bethesda, MD 20892

Table 9.2, *continued*

Organization/Agency	Topics covered	Address
National Heart, Lung, and Blood Institute	Cholesterol, heart disease, high blood pressure, smoking	NHLBI Bethesda, MD 20892
National Health Information Center	Referral to health information	NHIC P.O. Box 1133 Washington, D.C. 20013
National Kidney Foundation	High blood pressure control	Contact local affiliate
National Rural Health Network	Variety of topics to rural areas	NRHN 1800 Massachusetts Ave., N.W. Washington, D.C. 20036
National Wellness Institute, Inc.	Variety of areas	NWI, Inc. 1319 Fremont St. Stevens Pt., WI 54481
Office of Disease Prevention and Health Promotion	Variety of areas	ODPHP Health Information Center P.O. Box 1133 Washington, D.C. 20013-1133 1-800-336-4797
Planned Parenthood	AIDS, contraception, STDs	Contact local affiliate
Office on Smoking and Health	Smoking cessation	OSH Technical Information Center Park Building Room 1-10 5600 Fishers Lane Rockville, MD 20857
Society of Nutrition Education	Nutrition	SNE 1736 Franklin St. Suite 900 Oakland, CA 94612
State health department	All areas	Contact state health department
U.S. Department of Agriculture (USDA)	Nutrition	USDA Food and Nutrition Center National Agriculture Library Room 304 Beltsville, MD 20705

Table 9.2, *continued*

Organization/Agency	Topics covered	Address
U.S. Department of Agriculture Cooperative Extension Service	Nutrition	Contact county extension office or state land-grant university
U.S. Department of Transportation, National Traffic and Highway Safety Administration	Occupant safety, child safety seats, drunken driving, trauma prevention, and injury prevention	USDT National Traffic and Highway Safety Administration 400 7th St. S.W. Washington, D.C. 20590
Washington Business Group on Health	Worksite wellness	Washington Business Group on Health Institute for Organizational Health 229½ Pennsylvania Ave., S.E. Washington, D.C. 20003
Wellness Councils of America	Worksite wellness	WCA Historic Library Plaza 1823 Harney St. Suite 201 Omaha, NE 68102
YMCAs and YWCAs	Exercise	Contact local YMCA or YWCA

able. Most adults who enter smoking cessation programs are there because they do not want to smoke. Obviously this is not the case with teenagers who have been caught smoking. The approach taken with these two programs would have to be much different if they are to be successful. Another example of when use of a canned curriculum program would not be advisable is use of a program that was designed for upper-middle-class suburban adults in a program for low-income inner-city populations. The lifestyles of the two groups are just too different for the same curriculum to be appropriate in both situations.

Table 9.3 provides a selected list of canned programs that are currently available to program planners.

Canned programs often come attractively packaged and seemingly complete, but this does not mean they are well conceived and effective programs. Before adopting canned programs for use, planners should consider the following questions:

1.   Is the program based on sound theory and tested models? As noted in an earlier chapter, all programs should be based on sound theory and tested models.

Table 9.3 (pp. 143 – 145)
Selected list of canned health education programs

Organization/Agency	Type of program	Title of program
American Cancer Society	Breast cancer detection	Special Touch
	Cancer prevention	Taking Control
	High school cancer curriculum	Right Choices
	Involuntary tobacco	Where There's No Smoke
	Nutrition education	Changing the Course (for youth) Eating Smart (for adults)
	Smoking cessation	Freshstart Smart Move
	Smoking cessation for pregnant women	Special Delivery
American Heart Assn.	Cardiovascular risk reduction	Heart at Work
	Cooking course	Culinary Hearts Cooking Course
	Preschool health program	Heart Treasure Chest
American Institute for Preventive Medicine	Weight control and behavior modification for 8–18 year olds	The Body Shop
	Self-esteem	Self-Esteem and Positive Performance
	Smoking cessation	Smokeless
	Stress management	Systematic Stress Management
	Weight loss	Weight No More
	Weight loss for teens	Weight No More for Teens
American Lung Assn.	Smoking cessation self-help	Freedom from Smoking in 20 Days— A Self Help Quit Smoking Program
	Self-help smoking cessation for pregnant women	Freedom from Smoking for You and Your Baby
	Self-help smoking cessation maintenance	A Lifetime of Freedom from Smoking: A Maintenance Program for Ex-smokers
	Smoking cessation	Freedom from Smoking Clinics
	Stop-smoking videos	In Control
	Smoking cessation for worksites	Team Up for Freedom from Smoking (TUFFS)

Organization/Agency	Type of program	Title of program
American Red Cross	Risk assessment	On the Line
	Nutrition	Better Eating for Better Health
	High blood pressure	Lowdown on High Blood Pressure
	Measuring blood pressure	How to Measure Blood Pressure
Colorado State University	Nutrition	Healthy Heart Program: Eating and Your Heart
Control Data	General health	The StayWell Program
Health Insurance Assn. of America	Health promotion for school personnel	Wellness at the School Worksite
Johnson & Johnson	General health promotion	Live for Life
March of Dimes	Health promotion	Good Health is Good Business
National Center for Health Promotion	Weight and cholesterol reduction	The Leaner Weigh
	Physician supervised weight and cholesterol reduction	LiteFast...The Leaner Weigh
	Physical fitness	Personal Fitness
	Stress management	Personal Stress Management
	Smoking cessation	Smoke Stoppers
National Dairy Council	Eating and exercise habits for 9-11 year olds	Get Moving–Get Eating– Get Fit
	Eating and exercise habits for middle/junior high school students	Smart Moves
	Nutrition education	Nutrition & Your Busy Lifestyle
	Weight management	Lifesteps
Stanford Health Promotion Resource Center	Self-help smoking cessation	The Quit Kit
	Self-help nutrition	The Nutrition Kit
	Self-help weight control	The Weight Kit
	Self-help exercise	The Walking Kit
	Self-help exercise	The Jogging Kit

Table 9.3, *continued*

Organization/Agency	Type of program	Title of program
U.S. Department of Transportation, National Traffic Highway Safety Administration	Safety belts	The Great American Habit Plan (GAHP)
University of Minnesota	Smoking cessation	Quit & Win
Wellness Councils of America	Traffic safety education	Dare To Be Safe

2. Does the program include a long-term behavior modification component? There are no "quick fixes" with regard to health behavior change. If behavior modification is used, it should be based on sound health behavior practice over an appropriate time frame.

3. Is the program educational? Not only should the program be based on sound psychological and sociological theory, it should also be based on valid educational theory.

4. Is the program motivational? Health behavior change is not easy to accomplish, so all programs need to include activities that motivate people.

5. Is the program enjoyable? Planned programs should be enjoyable. Some people like hard work, but it is difficult to sustain hard work for a long time without some enjoyment.

6. Can the program be modified to meet the specific needs of the target population? As mentioned earlier, not all populations have the same needs and demographics.

SPACE

Another major resource needed for most health promotion programs is sufficient space—a place where the program can be held. Depending on the type of program and the intended audience, space may or may not be readily available. For example, an employer may make space available for a worksite program, or a school system may furnish space for a school program. If space is a problem, planners may locate inexpensive space in local schools, colleges, and universities, and in "community service rooms" of local businesses. It may also be possible to obtain space by trading for it. For instance, a planner might trade expertise, such as serving as consultant for a program, in return for the use of suitable space. Or it might be possible to trade one space for another, such as trading the use of classrooms for time in the local YMCA/YWCA pool.

EQUIPMENT AND SUPPLIES

Some programs may require a great deal of equipment and supplies. For example, first aid and safety programs need items such as CPR mannequins, splints, blankets, bandages, dressings, and video equipment. Other programs, such as a stress management program, may need only paper and pencils. Whatever the kinds and amounts of equipment and supplies required, planners must give advance thought to their needs so as to: (1) determine the necessary equipment and supplies to facilitate the program; (2) identify the sources where the equipment and supplies can be obtained; and (3) find a way to pay for the needed equipment and supplies.

FINANCIAL RESOURCES

To hire the individuals needed to plan, implement, and evaluate a health promotion program and to pay for the other resources required, planners must obtain appropriate financial support. Most programs are limited by the financial support available. In fact, few programs are financed at such a level that planners would say they have all the money they need. Because of this, the planners are often faced with making decisions about how to allocate the funds that are available. Some typical questions that planners generally must address are the following:

1.   Is it better to run an adequately financed program for a few people or to run a poorly financed program for more people?

2.   If funds are limited, where is the first place we should cut?

3.   Should we start a program knowing we will be short of funds, or should we wait until we have appropriate funding before we begin?

4.   Is it better to have fewer instructors or make do with fewer supplies?

Programs can be financed in several different ways. Some sources of financial support are very traditional, while others may be limited only by the creativity and imagination of those involved. We present here several established ways of financing programs.

Participant Fee

This method of financing a program requires the participants to pay for the cost of the program. Depending on whether or not the program is offered on a profit-making basis, this fee may be equal to expenses or may include a profit margin. Participant fees not only are a means by which programs can be financed, but they also help to motivate participants to stay involved in a program. If people pay to participate in a program, then they may be more likely to continue to participate because they have made an investment—that is, a commitment. This concept has also been referred to as ownership. Many participants who pay a fee feel like they are part "owners" of the program. However, it should be noted that not everyone shares in the ownership concept. There are some participants who still would prefer a free or almost free program that has been paid for by others—a fringe benefit, if you will.

Third-Party Support

Most individuals are familiar with insurance companies acting as third-party payers to cover the costs of health care. Although this is not a common means of paying for health promotion programs, it is sometimes used. By third-party, we mean someone other than participants (the first party) or program planners (the second party) paying for the program. Third-party payers that may cover the cost of health promotion programs are: (1) employers picking up the cost for employees, as is often the case in worksite health promotion programs; (2) agencies other than the groups sponsoring the program, for example, when local service or civic groups "adopt" a pet program; or (3) a professional association or union financially supporting a program. The money used by third-party payers can be generated from a special fund-raising event, from sale of concessions, or with money saved from reduced health care costs, absenteeism, or the remodeling of employee benefit plans.

Organizational Sponsorship

Many times the sponsoring organization (health department, hospital, or voluntary agency) bears the cost of the program as a part of its programming or operating budget. For example, the American Cancer Society offers its smoking cessation program free of charge. The program is paid for with the society's program-planning funds.

Grants and Gifts

Another means of financing health promotion programs is through gifts and grants from other agencies, foundations, groups, and individuals. This source of money is often referred to as **grant money**, external money, or **soft money**. The term *soft money* refers to the fact that grants and gifts are usually given for a specific period of time and at some point will be taken away. This is in contrast to **hard money**, which is an ongoing source of funds that is part of the operating budget of an organization from year to year.

Grant money is becoming more important to program planners because of limited resources dedicated to health promotion programming. It thus becomes necessary for program planners to develop adequate **grantsmanship** skills. These skills include (1) discovering where the grant money is located; (2) finding out how to get (apply for) the money; and (3) writing a proposal requesting the money.

Locating Grant Money

Those agencies, foundations, groups, and individuals that have money to give away can be found at three different levels—local, state, and national. Usually the organizations that have money to give away are businesses, foundations, service groups (such as Lion's Club and Jaycees), voluntary groups (such as United Way and American Heart Association), and other local groups specific to the locality. At the state and local levels the majority of grant money comes from foundations and governmental agencies.

To find out what funding agencies are available in a specific area requires some of the skills of a detective. Planners can check the Chamber of Commerce directories, call the Better Business Bureau, or look in the Yellow Pages. They can go to the library and read through a directory of foundations, *Directory of Research Grants* (1991), or *National Guide to Foundation Funding in Health* (Clinton, 1988). They may ask those who are familiar with the area, or just contact groups they think would be likely granters, in order to find out where money is available in their community. Planners should also be alert for **requests for proposals**, known as RFPs. Many times some funding agency would like to have a project conducted for it, so the group will issue an RFP. If you feel qualified to do the work, you can submit a proposal.

Submitting Grant Proposals

Most funding agencies have specific guidelines outlining who is qualified to submit a **proposal** (perhaps only nonprofit groups can apply, or only practitioners who hold certain certifications), and the format for making an application. Those seeking money can request or apply for the money by writing a proposal. A proposal can be thought of as a written document that represents a request for money. A good proposal is one that is well written and explains how the needs of the funding agency can be met by the group wishing to receive the money. To increase your chances of writing a good proposal, we recommend that you call the funding agency first to find out specifically what it is looking for and the format desired.

Because there is a great deal of competition for grant money, more than likely proposals will be read by a busy, impatient, skeptical person who has no reason to give any one proposal special consideration and who is faced with many more requests than he can grant, or even read thoroughly. Such a reader wants to find out quickly and easily the answers to these questions:

1. What do you want to do, how much will it cost, and how much time will it take?
2. How does the proposed project relate to the sponsor's interests?
3. What will be gained if this project is carried out?
4. What has already been done in the area of the project?
5. How do you plan to do it?
6. How will the results be evaluated?
7. Why should you, rather than someone else, conduct this project?

As noted, funding agencies request proposals in a variety of different forms. However, there are several components that are contained in most proposals no matter what the funding agency. Table 9.4 presents these components.

Table 9.4
The components of a grant proposal

1. **Title (or cover) page.** When writing title, be concise and explicit; avoid words that add nothing.
2. **Abstract or executive summary.** May be the most important part of proposal. Should be written last and be about 200 words long.
3. **Table of contents.** May or may not be needed, depending on the length of the proposal. It is a convenience for the reader.
4. **Introduction.** Should begin with a capsule statement, be comprehensible to the informed layperson, and include the statement of problem, significance of the program, and purpose of the program.
5. **Background.** Should include proposer's previous related work and the related literature.
6. **Description of proposed program.** Should include objectives, description of intervention, evaluation plan, and time frame.
7. **Description of relevant institutional/agency resources.**
8. **List of references.** Should include references cited in the proposal.
9. **Personnel section.** Should include the resumes of those who are to work with the program.
10. **Budget.** Should include budget needs for personnel (salaries and wages), equipment, materials and supplies, travel, services, other needed items, and indirect costs.

A Combination of Sources

It is not uncommon for a single program to be paid for by several groups. For example, many worksite health promotion programs are paid for through cost sharing among employees, employers, and unions.

SUMMARY

This chapter identified and discussed the most often used resources for health promotion programs: personnel, curriculum and other instructional materials, space, equipment and supplies, and funding. In addition, typical questions were covered regarding how to secure and allocate resources and to obtain funding.

QUESTIONS

1. What are the major categories of resources that planners need to consider when planning a health promotion program?
2. List and explain the different means by which health promotion programs can be funded.
3. Define the terms *ownership, flex time, vendor,* and *canned programs.*
4. What are the advantages and disadvantages of using internal resources? External resources?
5. How might program planners obtain free or inexpensive space for a program?

6.   What are some key questions that planners should ask vendors when they try to sell their product?

⬜ ACTIVITIES

1.   Identify and describe the resources you anticipate needing to carry out a program you are planning. Be sure to answer the questions below that apply to your program.

    a.   What personnel will be needed to carry out the program? List the individuals and the duties to be carried out.

    b.   What curriculum will you use in your program? Why did you select it?

    c.   What kind of space allocation will your program require? How will you obtain the space? How much will it cost?

    d.   What equipment and supplies do you anticipate using? How will you obtain them?

    e.   How do you anticipate paying for the program? Why did you select this method?

2.   Visit the local office of a voluntary agency and find out what type of resources it makes available to individuals planning health promotion programs. Ask for a sample of the materials. Also, ask if the agency offers any canned programs. If it does, find out as much as you can about the programs and ask for any available descriptive literature.

3.   Collect information on a single type of canned health promotion program (for example, smoking cessation or stress management) from vendors. Then compare the strengths and weaknesses of the programs.

4.   Through the process of networking and using the local telephone book, find where in your community there is free or inexpensive space available for health promotion programs.

5.   Call three different voluntary agencies and one hospital in your community and find out if they have a speaker's bureau. If they do, find out how to use the bureaus and what topics the speakers can address.

6.   Prepare a mock grant proposal for a program you are planning. Make sure it includes all the components noted in Table 9.4.

10

Marketing: Getting and Keeping People Involved in a Program

After reading this chapter and answering the questions at the end, you should be able to:

❑ Define *market, marketing, social marketing,* and *target marketing.*

❑ Explain the diffusion theory.

❑ Explain how the diffusion theory can be used in marketing a health promotion program.

❑ Identify the functions involved in the marketing process as outlined by Syre and Wilson (1990).

❑ Explain the relationship between a needs assessment and a marketing program.

❑ Explain the five Ps of marketing.

❑ Define *marketing mix.*

❑ Explain how the transtheoretical model can be useful in keeping people involved in a health promotion program.

❑ Name techniques for motivating program participants to continue in a program.

KEY TERMS

action stage

audience segmentation

contemplation stage

contingencies

diffusion theory

early adopters

early majority

external advertising

incentives

innovators

intangible

internal advertising

laggards

late majority

maintenance stage

market

marketing

marketing mix

market segmentation

placement

position the product

precontemplation stage

price

product

promotion

relapse

social marketing

social support

tangible

target marketing

After putting a great deal of work and energy into planning a health promotion program, planners naturally hope that the target population will want to participate in it. They also hope that, once involved in the program, the participants will want to continue with the program for its duration. Hoping is not enough, however. Planners must not just hope these things will occur, but work to make sure they occur. Planners need to have skills in marketing and psychology in order to get the target population involved and to keep them involved. Only when the participants continue the behavior learned in a health promotion program over a long period of time can the health goals of both the individual and program be met.

MARKET AND MARKETING

For the purposes of program planning, the people in the target population make up the market. Kotler and Clarke (1987, p. 108) have defined **market** as "the set of all people who have an actual or potential interest in a product or service." A key to getting and keeping these people involved in a health promotion program is to be able to market the program effectively. The process of **marketing** operates on the underlying concept of the exchange theory. "Marketing is the planned attempt to influence the characteristics of voluntary exchange transactions—exchanges of costs and benefits by buyers and sellers or providers and consumers. Marketing is considerably different from selling in that selling concentrates on the needs of the producer (to sell more products), whereas marketing, which may have the same ultimate objective, concentrates necessarily on the needs of the buyer or the public" (Pickett & Hanlon, 1990, p. 231).

Applying the definition of marketing to health promotion suggests that program planners would like to exchange cost and benefits with those in the target population. That is to say, program planners would like to exchange the benefits of participation in health promotion programs (the objectives or outcomes of the programs they planned) for the costs of the program, which come from the participants, such as time, money, and effort.

For this exchange to take place, program planners must have an understanding of marketing principles. Unfortunately, many health promotion planners have had to learn the hard way—by planning a program and then not have anyone sign up to participate in it. The principles of marketing are not difficult to learn, but application can be challenging. Applying marketing principles to health promotion programs is not as easy as applying them to the latest model of a car or a new line of clothing. Health promotion programs are social programs; as such they do not have material objects to market, but instead must market awareness, knowledge, skills, and behavior. The marketing of health promotion programs falls into a special type of marketing called social marketing.

Lefebvre and Flora (1988, p. 300) define **social marketing** this way: "Social marketing concepts and methods borrow heavily from traditional marketing literature. However, social marketing is distinguished by its emphasis on so-called `non-tangible' products—ideas, attitudes, lifestyle changes—as opposed to the more tangible products and services that are the focus of marketing in business, health-care, and non-profit service sectors." They continue, "For example, how does one buy a `healthier life'? The challenge is to begin to make these `intangibles' tangible in a way that appeals to the target audience" (Lefebvre & Flora, 1988, p. 306).

Table 10.1 compares the marketing of a **tangible** (product) and an **intangible** (a program that will improve the quality of life).

Table 10.1
Marketing a tangible vs. an intangible

Concern	Tangible	Intangible
Success	Increase sales 3-5%	Great enough to be cost-effective
Changes	One time sales	Lasting a life time
Target population	Most likely to respond	Least likely to respond

MARKETING AND THE DIFFUSION THEORY

One analytical tool that has been most useful in understanding the importance of marketing principles is the **diffusion theory** (Rogers, 1962). The theory provides an explanation for the diffusion of innovations (something new) in populations; stated another way, it provides an explanation for the pattern of adoption of the innovations. If we think of a health promotion program as an innovation, the theory describes a pattern the target population will follow in adopting the program. The pattern of adoption can be represented by the normal bell-shaped curve (Rogers, 1983) (Figure 10.1). Therefore, those individuals who fall in the portion of the curve to the left of minus 2 standard deviations from the mean (this would be between 2% and 3% of the target population) would probably become involved in the program just because they had heard about it and wanted to be first. These people are called **innovators**. They are venturesome, independent, risky, and daring. They want to be the first to do things, and they may not be respected by others in the social system.

The second group of people to become involved are those represented on the curve between minus 2 and minus 1 standard deviations. This group would include about 14% of the target population; they are called **early adopters**. These people are very interested in the innovation, but they are not the first to sign up.

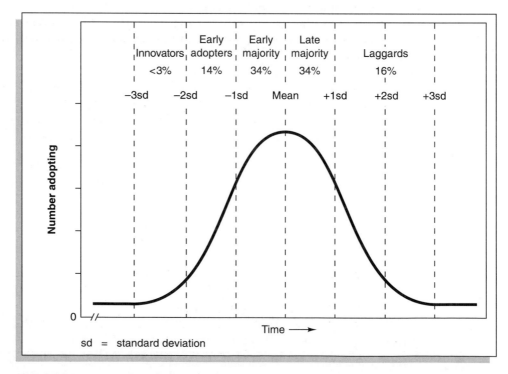

Figure 10.1
Bell-shaped curve and adopter categories (Adapted from *Diffusion of Innovations*, 3rd ed. (p. 247) by E. M. Rogers, 1983, New York: Free Press.)

They wait until the innovators are already involved to make sure the innovation is useful. Early adopters are respected by others in the social system and looked at as opinion leaders.

The next two groups are the **early majority** and the **late majority**. They fall between minus 1 standard deviation and the mean and between the mean and plus 1 standard deviation on the curve, respectively. Each of these groups comprises about 34% of the target population. Those in the early majority may be interested in the health promotion program, but they will need external motivation to become involved. Those in the early majority will deliberate for some time before making a decision. It will take more work to get the late majority involved, for they are skeptical and will not adopt an innovation until most people in the social system have done so. Planners may be able to get them involved through a peer or mentoring program, or through constant exposure about the innovation.

The last group, the **laggards** (16%), are represented by the part of the curve greater than plus 1 standard deviation. They are not very interested in innovation and would be the last to become involved in new health promotion programs. Some would say that this group will not become involved in health promotion programs at all. They are very traditional and are suspicious of innovations. Laggards tend to have limited communication networks so they really do not know much about new things.

As time passes, the number of adopters of an innovation increases. Figure 10.2 presents an s-shaped curve showing the cumulative prevalence of adopters at successive points in time.

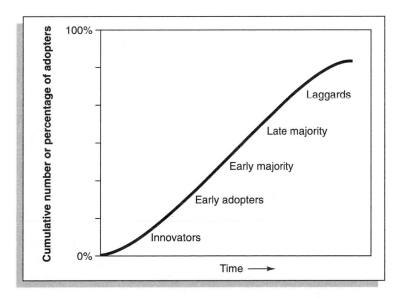

Figure 10.2
S-shaped curve and cumulative adoption (Adapted from *Diffusion of Innovations*, 3rd ed. (p. 95) by E. M. Rogers, 1983, New York: Free Press.)

The real plus of using the diffusion theory when trying to market a health promotion program is that "the distinguishing characteristics of the people who fall into each category of adopters from `innovators' to `early adopters' to middle majority categories to `late adopters' [laggards] tend to be consistent across a wide range of innovations" (Green, 1989, March). Therefore, different marketing techniques can be used depending on the type of people the program planners are trying to attract to a program. For example, smoking cessation programs have been around for many years. In the last 20 years, the percentage of adult smokers in the United States has dropped from just over 50% to less than 30%. Thus, taking into account that there will always be some new smokers, one could safely assume that the majority of smokers in the United States today are probably not innovators, early adopters, or early majority, at least with regard to smoking cessation programs. Instead, they are likely to be those who would be much more difficult to reach—late majority and laggards. Therefore, according to the diffusion theory, the marketing techniques that were used to get people to stop smoking right after former surgeon general Terry's report in 1964, probably would be less effective if used today.

Table 10.2 lists some generalizations drawn from the work of various researchers on innovations and reported in Rogers (1983). These generalizations could have an application to the innovation of health promotion programs.

The application of the diffusion theory to health promotion programs is quite common now. To learn more about the concept and its application to health promotion programs, you should review some other references to see how they have applied the concept in a variety of health promotion and health education settings (Anderson & Portnoy, 1989; Basch, 1984; Basch & Sliepcevich, 1983; Dishman, 1988; Kolbe & Iverson, 1981; Monahan & Scheirer, 1988; Orlaldi, 1986; Parcel, Erickson, Lovato, Gottlieb, Brink & Green, 1989; USDHHS, 1987).

THE MARKETING PROCESS AND HEALTH PROMOTION PROGRAMS

If everyone in a given population were an innovator or early adopter there would be no need for marketing plans. Since that is not the case, there is a need for program planners to understand the marketing process and be able to apply its principles.

Syre and Wilson (1990) have identified five distinct functions of the marketing process as they relate to the health care field. These include: (1) using marketing research to determine the needs and desires of the present and prospective clients from the target population; (2) developing a product that satisfies the needs and desires of the clients; (3) developing informative and persuasive communication flows between those offering the program and the clients; (4) ensuring that the product is provided in the appropriate form, at the right time and place, and at the best price; and (5) keeping the clients satisfied and loyal after the exchange has taken place. We will discuss each of these functions below.

Using Marketing Research to Determine Needs and Desires

Stated another way, this particular function involves conducting a needs assessment. Since the needs assessment process was discussed in detail in Chapter

4, we will not repeat the discussion here. However, we would like to point out that when conducting a needs assessment, if appropriate, planners might include marketing questions. If planners collect primary data as a part of the needs assessment process, they could easily include questions that would later prove helpful in marketing the program. Examples of such questions would be:

1. What type of health promotion programs would you participate in if they were offered in the community?
2. Where would you like the program offered?
3. On what days of the week would you like the program offered?
4. At what time of the day would you like the program offered?

Table 10.2
Generalizations about selected variables and innovation

Socioeconomic Characteristics

1. Earlier adopters have more years of education than later adopters have.
2. Earlier adopters are more likely to be literate than are later adopters.
3. Earlier adopters have higher social status than do later adopters.
4. Earlier adopters have a greater degree of upward social mobility than do later adopters.
5. Earlier adopters are more likely to have a commercial (rather than a subsistence) economic orientation than are later adopters.

Personality Variables

1. Earlier adopters have a greater ability to deal with abstractions than do later adopters.
2. Earlier adopters have a more favorable attitude toward change than later adopters have.
3. Earlier adopters are more able to cope with uncertainty and risk than are later adopters.
4. Earlier adopters have a more favorable attitude toward education than do later adopters.
5. Earlier adopters have a more favorable attitude toward science than do later adopters.
6. Earlier adopters have higher levels of achievement motivation than do later adopters.
7. Earlier adopters have higher aspirations (for education, occupations, and so on) than later adopters have.

Communication Behavior

1. Earlier adopters have more social participation than do later adopters.
2. Earlier adopters are more highly interconnected in the social system than are later adopters.
3. Earlier adopters are more cosmopolitan than later adopters are.
4. Earlier adopters have more change agent contact than do later adopters.
5. Earlier adopters have greater exposure to mass media communication channels than do later adopters.
6. Earlier adopters have greater exposure to interpersonal communication channels than later adopters have.
7. Earlier adopters have a higher degree of opinion leadership than later adopters have.
8. Earlier adopters are more likely to belong to highly interconnected systems than are later adopters.

Source: Adapted from *Diffusion of Innovations*, 3rd ed. (pp. 251–59) by E. M. Rogers, 1983, New York: Free Press.

5.   How much would you be willing to pay to attend the program?

6.   What might be the best way to notify you of future programs?

7.   Do you think other members of your family would like to attend these programs? If yes, which members?

Developing a Product That Satisfies the Needs and Desires of the Clients

The steps involved in developing a high quality, marketable product (health promotion program) were discussed in earlier chapters. One key to developing a marketable product is knowing as much as possible about the target population. The more they know about a population, the better program planners can describe the population. By describing the population, planners are then able to divide the population based upon certain characteristics, a process called **audience segmentation** or **market segmentation**. Figure 10.3 shows the concept of market segmentation, identifying black teenagers for a dietary excess intervention. "Audience segmentation has two major goals: (1) define homogeneous subgroups for message and product design purposes, and (2) identify segments that

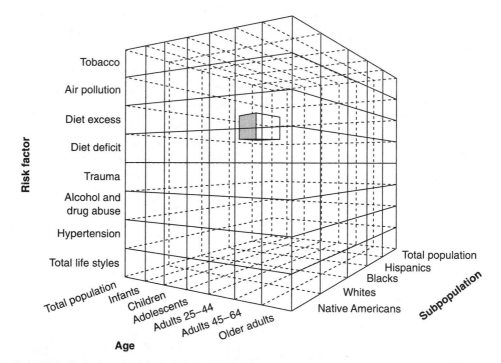

Figure 10.3
Example of market segmentation, identifying black teenagers for a dietary excess intervention

Source: From *Integration of Risk Factor Interventions* (p. 41) by U.S. Dept. of Health and Human Services, Public Health Service, Office of Disease Prevention and Health Promotion, 1986b, Washington, DC: Government Printing Office.

will target distribution and communication channel strategies" (Lefebvre & Flora, 1988, p. 303). Segmentation permits planners to develop programs that will meet the specific needs and desires of the target population, thus greatly increasing the chances for an exchange between the two parties. Segmentation is especially useful when trying to reach "high risk" and "hard to reach" groups. This type of marketing is referred to as **target marketing** and allows program planners to strongly **position the product** (health promotion program) in the community by focusing on the needs and wants of a particular group. Figure 10.4 outlines the steps in market segmentation and target marketing.

Planners can carry out the segmentation of groups of people before surveying them (a priori) by examining demographic variables, such as age, gender, income, marital status, occupation, religion, ethnicity, and socioeconomic status,

Figure 10.4
Steps in segmenting and targeting the market

Source: Adapted from *Strategic Marketing for Nonprofit Organizations*, 4th ed. (p. 168) by P. Kotler & A. R. Andreasen, 1991, Englewood Cliffs, NJ: Prentice-Hall. Reprinted by permission of Prentice-Hall, Inc., Englewood Cliffs, NJ 07632.

Market segmentation

1. Identify bases (variables) for segmenting the market (those whom you would like to reach)

2. Using appropriate variables, develop profiles of resulting segment(s) (sub-groups)

3. Develop measures of segment attractiveness

Target marketing

4. Select the target market(s) (specific groups you want to reach and think you can reach)

5. Develop positioning for each target market

6. Develop marketing mix (5 Ps) for each target market

or on the basis of a relevant model or theory. Or planners can conduct segmentation after surveying (a posteriori) the target population and collecting data, such as psychographics (attitudes, values, and lifestyle), risk factors, health history, or personal health behaviors. For example, the National Cancer Institute (NCI) used attitudes and lifestyle to identify different segments of the target population for communications about cancer. They found that one group, which they called the naive optimists, were generally optimistic, self-involved, and complacent about their health. They did not make any effort to stay healthy or seek health information and did not worry about their health. This group of people was young with high incomes and made up about 12% of the population (Freimuth & Mettger, 1990). Segmentation is thus most helpful in developing a market plan for this group of people.

Kotler and Clarke (1987, p. 236) have indicated that "there is no one, or right, way to segment a market." Program planners will need to experiment with the various variables to determine what works best for them. Table 10.3 includes many of the major segmenting variables identified by Kotler and Clarke (1987). Figure 10.5 presents an example of a possible segmenting matrix for worksite health promotion programs, using some of the segmenting variables.

Figure 10.5
Example of worksite health promotion program segmenting matrix

Table 10.3
Segmentation and variables

1. Geographic segmentation
    a. Nations
    b. States
    c. Regions
    d. Service areas
    e. Counties
    f. Cities, towns, villages
    g. Neighborhoods
2. Demographic segmentation
    a. Age
    b. Stage of life cycle
    c. Disease or diagnostic category
        ❑ Health history
        ❑ Risk factors
    d. Gender
    e. Health insurance
    f. Income
    g. Education
3. Psychographic segmentation
    a. Social class
        ❑ Upper upper (less than 1% of population)
        ❑ Lower upper (2%)
        ❑ Upper middle (12%)
        ❑ Lower middle (30%)
        ❑ Upper lower (35%)
        ❑ Lower lower (20%)
    b. Lifestyle
    c. Attitudes
    d. Values
    e. Personality
        ❑ Self-image
        ❑ Self-concept
4. Behavioristic segmentation
    a. Purchase occasion
    b. Benefits sought
    c. User status
    d. Usage rate
    e. Loyalty status
    f. Stages of buyer readiness
    g. Health behavior
5. Multivariable segmentation (i.e., males age 42 living in Indiana)

Transtheoretical Model

One model that is relevant to segmentation is the transtheoretical model (DiClemente & Prochaska, 1982; Prochaska, 1989; Prochaska & DiClemente, 1982, 1983; Prochaska, DiClemente, Velicer, Ginpil & Norcross, 1985). This model is relevant to marketing strategies because it allows for the fact that there may be a variety of reasons why individuals are attracted to a program, thus allowing for greater segmentation. This model was discussed in greater detail in Chapter 6, but here it is applied to marketing.

There may be a few individuals who enroll in a program when they are in the **precontemplation stage**. They really do not want to be in the program, but they may be attending because someone else—such as a significant other—wants them to enroll. In most health promotion programs, there will be some who are in the **contemplation stage**. These are usually individuals who want to find out more about a contemplated change. Most of the people enrolled in the program should be individuals who are in the **action stage** and are ready for change. Some of these people will be entering their first attempt at changing a behavior, while others will have experienced **relapse** and will be trying again to make a change. Program planners may also find some individuals who are in the **maintenance stage** of change enrolled in their programs. These people may have entered the program to gain needed social support, reinforcement, or additional motivation.

Developing Informative and Persuasive Communication Flows and Ensuring That the Product Is Provided in an Appropriate Manner

The third and fourth marketing functions outlined by Syre and Wilson (1990) can best be explained by McCarthy's (1978) four Ps—product, price, placement, and promotion. The particular blend of these four marketing variables that planners use to achieve their objective(s) in the target market is referred to as the **marketing mix** (Kotler & Andreasen, 1991; Kotler & Clarke, 1987; Wilson & Olds, 1991).

Product

Product refers to the actual program you are planning: the program is your product. A goal for all planners is to develop the best product possible with the resources available.

Price

"Prices can be thought of in a variety of ways; in addition to economic reasons, there are social, behavioral, psychological, temporal, structural, geographic, and physical reasons for exchanging or not exchanging" (Lefebvre & Flora, 1988, p. 307). From an economic standpoint, **price** refers to charging the appropriate amount for the product (program) being provided. As was mentioned in Chapter 9, there are many ways to finance a program. If you are "selling" participation in the program, then the price must match the participants' ability to pay.

When considering the amount to be charged for a product (program), planners should determine the following:

Who are the clients?

What is their ability to pay?

Are copayers involved?

Is the program covered under an insurance program?

What is the mission of the planner's agency?

What are competitors charging?

What is the demand for the program?

The price of a program and who pays for it help determine how a program should be marketed. Whether or not the program is intended to make a profit will have a great impact on the price. Does the program have to make money? Break even? Or can it lose money? It is a real art not to overprice or underprice the program. Demand and location (placement) will also influence price. If a program is in high demand, obviously the price can be higher than if it is not. For example, a stress management program in a large metropolitan area may be able to command a higher price than one located in a small rural area.

In addition to the economic price of a program, there are also noneconomic prices, such as physical and social prices. A physical price is one that physically hurts the participant, while a social price is one that affects the participant in a social setting. Bensley (1989, p. 20) gives some examples of physical and social prices by stating that "sacrifice may include physical withdrawal symptoms, or even a social price which is particularly high among young people when they resist the pressures from their peer group."

Placement

The third P of marketing is **placement**, which can be thought of as distribution. Where is the best place to offer the program? How large is the service area? How many distribution points should there be? One of the major reasons that worksite health promotion programs have been so successful is that they are offered at the workplace: they are convenient. Accessibility to programs is very important. People do not have to make a special trip to participate in a worksite program. It is much easier to walk down the hall to a program than to drive across town to attend one. It is important to avoid areas where people do not normally go or places where they would not feel comfortable or safe.

The timing of a program is closely associated with its placement. When is the program best offered? If a worksite program were offered in the evenings, so that the workers had to return to the worksite after dinner, that probably would not be much different than driving across town from work to attend a program. Offering a program right after a shift or on a lunch hour would be much more appealing to most workers. Obviously, planners should be concerned about placing their program in a desirable locale (where they are wanted and needed) at the best possible time.

Promotion

The fourth P of marketing is **promotion**. This deals with both the oral and written communication that program planners use to attract those in the target population to become involved in a program. This means taking the necessary steps to make people aware that you have a product (program) in which they would be interested. Such communication should be both informative and persuasive. The choice of a title for a program is an important element in its promotion, since the title can make a difference in whether or not someone from the target population will be interested in a program. Which of these program titles do you think would attract more attention, "Alcohol and You" or "Not Knowing Your Company's Drug Policy Can Cost You Your Job"?

Promotion can be thought of as advertising the program. As with product development, planners should consider the segmentation of the target population when promoting the program. For example, advertising a program to reach high-risk new mothers would be much different than for one intended for all new mothers. Depending on the type of program planned and the setting for the program, the techniques of advertising the program will vary. If the program is being promoted through **internal advertising**—that is within an organization, say for the employees of a business or for the faculty and staff of a school—promotion might include such elements as posters, bulletin boards, brochures, displays, table tents, newsletters, envelope stuffers, and announcements made through groups that represent the target population, such as unions or professional organizations. If the program is being promoted through **external advertising**—that is, not within an organization but in a community at large—some of the same techniques can be used. Posters, bulletin boards, brochures, and displays are also useful when trying to attract members of a larger community. Other useful techniques for external advertising might include: (1) advertising through the mass media (newspapers, television, and radio); (2) direct contact with specific groups that might be at high risk and in need of the programs (contacting recent heart attack patients about a program on the need to eat in a "heart healthy" way); and (3) contact with specific professionals who would be in a position to make referrals to your program.

Of these techniques, the first, advertising through the mass media, requires a special set of skills in order to be used effectively. High on the list of these skills is the ability to interact with media representatives (newspaper reporters and television or radio journalists, and advertising staff). Before a program is ready to be marketed, planners should meet with the advertising staff, the health editor and/or writers, and the health/consumer reporters. These people can provide insight into the type of advertising to be used. They know what attracts their readers, listeners, and watchers to an advertisement. They can also provide additional insight into how to prepare news releases and stage newsworthy activities that can lead to stories and articles in the media. Such stories can be thought of as free advertising, since the space or time is not paid for.

Other techniques that can be useful in promoting a program either internally or externally are: (1) providing incentives for people to become involved, such as free tee shirts, extra vacation time, a free introductory offer, free health appraisal, flex time, or money; (2) gaining the endorsement of key people in an organization (those who are admired, a supervisor or the boss) or a famous person or someone well known in the community; (3) distributing mailbox or door-to-door stuffers; (4) making a personal contact with an individual, such as a friend already involved or a superior or boss who is involved; (5) setting up a mentoring program where someone already in the program works with a beginner; and (6) a special kick-off, countdown, ribbon-cutting, or health party to get a program started.

Person

Although McCarthy (1978) proposed only four Ps—product, price, placement, and promotion—we have added a fifth P, which stands for *person*. Too often program planners become so wrapped up in the development and marketing of their program that they forget the personal element—the people involved. Remember, marketing is an exchange process between those who have developed the product and those who are in need of it. Do not lose sight of the importance of the person and his or her needs when marketing the product.

Keeping the Clients Satisfied and Loyal

Keeping clients satisfied and loyal involves two key concepts. The first is that satisfied and loyal clients can add much to future marketing efforts by providing word-of-mouth advertising. They can provide a lot of favorable advertising, free of charge. Second, and more important, is the value of keeping the target population involved in the health-enhancing behavior that they began as a result of being involved in the health promotion program. Becoming involved in a program is important, but maintaining a health-enhancing behavior is a more important objective. There is strong evidence that people are not very likely to maintain health behavior change over a long period of time. The problem of recidivism to past behaviors, such as substance abuse, has been known for quite a while (Hunt, Barnett, & Branch, 1971). More recently, however, researchers have warned health education and health promotion program planners of recidivism and dropout problems associated with exercise (Dishman, Sallis & Orenstein, 1985; Horne, 1975), weight loss (Stunkard & Braunwell, 1980), and smoking cessation (Leventhal & Cleary, 1980; Marlatt & Gordon, 1980). (A detailed discussion of relapse can be found in Chapter 7.)

Why do people behave the way they do? Why do some people begin and continue with health promotion programs, while others make a strong start but drop out, and still others never begin? Research has shown that the reasons are many and varied. Participation in health promotion programs may be influenced by a variety of factors, including demographic, behavioral, and psychosocial variables, and program structure.

Motivation

A key element for initial involvement and continued participation in a health promotion program seems to be motivation, which has been described as a concept that is both simple and complex. "The concept of motivation....is simple because the behavior of individuals is goal-directed and either externally or internally induced. It is complex because the mechanism which induces behavior consists of the individual's needs, wants, and desires and these are shaped, affected, and satisfied in many different ways" (Rakich, Longest & O'Donovan, 1977, p. 262). Feldman (1983) has suggested a variety of ways in which participants may be motivated to adopt a new health behavior. These means are seldom independent of each other, but from a planning standpoint they are usually viewed separately. In our opinion, the key to motivation is matching the means of motivating with those things that seem to reinforce the individual program participants. What motivates one individual may not be the least bit motivating to another individual and vice versa.

Two approaches are commonly used. The first is to include questions about motivation as part of any needs assessment conducted in program planning. For example, if the planners are surveying a target population regarding their needs, they could include questions on reinforcers, such as "What incentives would entice you to participate in the exercise program?" or "What would it take to get you to participate in this program?" or "What would it take to keep you involved in a program?" The responses to these questions should provide some direction concerning the type of reinforcers that would be most useful for the target audience. The second is the "shotgun" approach based upon a planner's previous experience or the experience reported by others. Using the "shotgun" approach, a program planner would offer a variety of reinforcers to meet the needs of a large percentage of the program's target population. We recommend the former approach in most cases, but sometimes motivation is not considered when a needs assessment is completed. In such a case the latter approach is used. The remaining portions of this chapter provide ideas for motivating program participants.

Using Contracts to Motivate.   A contract is an agreement between two or more parties that outlines the future behavior of those parties. Contracts are a common part of everyday living. We enter into contracts when we sign a lease for an apartment or a residence hall agreement, take out an insurance policy, borrow money, or buy something over a period of time. The same concept can be applied to getting and keeping people motivated in health promotion programs. Each program participant would enter into a contract with another person (the program facilitator, a significant other, or a fellow participant) and then work toward an objective or agreement specified in the contract. The contract would also specify **contingencies**—that is, what happens as a result of the contract either being met or not being met.

For an exercise program, this system might work as follows. The program participant and program facilitator would draw up a contract based upon the participant's present status in the program (exercising for 20 minutes once a week) and upon what would be a reasonable goal for the near future—say, eight weeks. Thus the contract might state that the participant will exercise for 20 minutes twice a week for the first week, 20 minutes three times a week for the second week, and so forth, thus building up gradually to the final goal of exercising for 50 minutes three or four times a week at the end of eight weeks. The outcome should focus on a behavior that can be maintained at the end of the contract period. For a weight loss program, the goal might be written as eliminating snacking in the evening, increasing fruits and vegetables in the diet to three servings per day, and walking for 20 minutes three times a week. These are behaviors that can reasonably be maintained after the weight loss.

The parties to the contract then decide upon what the contingencies will be. Thus the participant might offer to make a contribution to some local charity or state that she will continue in the program for another eight weeks if she does not meet the contract goal. The facilitator might promise the participant a program tee shirt if she fulfills the contract during the specified eight-week period. Other ideas for contingencies might include granting a kickback on fees for completing a certain percentage of the classes, or earning points towards products or services. No matter what the contingencies are, it seems to help if the contract is completed in writing. A sample contract is presented in Appendix J.

Using Social Support to Motivate.   It has long been recognized that whatever the behavior may be, it is almost always easier to do if people have the support of those around them. Long-standing examples of the concept of **social support** in the area of health education and health promotion are programs like Weight Watchers and Alcoholics Anonymous. They are based upon the support of others who are experiencing the same behavior change. One of the key reasons why worksite health promotion programs are so effective is that the working environment lends itself to social support. Being around other individuals who are engaging in the same behavior change provides a good support system.

Another means of helping program participants develop the necessary support system might be to pair them with other participants in a "buddy" arrangement. People find it harder to let others down than to disappoint themselves. Another technique that is being used increasingly is to incorporate the help of family members or significant others to provide the needed motivation. It is easier for someone to quit smoking if all members in the household try quitting at the same time, than to "go it alone" while others in the household continue to smoke.

Using Media to Motivate.   Another technique for keeping people motivated to continue in a health promotion program is to recognize them publicly through some medium available to those in the program. Examples of such media include organization newsletters or newspapers, community newspapers, local television and radio stations, bulletin boards at the location where the program is being offered or public bulletin boards elsewhere, and letters sent to the significant others of the participants (family members, job superiors, and so forth) noting the participants' progress in the program.

It is important for program planners to exercise caution when recognizing people through the different types of media. Not everyone likes to see their name publicized. Before you publicly acknowledge individual participants, make sure they do not mind if you do so.

Using Incentives to Motivate.   In Chapter 7, **incentives** were discussed as an intervention strategy, but they are also useful in keeping people involved in programs (Jason, Jayaraj, Blitz, Michaels & Klett, 1990). Dunbar, Marshall, and Howell (1979) state that reinforcement may be any consequence that would increase the probability of a behavior being repeated. Wilson (1990, p. 33) defined incentive as "some reward for achieving a level of performance or goal." It has been reported (Frederiksen, 1984) that incentives seem to be most effective if they are provided in small quantities, are frequent in nature, are tailored to those in the target population, address behaviors over which the individual has control, and do not conflict with any organizational policies.

To give program planners some ideas for appropriate incentives, we offer the following list. The ideas included in it have been reported in the literature; shared with us by current practitioners or students; or created by McKenzie, Luebke, and Romas (1992). No attempt has been made to identify which incentives would be best used to entice people to enroll in a program, and which ones would be best to keep people participating after they are enrolled. Thus the list could be used to encourage individuals to start a program, to induce them to continue participating in a program, or to help them meet an individual, group, or program goal. The incentives listed have been categorized into two types of reinforcers defined by Feldman (1983)—social reinforcers and material reinforcers—with a third category of miscellaneous reinforcers.

I.   Social reinforcers (Feldman, 1983; Shepard, 1985)

   1.   Special attention or recognition from instructors, peers, classmates, or coworkers

   2.   Praise/verbal reinforcement

   3.   Public and other recognition (name in newsletter, name on bulletin board)

   4.   Encouragement

   5.   Friendship

   6.   Inclusion of family members in the program

II. Material reinforcers

   1.   Inexpensive "token" incentives

      a.   Tee shirts, hats, caps, visors, warm-up jackets, calendars, key chains, flashlights, pens, windshield scrapers, wallets, tape measures, vacuum bottles, mugs, home fire extinguishers, smoke detectors, and auto safety kits (Cinelli, Rose-Colley & Hayes, 1988; Kendall, 1984)

        b.   Certificates

        c.   Pins, buttons, patches, decals that can be worn, and plaques or markers that can be displayed in the work area

        d.   Towels, lockers

        e.   Preferred or free parking

2.   Program cost sharing between employer and employee

        a.   Cost of registering for a program (Pollock, Foster, Salisburg & Smith, 1982)

        b.   Membership at a fitness center/club

        c.   Sliding-scale fee based upon the ability to pay

        d.   Refund of part or all of program fee upon participant's completion

3.   Health insurance

        a.   Sharing between employer and employee of money saved on health insurance from one year to the next (Toufexis, 1985)

        b.   Alteration of fringe benefit package to reward good health practices

        c.   Employer picking up more of the insurance costs to reward good health practices (Toufexis, 1985)

        d.   Provision of a fund for each employee to pay for the person's health care costs during the year, with any unused money from this account given to the employee at the end of the year (Hosokawa, 1984; Toufexis, 1985)

        e.   Lower premiums for employees with fewer health risks (nonsmoker or exerciser) (Hosokawa, 1984)

4.   Monetary items

        a.   Tokens, Monopoly-style dollars, stamps, coupons, or points that are redeemable at a company store, at retail stores, or for catalog shopping for prizes or merchandise (Kendall, 1984; Piniat, 1984; Toufexis, 1985)

        b.   Drawings, lotteries, and raffles open to those who have participated or met a goal (Cinelli et al., 1988; Toufexis, 1985; Health Insurance Association of America, 1983)

        c.   Bonus, extra pay, or just plain pay for completion of contract, participation, not smoking on the job, or quitting (DiBlase, 1985; Toufexis, 1985)

        d.   Financial rewards for both individuals and groups who have fewer and/or no work accidents during the year (DiBlase, 1985)

        e.   "Well pay" for unused sick days (DiBlase, 1985)

        f.   Gift certificates, from a small one such as a free ice cream cone to something of greater value, such as a U.S. savings bond (Kendall, 1984)

   5.   Work hours

        a.   Flex time (flexible work hours) in order to participate

        b.   Released time to participate

        c.   Time off (Cinelli et al., 1988)

   6.   Contracts

        a.   Contract (competition) with a buddy

        b.   Contract with instructor to reach a specific goal, with a material incentive provided by instructor

        c.   Forfeiture of money or time to charity for not fulfilling a contract (Bloomquist, 1981)

        d.   Contract with instructor, in which money is withheld (via payroll deduction) while the person is enrolled in the program, so that if goal is met the money is refunded, if not it is forfeited (Forster, Jeffery, Sullivan & Snell, 1985)

III.   Miscellaneous

   1.   Special medical examinations and screenings for those who participate

   2.   Special events, such as contests or luncheons (Kendall, 1984; Patton et al., 1986)

Finally, we offer this advice for program planners who choose to use incentives:

1.   Make sure everyone can receive one, whatever the incentive may be (Kendall, 1984).

2.   Make the incentives useful and meaningful (Kendall, 1984).

3.   Ensure that the ground rules are fair, understandable, and followed by everyone (Kendall, 1984).

4.   Make a big deal of awarding the incentive.

5.   Use incentives that are consistent with health promotion philosophies. For example, avoid incentives of alcoholic beverages, high-fat or high-sugar foods, or other mixed-message prizes.

Competition as a Means of Motivating.   Wilson (1990, p. 33) has reported that competitions have been a useful means of "introducing and promoting health promotion programs and achieving significant initial participation rates." A competition can be described as a contest between two teams (groups) or individuals in which the object is to try to out perform the other competitor. In a health promotion context, this could mean competing to lose the most pounds, smoke fewer cigarettes, walk the most miles, swim the most laps, or plan the most nutritious meals. Wilson (1990) further stated that competitions can vary in method and design, and that they work best with weight loss and smoking cessation programs. In Wilson's view, competitions are a good method of introducing a health promotion program but are probably not useful as an ongoing recruitment tool.

Final Comment on Marketing

Planners who intend to use a canned program should be sure to ask the vendor if there is a marketing plan that goes along with the program. The good programs will usually include some useful marketing strategies if not an entire plan. A word of caution about the marketing materials: like the canned programs themselves, they are usually aimed at a general target population, not one that has been segmented. Therefore they may have to be adapted to meet local needs.

SUMMARY

An important aspect of any health promotion program is being able to attract participants initially and to keep them involved once they have begun the program. An understanding of the diffusion theory is helpful in determining strategies for marketing a program. The actual marketing mix for a program should take into account the five Ps of marketing: product, price, placement, promotion, and person. Special attention should be given to segmenting the target population. Once people are enrolled in a program, they need to be motivated to remain involved. Strategies of contracts, social support, media recognition, incentives, and competition can be most helpful in motivating people to continue their participation in a program.

QUESTIONS

1. Define the following terms: *market, marketing, social marketing, target marketing*.
2. What is the relationship between marketing and needs assessment?
3. How does the diffusion theory relate to marketing a program?
4. What are the five different groups of people described in the diffusion theory? When would each group most likely join a health promotion program?
5. What is the difference between marketing a tangible product versus an intangible product?
6. What are the five Ps of marketing? Explain each one.
7. What is meant by *marketing mix*?
8. Explain how the transtheoretical model applies to marketing.

9.   What are five techniques for motivating people to stay involved in a health promotion program?

⬜ ACTIVITIES

1.   Respond to the following statements/questions with regard to a program you are planning.

   a.   Describe your product.

   b.   Describe your segmented population.

   c.   How much will you charge for the program? Explain the rationale on which you based your decision. What other "prices" do you see for this program?

   d.   Where will you place your program (location, days, and time)? Why are you placing it this way?

   e.   How will you promote your program? How, when, where will you advertise?

2.   Create a marketing plan for a health promotion program you are developing or another program described by your professor. Use the outline below [a modification of the work of Kotler and Clarke (1987) and Syre and Wilson (1990)] for presenting your plan.

   I.   Executive summary or abstract of the plan (written as a paragraph)

   1.   Product (program) to be offered (describes the program and who it is for)

   2.   Summary of main marketing goals (what will be accomplished by marketing the program)

   3.   Summary of recommendations of marketing plan (how the program will be marketed)

   4.   Budget summary (including both expected income and expenses)

   II.   Situational analysis

   1.   Needs and desires assessment (including marketing questions: What did you find to be the needs and desires of the target group? What questions did you use to find this out?)

   2.   Program strengths and weaknesses

   3.   Competition from other programs (including their strengths and weaknesses: What other programs will you be competing against for those in the target group? What are their strengths and weaknesses?)

   III.   Marketing objectives

   1.   Target market (Whom do you hope to reach?)

   2.   Market share expected (What percentage of the market do you want to use your product?)

    3.   Outcomes expected from the program (What will happen because of the marketing process?)

   IV.   Marketing strategies/Mix

    1.   Price (What must those in the market give up to be involved in your program? Consider economic, physical, and social prices)

    2.   Placement (Where will the program be offered?)

    3.   Promotion (communication channels)

        a.   Oral (electronic media, word of mouth)

        b.   Written

   V.   Time line (when and in what sequence will the marketing events take place?)

   VI.   Exhibits supporting the plan (brochures, flyers, table tents, PSAs, and ads)

3.   Create a one-page advertisement that could be used as a table tent, newspaper ad, or a poster for your program.

4.   Give an example of how you could use each of the four methods described in the chapter for motivating program participants to stay in a program.

11

Implementation: Strategies and Associated Concerns

After reading this chapter and answering the questions at the end, you should be able to:

❑ Define *implementation.*

❑ Identify several different strategies for implementing health promotion programs.

❑ List the concerns that need to be addressed before implementation can take place.

KEY TERMS

beneficence	nonmaleficence
commission	omission
implementation	phased in
informed consent	pilot testing
liability	prudent
logistics	

Once a program has been planned and marketed, it must then be implemented. Ross and Mico (1980, p. 225) have stated that **implementation** "consists of initiating the activity, providing assistance to it and to its participants, problem-solving issues that may arise, and reporting on progress." To accomplish all of this, program planners must select the most appropriate implementation strategy and see that any special concerns associated with implementation are handled properly.

STRATEGIES FOR IMPLEMENTATION

Planners decide on the best way to implement the program they have planned based upon the resources available and the setting for which the program is intended. Two models for implementing a program are presented here. The first combines some of our ideas with those of Parkinson and Associates (1982). The second model was developed by Borg and Gall (1989) for research and development projects. Both models are flexible and can be modified to meet the circumstances of different programs.

First Implementation Model

Parkinson and Associates (1982) have suggested three major ways of implementing a program: by using a piloting process; by phasing it in, in small segments; or by initiating the total program all at once. We think these three strategies are best explained by using an inverted triangle, as shown in Figure 11.1. The triangle represents the number of people from the target population who would be involved in the program based upon the implementation strategy chosen. The wider portion of the triangle at the top would indicate offering the program to a larger number of people than is represented by the point of the triangle at the bottom.

We see these three different implementation strategies as an implementation hierarchy. It is our opinion that all programs should go through all three of the strategies, starting with piloting, then phasing in, and finally implementing the total program.

Advantages

- More people involved
- Evaluation more meaningful
  with larger group

- Easier to cope with workload
- Gradual investment

- Opportunity to test program
- Close control of program

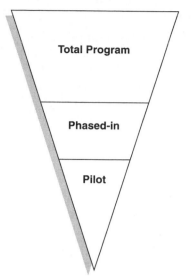

Disadvantages

- Big commitment
- No chance to
  test program

- Fewer people
  involved

- Very few involved
- Not meeting all needs
- Hard to generalize
  about results

Figure 11.1
Implementation strategies

Pilot Testing

Pilot testing (or piloting or field testing) the program is a crucial step. Even though planners work hard to bring a program to the point of implementation, it is important to try to identify any problems that might exist with the program. Pilot testing allows planners to work out any bugs before the program is offered to a larger segment of the target population, and also to validate the work that has been completed up to this point. For the most meaningful results, a newly developed program should be piloted in a similar setting and with people like those who are eventually to use the program. Use of any other group may fail to identify problems or concerns that would be specific to the target population. As an example of the piloting process, take the case of a hospital developing a work-site health promotion program. It would be best if the program were piloted on a worksite group before it was marketed to worksites in the community. The hospital could look for a company that might want to serve as a pilot group, or it might use its own employees.

As part of piloting the program, planners should check to make sure that: (1) the intervention strategies work as planned; (2) adequate program logistics have been worked out; and (3) the program participants are asked to evaluate the program. It is important to have the program participants critique such aspects of the program as content, approaches used, instructor's effectiveness, space, accommodations, and other resources used. Such feedback will give planners insight as to how to revise the program. If many changes are made in the program as a result of piloting, planners may want to pilot it again before moving ahead. This evaluation process during the piloting phase is part of process or formative evaluations and will be discussed further in Chapter 12.

Phasing In

Once a program has been piloted and revised, we believe the program should be **phased in** as opposed to implementing in its entirety. Phasing in allows the planners to have more control over the program and helps to protect planners and facilitators from getting in over their heads.

There are several ways in which to phase in a program: (1) by different program offerings; (2) by a limit on the number of participants; (3) by choice of location; and (4) by participant ability. Say a comprehensive health promotion program was being planned for Blue Earth County, Minnesota. To phase in the program by different offerings, planners might offer stress management classes the first six months. During the next six-month period, they could again offer stress management but also add smoking cessation programs. This process would continue until all offerings were included.

If the program were to be phased in by limiting the number of participants, planners might limit the first month's enrollment to 25 participants, expand it to 35 the second month, to 45 the third month, and so on until all who wanted to participate were included. To phase in the program by location, it might initially be offered only to those living in the southwest portion of the county. The second year, it might expand to include those in the southeast, and continue in the same manner until all were included. A program planned for a college town might be offered first on campus, then off campus to the general public. A program phased in by participant ability might start with a beginning group of exercisers, then add an intermediate group, and finally include an advanced group.

Total Implementation

We believe that implementing the total program all at once is the wrong way to proceed. It is our opinion that planners should work toward total implementation through the piloting and phasing-in processes. The only exception to this might be "one shot" programs, such as programs designed around a single lecture. Another possible exception would be screening programs, but even then piloting would probably help.

Second Implementation Model (Borg and Gall)

The second model for implementation provides program planners with another way of approaching implementation. Borg and Gall (1989) have presented a 10-step research and development cycle, of which the last 7 steps can be used as an implementation model for health promotion programs. Table 11.1 lists the major steps in the model.

The implementation portion of the model begins with the fourth step in the process—the preliminary field test. This step is performed "to obtain an initial qualitative evaluation" (Borg & Gall, 1989, p. 790). Only a very small number from the target population would participate in this test. The fifth step deals with the revision of the program based on information gained from the preliminary testing. All aspects of the program would be reviewed and revised as appropriate. The revised program would then be tested again with a slightly larger group from the target population. This second testing of the program makes up step 6 and is called the main field test. The purpose of the main field test is to determine whether the program under development meets the program objectives set forth in the earlier stages of planning. If it was found that the program did not meet the objectives, it would be revised accordingly and the main field test would be repeated. In practice, if the program did not meet the objectives during this second main field test, it would more than likely be abandoned. However, if it met the objectives minor adjustments would be made (step 7), and the program would be readied for the eighth step—operational field testing (Borg & Gall, 1989).

The purpose of the first eight steps is to determine whether the program is fully ready for implementation without the presence of the program planner. In order to be fully ready for use, the program must be completely and thoroughly tested in every respect. In step 9, the final program is revised based on the operational test. The tenth step would include dissemination and final implementation. This includes distributing the program to those who are to use it and helping them to use it properly (Borg & Gall, 1989).

Remember Borg and Gall's model was originally presented as a research and development cycle and not as an implementation model. We have found, however, that the last seven steps of the cycle make up a well-conceived and thorough implementation model. Some might say this model is too thorough because it requires so much testing before implementation and does not take into account the frequent lack of time and money for program development. We suggest, however, that planners should modify the model as needed to meet specific needs and available resources.

Table 11.1
Major steps of Borg and Gall's research and development cycle applied to creating a health promotion program

---

1. Research and information collecting—includes needs assessment, review of the literature, small-scale research studies, and preparation of report on the state of the art.

2. Planning—includes defining skills to be learned, stating and sequencing the objectives, identifying learning activities, and small-scale feasibility testing.

3. Development of preliminary form of program—includes preparation of instructional materials, procedures, and evaluation instruments.

4. Preliminary field testing—program given to just a few individuals from the target population. Interview, observational, and questionnaire data collected and analyzed.

5. Main program revision—based on results of preliminary field test.

6. Main field testing—program given to approximately twice as many as in preliminary field test. Pre- and postprogram quantitative data on participants collected; results examined with respect to program objectives and compared to control/comparison group, when possible.

7. Operational program revision—based on results of the main field test.

8. Operational field testing—program given to approximately twice as many as in main field test. Interview, observational, and questionnaire data collected and analyzed.

9. Final program revision—based on results of the operational field test.

10. Dissemination and implementation—program shared with others and implemented where appropriate.

Source: Adapted from *Educational Research: An Introduction*, 5th ed. (pp. 784–85), by W. R. Borg and M. D. Gall, 1989, New York: Longman.

First Day of Implementation

No matter what implementation model or strategy the planners choose, there will be a "first day" for the program. The first day of the program is just an extension of the fourth P of marketing, promotion (see Chapter 10). The purpose of promotion is to make the target population aware of the health concern that is the focus of the program. This leads to the initiation of the program. The first day of the program might include some special event, such as a ribbon cutting, appearance by a celebrity, or some other event that starts off the program on a positive note. Consideration should be given to obtaining news coverage (print and/or broadcast) for the first day to further publicize the program.

Dealing with Problems

With the program up and running, the task of the planners is to deal with problems that might arise and to do so in a constructive manner (Ross & Mico,

Tasks Year 1	Months											
	J	F	M	A	M	J	J	A	S	O	N	D
Develop program rational	✔	✔										
Conduct needs assessment			✔									
Develop goals and objectives				✔								
Create intervention					✔							
Conduct formative evaluation						✔						
Assemble necessary resources						✔						
Market program						✔	✔					
Pilot test program								✔				
Refine program									✔			
Phase in program #1										✔		
Phase in program #2											✔	
Phase in program #3												✔

Figure 11.2
Sample planning and implementation timetable

1980). Even if a program has been piloted, problems can still arise. The problems that could be encountered can range from petty concerns to matters of life and death. Problems might involve **logistics** (room size, meeting time, or room temperature), participant dissatisfaction, or an emergency. Whatever the problem, it should be worked out as much as possible to the satisfaction of all concerned. If there is a question of whether to accommodate a program participant or the program personnel, 99% of the time the participants should be satisfied. They are the life blood of all programs. As a part of this step of implementation, it might be a good idea to conduct a one-month evaluation asking questions similar to the ones asked in the piloting evaluation.

Reporting and Documenting

Planners need to give attention to reporting or documenting the ongoing progress of the program to interested others (Ross & Mico, 1980). Planners should keep others informed about the program for several different reasons including: (1) accountability; (2) public relations; (3) motivation of present participants; and (4) recruitment of new participants. The exact nature of the reporting or documenting will vary, but it is important for planners to be able to communicate well both in writing and in speaking.

Implementation Timetable

To provide some guidance in implementing a program, it is helpful to compile a tentative timetable for implementation. It might even be useful to include the entire planning process. Figure 11.2 presents an example of a planning and implementation timetable.

Tasks Year 2	Months											
	J	F	M	A	M	J	J	A	S	O	N	D
Phase in program #4	✔											
Total implementation		✔	✔	✔	✔	✔	✔	✔	✔	✔	✔	✔
Summative evaluation			✔									
Prepare evaluation report				✔								
Distribute report					✔							
Continue with follow-up for long term evaluation						✔	✔	✔	✔	✔	✔	✔

Figure 11.2, *continued*

CONCERNS ASSOCIATED WITH PLANNING

There are many matters of detail to be considered before the implementation actually takes place. The exact order in which they are considered is not as important as just making sure that they have been taken care of. Therefore, we list and describe these items in no specific order.

Legal Concerns

Liability is on the mind of many professionals today because of the concern over lawsuits. With this in mind, all personnel connected with the planned health promotion program, no matter how small the risk of injury to the participants (physical or mental), should make sure that they are adequately covered with liability insurance. In addition, program personnel should have an understanding of informed consent, negligence, and approval of appropriate professional groups (see Chapter 7 for information about guidelines from professional groups).

Informed Consent

No one should be allowed to participate in any health promotion program without giving his **informed consent**. As a part of the process of obtaining informed consent from participants, program facilitators should:

1.   Explain the nature and purpose(s) of the program.
2.   Inform program participants of any inherent risks or dangers associated with participation and any possible discomfort they may experience.
3.   Explain the expected benefits of participation.
4.   Inform participants of alternative programs (procedures) that will accomplish the same thing.
5.   Indicate to the participants that they are free to discontinue participation at any time.

In addition, planners must "ask if they have any questions, answer any such questions, and make it clear they should ask any questions they may have at any time during the program. Informed consent forms should be signed by participants before they enter the program" (Patton et al., 1986, p. 236).

Program planners must be aware that informed consent forms (or waiver of liability or release of liability as some refer to them) do not protect them from being sued. There is no such thing as a waiver of liability. If you are negligent you can be found liable. However, informed consent forms do make participants aware of special concerns. Further, because people must sign the forms, they may not consider legal action even if they have a case, feeling they were duly warned. Appendix K provides sample consent forms.

Negligence

Negligence is failing to act in a **prudent** (reasonable) manner. If there is a question whether someone should or should not do something, it is generally best to err on the side of safety. Negligence can arise from two types of acts—omission and commission. An act of omission is not doing something when you should, such as failing to warn program participants of the inherent danger in participation. An act of commission is doing something you should not be doing, such as leading an aerobic dance program when you are not trained to do so.

Reducing the Risk of Liability

The real key to avoiding liability is to reduce your risk by planning ahead. Patton et al. (1986, p. 236) offer the following tips for reducing legal problems in exercise programs; however, similar advice would apply to all types of health promotion programs. We have added the words in brackets.

1. Be aware of legal liabilities.
2. Select certified instructors [in the activity and emergency care procedures] to lead classes and supervise exercise equipment [and for that matter all types of equipment].
3. Use good judgment in setting up programs and provide written guidelines for medical emergency procedures.
4. Inform participants about the risks and danger of exercise [or other activities] and require written informed consent.
5. Require that participants obtain medical clearance before entering an exercise program [or other strenuous programs].
6. Instruct staff not to "practice medicine" but instead to limit their advice to their own area of expertise.
7. Provide a safe environment by following building codes and regular maintenance schedule for equipment.
8. Purchase adequate liability insurance for all staff.

Medical Concerns

Does the program put the participants at any special medical risk so that they would need medical clearance (for example, cardiovascular exercise programs)? If so, the necessary steps need to be taken so that the participants can provide proof of clearance. Also, it may be necessary to develop a plan for first aid. Appendix L presents an example of a medical clearance form.

Program Registration and Fee Collection

If the program you are planning requires people to sign up and/or pay fees, you will need to establish registration procedures. Program registration and fee collection may take place before the program (preregistration), by mail, in person, via an indirect method like payroll deduction, or at the first session. Planners should also give thought to the type of payment that will be accepted (cash, credit card, or check).

Procedures for Recordkeeping

Almost every program requires some records to be kept. Items such as information collected at registration, medical information, data on participant progress, and evaluations must be accounted for. In addition, planners must decide whether participant files will be kept in a traditional way, with paper and pencil, or using some type of computer program. It is not unusual today to find participants in health promotion programs "logging in" and out on computers for purposes of keeping records of attendance and daily activities.

Program Logistics

Before implementation, program planners need to make sure that arrangements are made for a number of small but important program details. These are often referred to as program logistics. Logistics has been defined as the procurement, maintenance, and transportation of materials, facilities, and personnel (Woolf, 1979). Reserving space where the program is to be held, making sure audiovisual equipment is available when requested, and ordering the correct number of participant education packets are examples of program logistics that are important to the success of the program.

Program Budget

Program planners need to put together a budget for the program. As noted in Chapter 9, the budget will depend on whether the program is being offered to make a profit or not. As with any budget, details of expenses and expected income should be outlined. Figure 11.3 presents a sample budget sheet that lists some of the line items that might be considered.

Moral and Ethical Concerns

There are times when certain behavior is legal but not moral or ethical. Program planning and evaluation provide the health educator with almost daily opportunities to make decisions that affect other people. There are times when these decisions are easy to make and other times when there is a question of what is the right or wrong decision. In other words, because of the nature of health promotion, program planners are confronted with many moral and ethical decisions.

One might ask, Who is to judge what is right and wrong? Most often these decisions are compared to a standard of practice that has been defined by other professionals in the same field. For health promotion planners, the standard of practice is outlined in the Code of Ethics of the Society for Public Health Education (SOPHE) (see Appendix M). However, even a code of ethics cannot spell out all the rights and wrongs of the many decisions that must be made. The interpretation of the code still creates some gray areas. Although the purpose of

Income	Amount
Contribution from sponsors	_____
Gifts	_____
Grants	_____
Participant fee	_____
Sale of curriculum materials	_____
Total income	_____
Expenses	
Curriculum materials	_____
Equipment	_____
Marketing	_____
Print advertising	_____
Other media	_____
Personnel	_____
For planning	_____
Program facilitators	_____
Clerical	_____
Evaluator(s)	_____
Participants	_____
Postage	_____
Space	_____
Supplies	_____
Travel	_____
Total expenses	_____
Balance	_____

Figure 11.3
Sample budget sheet

this section is not to say what is right or wrong, we do want to alert health promotion planners to some of the more common ethical issues that they will face.

The first is respect. Even though one may not agree with the values,
behavior, and goals of others, it is important to respect them. The program planner's role is not to judge but to facilitate. Fennell and Beyrer (1989) have written
a thought-provoking article on some ethical issues concerning AIDS and the
health educator.

Autonomy is another issue with which program planners must deal.
Should letting people voluntarily adopt health behavior be the guiding princi-
ple? Or is there a place for manipulation and coercion in health promotion?
Table 11.2 presents a hierarchy of autonomy.

Table 11.2
Hierarchy of autonomy

A. Facilitation—assist in achieving objectives set by a target group. Examples: putting safety belts in cars or teaching people the skills necessary to perform CPR.

B. Persuasion—argue and reason. Examples: tell about the importance of wearing safety belts or taking blood pressure medicine.

C. Manipulation—modify the environment around a person or the psychic disposition of the person. Example: automatic safety belts.

D. Coercion—threat of deprivation. Example: safety belt or motorcycle helmet laws and fine.

A third issue concerns informed consent. Although this was discussed earlier with regard to legal concerns, it is often also an ethical concern. Program planners are faced with questions such as these: Even though the benefits outnumber the risks, do we scare people away by telling them the risks? Is it okay to withhold information if it could affect the results of an evaluation?

Program planners also have to consider the concept of **nonmaleficence**—not causing harm or not doing evil. For example, is it permissible to use an aversive behavior technique to get someone to stop smoking? Which is worse, smoking cigarettes or receiving some physical punishment for doing so?

The concept of **beneficence**—that is, bringing about or doing good—can also be related to ethical issues. Can there be any question whether it is right to do good? If the good comes at the expense of another, then it raises ethical concerns.

Justice and fairness are also involved in ethical issues. For example, the question of fairness might arise in pricing a program. The program needs to show a profit, but the clients cannot afford the price that would be necessary to achieve a profit. (Legal concerns can enter into this area, too.) Issues of sexism and racism also involve concepts of justice and fairness.

Finally, the concepts of confidentiality and privacy are involved in ethical issues. Should a program planner release information about a person without his consent, even though it will benefit him? Consider a high school sophomore who approaches the health teacher with confidential information that she is pregnant. Should the health teacher tell anyone else, such as the girl's parents?

The opportunities for dealing with ethical issues are many, and program planners need to be prepared to handle them.

Procedural Manual and/or Participant's Manual

Depending on the complexity of a program, there may be a need to develop manuals, or to purchase them from a vendor. Manuals may outline procedures for program facilitators; some refer to these as training manuals. Manuals may also provide the participants with detailed information. Developing either type of manual in-house would be a major task; therefore, adequate resources and time need to be given to developing manuals.

Training for Facilitators

If a program that is being planned needs a specially qualified person (certified or licensed) to facilitate it, every effort should be made to secure such a person. This may mean having to hire a vendor to provide such a service. If funds are not available to hire one, others will need to be trained appropriately. This may mean running your own training program, or sending people to other training classes to become qualified facilitators.

Program Safety

The necessary steps need to be taken to ensure the health and safety of those participating in the program and all staff members. Providing a safe environment includes finding a safe program location (low-crime area), ensuring that classrooms and laboratories are free of hazards, providing qualified facilitators, supplying first-aid equipment, and developing an emergency care plan.

☐ SUMMARY

Much work goes into developing a program before it is ready for implementation. The process used to implement a program may have much to say about its success. This chapter presents two models for program implementation. The first, a modification of the Parkinson and Associates (1982) model, includes three commonly used strategies—piloting, phasing in, and total implementation. The second, Borg and Gall's (1989) research and development cycle, can be modified to provide a thorough implementation strategy. Also presented in this chapter are matters that need to be considered and planned for prior to implementation.

☐ QUESTIONS

1. What is meant by the term *implementation*?
2. What are three strategies from the modified model of Parkinson and Associates (1982) for implementing health promotion?
3. Why are the final seven steps of Borg and Gall's (1989) research and development cycle considered a thorough implementation model?
4. Name the fourth P of marketing and explain how it leads into implementation.
5. What are the legal concerns planners need to be aware of when implementing a program?
6. What is logistics and why is it important to program planners?
7. What is the difference between an act of omission and an act of commission?
8. What role does autonomy play in the ethical decisions a program planner must make?

☐ ACTIVITIES

1. Explain how you would implement a program you are planning using a pilot study, phasing in, and total implementation. Also explain what you plan to do to "kick off" the program.

2. Explain how you would implement a program you are planning using the final seven steps of the Borg and Gall (1989) research and development cycle.

3. Develop an informed consent form that outlines the risks inherent in a program you are planning. Make sure the form includes a place for signatures of the participant and a witness and the date.

4. In a one-page paper, identify what you see as the biggest ethical concern of health promotion programming, and explain your choice.

5. Outline the major sources of income and expenses that would be associated with the program you are planning, by preparing a budget sheet.

Part III
Evaluating a Health Promotion Program

12
Evaluation: An Overview

After reading this chapter and answering the questions at the end, you should be able to:

❑   Compare and contrast the various types of evaluation.

❑   Identify some of the problems that may hinder an effective evaluation.

❑   List reasons why evaluation should be included in all programs.

❑   Explain the difference between internal and external evaluation.

❑   Describe several considerations in planning and conducting an evaluation.

☐ KEY TERMS

baseline data	internal evaluation
evaluation	process evaluation
external evaluation	outcome evaluation
formative evaluation	stakeholders
impact evaluation	summative evaluation

Whether they realize it or not, program planners are constantly evaluating their health promotion efforts by asking questions such as: Did the program have an impact? How many people stopped smoking? Were the participants satisfied with the program? Properly conducted, an evaluation can provide objective answers to these types of questions; however, the usefulness of an evaluation can be limited by a variety of biases and/or inadequate design.

Evaluation is critical for all health promotion programs. It is important to have accurate information to determine the impact of programs and to make decisions about their future. For example, evaluation can help a program planner determine whether participants were satisfied with a weight loss program, whether a smoking cessation workshop actually changed smoking behavior, or whether an exercise program should continue or not. Without adequate evaluation, accurate information is not gained, and decisions are based on speculation.

In order to generate useful and meaningful data about programs, the evaluation must be designed early in the process of program planning. As mentioned in an earlier chapter, evaluation begins when the program goals and objectives are being developed. Evaluation can help not only to determine whether program goals and objectives are met but also to answer questions about the program as it is being implemented. If the evaluation is not designed until the program has ended, the information cannot be used to improve the program as it progresses. For example, low enrollment in a stress management workshop might reflect an inadequate setting, inconvenient hours, or lack of publicity. All of these problems could be reduced or eliminated if evaluation was conducted in the planning stage.

The process of designing an evaluation should be a collaborative effort of all program **stakeholders** (those individuals who have something to gain or lose from the evaluation results). Program planners, administrators, program facilitators, and the representatives from the funding source all have specific questions they would like answered regarding the program's development and outcome. Program planners may want to know if the program met the needs of the target population; program administrators may want to know if the program is making any money; program facilitators may want to know if participants changed their behavior as a result of the program; and representatives from the funding source may be interested in knowing if the program was cost-effective. These questions can all be answered if the evaluation is properly planned and implemented.

BASIC TERMINOLOGY

A variety of definitions of the term *evaluation* have been written; most include the concept of determining the value or worth of the object of interest (the health promotion program) against a standard of acceptability. Table 12.1 lists commonly used standards of acceptability for evaluating health promotion programs.

When determining the value of a program, planners can use several types of evaluation. The type of evaluation reflects whether the results are needed to improve a program before or during implementation, to assess the effectiveness of a program, or to determine whether the program met the goals and objectives.

Evaluations generally use one of two sets of evaluation terms. Some authors use the terms *process, impact,* and *outcome* to identify types of evaluation used to determine the value of a program. Other authors use the terms *formative* and *summative* to describe the evaluation that occurs during the program and after the program, respectively.

> **Process evaluation:** Provides documentation during program implementation to make adjustments for improvement of the program, for example, getting reactions from participants about the times programs are offered or about speakers in a workshop. This could be accomplished with a short questionnaire or with information gained from a focus group.

> **Impact evaluation:** Assesses the overall effectiveness of a program in producing favorable knowledge, attitudes, behaviors, health status, and/or skills in the target population; indicates immediate effects, such as a change in behavior or an increase in knowledge. For example, how many people stopped smoking? How many people can perform CPR? How much do people know about AIDS?

Table 12.1
Standards of acceptability

Standard of acceptability	Examples
Mandate (policies, statues, laws) of regulating agencies	Percent of children immunized for school
	Percent of target population wearing safety belts
Target population health status	Rates of morbidity and mortality compared to state and national norms
Values expressed in the local community	Type of school curriculum expected
Standards advocated by professional organizations	Passing scores, certification, or registration examinations
Norms established via research	Treadmill tests or percent body fat
Norms established by evaluation of previous programs	Smoking cessation rates
Comparison or control groups	Used in experimental or quasi-experimental studies

Outcome evaluation: Determines whether the program met the stated long-term goals and objectives, such as a reduction in morbidity or mortality rates of the target population or an improvement in quality of life.

Formative evaluation: Provides immediate feedback during program planning and implementation to improve and refine the program. It is more comprehensive than process evaluation since information is collected from a variety of sources (such as program participants or program providers) both before and during program implementation.

Summative evaluation: Determines achievements, such as numbers of individuals who changed their behavior or whether other program objectives were reached. It is conducted at the end of the program.

Both sets of evaluation (process, impact, and outcome; formative and summative) take into account the need to conduct evaluation before and/or during the program, and at the end of the program. All types of evaluation should be in place before or during program implementation.

RATIONALE FOR EVALUATION

Basically, there are two reasons for evaluating a program: to improve it or to determine its effectiveness (Fink & Kosecoff, 1978). The types of evaluation are distinguished by how the information is going to be used. The information may be used by program planners during the implementation of a program to make improvements in services (process evaluation). It may be used to see if certain immediate outcomes, such as knowledge, attitude, skills, and behavior change have occurred (impact evaluation). It may be used at the end of a program to determine whether long-term goals and objectives have been met (outcome evaluation). Within this general rationale for evaluation, several additional reasons can be found for evaluating a program:

1. *To demonstrate the worth of a program.* An evaluation can help to determine whether the program is moving in the right direction, is justifying past or projected expenditure, is providing a positive change in conditions or behavior, or is cost effective. Evaluation can document whether the health needs of the target population have been met. Information about the worth of a program can be used to make decisions about the fate of the program.

2. *To compare different types of programs.* Different types of programs, methods, or approaches can be compared to determine which are the most effective in meeting initial goals. For example, if the goal is to reduce the number of smokers in a corporation, smoking rates of those who completed a smoking cessation workshop could be compared to those who completed a self-directed program. An evaluation can also test innovative ideas to determine whether the effort should be duplicated. A cost-benefit

or cost-effectiveness analysis could be completed to compare the economic aspects of different programs.

3.   *To meet requirements of the funding source.* Many times the funding source requires an evaluation to determine whether the goals and objectives of a program have been met, to document that the program is cost-effective, to make decisions about the fate of the program (whether it should be continued, duplicated, expanded, or discontinued), or to determine whether mandates of regulatory agencies have been met, as in the case of immunizations or environmental standards.

4.   *To provide information about the program.* When information is provided to the media, the evaluation results often increase the program's visibility and public support; it may be possible to use the results as a marketing technique to "sell" the program. Information about the program can also be provided to select groups, such as the program staff, participants, and potential participants. Providing information to professional colleagues can increase the knowledge base and avoid duplication of efforts when designing and implementing health promotion programs in the future.

THE PROCESS FOR EVALUATION

The process of evaluating a program or activity begins with the initial program planning. Those involved in developing new programs need to be aware of the importance of a well-defined evaluation plan. The evaluation process consists of several steps. The following list provides guidelines for planning and conducting an evaluation.

Planning

❑   Review the program goals and objectives.

❑   Meet with the stakeholders to determine what general questions should be answered.

❑   Determine whether the necessary resources are available to conduct the evaluation; budget for additional costs.

❑   Hire an evaluator, if needed.

❑   Develop the evaluation design.

❑   Decide which evaluation instrument(s) will be used and, if needed, who will develop the instrument.

❑   Determine whether the evaluation questions reflect the goals and objectives of the program.

❑   Determine whether the questions of various groups are considered, such as the program administrators, facilitators, planners, participants, and funding source.

❑   Determine when the evaluation will be conducted; develop a time line.

Data Collection

❑ Decide how the information will be collected: survey, records and documents, telephone interview, personal interview, observation.

❑ Determine who will collect the data.

❑ Plan and administer a pilot test.

❑ Review the results of the pilot test to refine the data collection instrument or the collection procedures.

❑ Determine who will be included in the evaluation—for example, all program participants, or a random sample of participants.

❑ Conduct the data collection.

Data Analysis

❑ Determine how the data will be analyzed.

❑ Determine who will analyze the data.

❑ Conduct the analysis, and allow for several interpretations of the data.

Reporting

❑ Determine who will receive the results.

❑ Choose who will report the findings.

❑ Determine how (in what form) the results will be disseminated.

❑ Discuss how the findings of the process or formative evaluation will affect the program.

❑ Decide when the results of the impact, outcome, or summative evaluation will be made available.

❑ Disseminate the findings.

Application

❑ Determine how the results can be implemented.

PRACTICAL PROBLEMS IN EVALUATION

Certain problems may exist, which may impede an effective evaluation. Solomon (1987, pp. 366–68) identifies seven types of problems that can hinder an effective evaluation:

1. Planner failed to build evaluation into program planning.

2. Adequate procedures cost time and resources.

3. Changes in adults come slowly.

4. Some changes do not last.

5. It is often difficult to distinguish between cause and effect.

6. Conflict can arise between professional standards and "do it yourself" attitudes.

7. Sometimes people's motives get in the way.

Awareness of these problems and development of strategies to deal with them may improve the accuracy of program evaluation. We discuss many approaches that can help minimize these problems, such as including evaluation in the early stages of program planning, determining who will conduct the evaluation, carefully considering the evaluation design, increasing objectivity, and developing a plan to use the evaluation results.

EVALUATION IN THE PROGRAM-PLANNING STAGES

As we have mentioned, to be most effective the evaluation must be planned in the early stages of program development. Results from evaluations conducted early in the program-planning process can assist in improving the program. Having a plan in place to conduct an evaluation before the end of a program will make collecting information regarding program outcomes much easier and more accurate.

We will discuss how evaluation plans can be included in program planning by using the examples of formative and summative evaluations. The formative evaluation should provide feedback to the program administrator, with program monitoring beginning in the early stages. Collecting and communicating information to the administrator quickly allows for the program to be modified and improved.

Data reflecting the initial status or interests of the participants (**baseline data**) or data from a needs assessment can be used for comparison to the early data collected from program participants. Additional information from the formative evaluation may indicate that the necessary staff have been hired, the program sites are available, brochures have been printed, participants are satisfied with the times the programs are offered, and classes are offered with the needs of the prospective participants in mind.

Early data regarding the program should be analyzed quickly to make any necessary adjustments to the program. This type of evaluation can improve both new and existing programs. Information from the formative evaluation can be useful in answering questions, such as whether the programs are provided at convenient locations for the community members, whether the necessary materials arrived on time, and whether people are attending the workshops at all the various times they are offered.

By developing the summative evaluation plan at the beginning of the program, planners can ensure that the results will be less biased. Early development of the summative evaluation plan ensures that the questions answered reflect the original objectives and goals of the program. This type of evaluation can provide answers to many questions, such as whether the group approach or the individual approach was more effective in reducing tobacco use among the participants in a smoking cessation program, whether the participants in a weight loss program lost weight and kept the weight off, and how many people in the target population participated in a given program.

WHO WILL CONDUCT THE EVALUATION?

At the beginning of the program, planners must determine who will conduct the evaluation. The program evaluator must be as objective as possible, and should have nothing to gain from the results of the evaluation. The evaluator may be someone associated with the program or someone from outside.

If someone trained in evaluation and personally involved with the program conducts the evaluation, it is called an **internal evaluation**. An internal evaluator would have the advantage of being closer to the program staff and activities, making it easier to collect the relevant information. Conducting an internal evaluation is also less expensive than hiring additional personnel to conduct the evaluation. The major drawback, however, is the possibility of evaluator bias or conflict of interest. Someone closely involved with the program has an investment in the outcome of the evaluation and may not be completely objective. After all, a positive evaluation of the program may result in future funding that would secure the positions of the staff members.

An **external evaluation** is one conducted by someone who is not connected with the program. This type of evaluator is somewhat isolated, lacking the knowledge and experience of the program that the internal evaluator possesses. This type of evaluation is also more expensive, since an additional person must be hired to carry out the work. However, this type of evaluation can provide a more objective outlook and a fresh perspective, and it helps ensure an unbiased outcome evaluation.

Whether an internal or external evaluator conducts the program evaluation, the main goal is to choose someone with credibility and objectivity. The evaluator must have a clear role in the evaluation design, accurately reporting the results regardless of the findings.

EVALUATION RESULTS

The question of who will receive the evaluation results is also an important consideration. The evaluation can be conducted from several vantage points, depending on whether the results will be presented to the program administrator, the funding source, the organization, or the public. These stakeholders may all have different sets of questions they would like answered. The evaluation results must be disseminated to groups interested in the program. Different aspects of the evaluation can be stressed, depending on the group's particular needs and interests. A program administrator may be interested in which approach was more successful, the funding source may want to know if all objectives were reached, and a community member may want to know if participants felt the program was beneficial.

The planning process of the evaluation should include a determination of how the results will be used. It is especially important in process and formative evaluation to implement the findings rapidly to improve the program. However, an action plan is needed in summative, impact, and outcome evaluation to ensure that the results are not filed away but are used in the provision of future health promotion programs.

SUMMARY

Evaluation can be thought of as a way to make sound decisions regarding the worth or effectiveness of health promotion programs, to compare different types of programs, to meet requirements of funding sources, or to provide information about programs. The evaluation process takes place before, during, and after program implementation. If the evaluation is well designed and conducted, the findings can be extremely beneficial to the program stakeholders.

QUESTIONS

1. Give an example of a question that could be answered in a process evaluation, impact evaluation, and outcome evaluation.
2. What are some of the general reasons for evaluating a program?
3. Why types of problems can block an effective evaluation?
4. What different types of information could an evaluation provide for the various stakeholders (program planners, the funding source, the administrators, and the participants)?
5. Why is it important to begin the evaluation process in the program-planning stages?
6. Explain how feedback from an evaluation can be used in program planning.
7. What are some of the steps in evaluation planning, data collection, data analysis, and reporting?
8. In what type of situation would an internal evaluation be more appropriate than an external evaluation?

ACTIVITIES

1. Describe how process, impact, and outcome evaluation could be used in a stress management program for college students. Describe how formative and summative evaluation could be used.
2. Write a rationale to a funding source for hiring an external evaluator.
3. Review the evaluation component from a health promotion program in your community and/or discuss an evaluation plan with a program planner or evaluator. Look for the planning process used, the rationale for the data collection method, and how the findings were reported.
4. Assume you are responsible for selecting an evaluator for a health promotion program you are planning. Would you select an internal or external evaluator? Explain your rationale. If you select an external evaluator, where do you think you could find such a person?

13

Evaluation Models

After reading this chapter and answering the questions at the end, you should be able to:

❑ Define the term *model,* and discuss the rationale for the use of a model in evaluation.

❑ Describe the various evaluation models outlined.

❑ Explain the components of the five models emphasized in this chapter and discuss their strengths and limitations.

❑ Explain why it is difficult to categorize models, and discuss the classification used by Popham (1988).

KEY TERMS

behavioral objectives model

cost-benefit analysis

cost-effectiveness analysis

decision-making model

goal-attainment model

goal-based model

goal-free model

model

naturalistic model

systems analysis model

A **model** can be thought of as a framework or plan that can be used to conduct an evaluation. This concept of a model is similar to the one given in Chapter 2, in the discussion of models for program planning. In this chapter, various evaluation models are presented, which evaluators can select based on their requirements and those of the stakeholders. Washington (1987) indicates that each model represents a certain way of thinking, which defines what evaluation questions should be asked. For example, the evaluation questions may focus on the goals and objectives of the program, the effects of the intervention, the cost-benefit ratio of the program, and the behavior of the participants.

This chapter provides an overview of evaluation models, emphasizing those commonly used in health promotion programs. Alternative approaches are also included, since different authors classify the various models differently and may call similar approaches by different names. It is important for the evaluator to select a model or portions of models to use in structuring an evaluation; models do not have to be used in their pure form.

MAJOR EVALUATION APPROACHES

This overview includes eight major approaches used in evaluation. As previously mentioned, the models may be called by more than one name, or one model may have slight variations in approach. With this in mind, the evaluation models most commonly found are presented here, using categories chosen by House (1980).

Systems analysis uses output measures, such as test scores, to determine if the program has demonstrated the desired change. It also determines whether funds have been efficiently used, as in cost-benefit analysis.

Behavioral objectives, or goal-based evaluation, uses the program goals and collects evidence to determine whether the goals have been reached.

Decision making focuses on the decision to be made and presents evidence about the program to the decision maker (manager or administrator).

Goal-free evaluation does not base the evaluation on program goals; instead, the evaluator searches for all outcomes, often finding unintended side effects.

Art criticism uses the judgment of an expert in the area to increase awareness and appreciation of the program in order to lead to improved standards and better performance.

Professional review uses professionals to judge the work of other professionals; the source of standards and criteria is the professionals conducting the review.

Quasi-legal evaluation uses a panel to hear evidence; a quasi- legal procedure is used for both evaluating and policy making.

Case study uses techniques such as interviews and observations to examine how people view the program.

Table 13.1 presents a taxonomy of these major approaches to evaluation, developed by House (1980). It is very helpful in identifying the audience of the evaluation, the points on which the model assumes consensus, the methodology most commonly used, the outcome, and typical evaluation questions that could be answered.

Difficulty in Categorizing Evaluation Models

Due to the number of evaluation models and the various names used for similar models, classification is difficult. The development of many models in the late 1960s and early 1970s led to overlap, as new models incorporated parts of earlier models. Popham (1988) has discussed the difficulty in classification of models and has offered a five-category set of descriptors to classify the variety of models. These categories may be summarized as follows:

Goal-attainment models focus on the degree to which goals were achieved.

Judgmental models emphasizing inputs give major attention to professional judgment and are based on intrinsic or process criteria, with the evaluator's judgment having a strong influence on whether the evaluation results are positive or negative.

Judgmental models emphasizing outputs use extrinsic or product criteria, with the evaluator offering a judgment on the program.

Decision facilitation models are intended to serve decision makers; information is collected by the evaluator and presented to someone else to judge its worth and then make a decision.

Naturalistic models use program participants to form judgments about the program, or else evaluators conduct observations to form judgments.

In addition to using descriptors to classify models, Popham suggested an eclectic approach to alternative strategies for education evaluation. He believes that models can rarely be used in their pure form, so that choosing parts of models or categories may be more beneficial to the evaluator.

MODELS COMMONLY USED IN HEALTH PROMOTION EVALUATION

Not all types of evaluation models are commonly used in evaluating health promotion programs. Five of the models most often used are discussed in greater detail in this section.

Behavioral Objectives/Goal-Attainment/Goal-Based Model

One of the most commonly used types of evaluation models is the **behavioral objectives model**, which focuses on the stated goals of the program. Models using this type of goal directed focus are also known as **goal-attainment models** or **goal-based models**. Data are collected to determine whether the predetermined goals have been met. Success or failure is measured by the relationship between

Table 13.1

A taxonomy of major evaluation approaches

Model	Major audiences or reference groups	Assumes consensus on
Systems analysis	Economists, managers	Goals, know cause and effect, quantified variables
Behavioral objectives	Managers, psychologists	Prespecified objectives, quantified outcome variables
Decision-making	Decision-makers, especially administrators	General goals, criteria
Goal-free	Consumers	Consequences, criteria
Art criticism	Conoisseurs, consumers	Critics, standards
Professional review	Professionals, public	Criteria, panel, procedures
Quasi-legal	Jury	Procedures and judges
Case study	Client, practitioners	Negotiations, activities

Source: From *Evaluating with Validity* (p. 23) by E. R. House, 1980, Beverly Hills, CA: Sage Publications. Reprinted by permission of Sage Publications, Inc.

the outcome of the program and the stated goals. This type of model is based on behavior, and the dependent variable is defined in terms of behaviors the program participant should be able to demonstrate at the end of the intervention.

In the behavioral objective model, the program goals serve as the standards for evaluation. This type of evaluation was first used in education, to assess student behaviors. Competency testing is an example of goal-attainment evaluation, determining whether a student is able to pass an exam or advance to the next grade. Goal attainment was later used in other fields, and more emphasis was placed on how objectives are to be measured. This model is also found in business, where organizations use "management by objectives" to determine how well they are meeting their objectives.

This model was used in public health by Suchman (1967), who identified the evaluation process as circular (see Figure 13.1). Evaluation starts with a

Methodology	Outcome	Typical questions
Planning, programming, and budgeting system (PPBS), linear programming, planned variation, cost-benefit analysis	Efficiency	Are the expected effects achieved? Can the effects be achieved more economically? What are the *most* efficient programs?
Behavioral objectives, achievement tests	Productivity, accountability	Is the program achieving the objectives? Is the program producing?
Surveys, questionnaires, interviews, natural variation	Effectiveness, quality control	Is the program effective? What parts are effective?
Bias control, logical analysis, modus operandi	Consumer choice, social utility	What are *all* the effects?
Critical review	Improved standards, heightened awareness	Would a critic approve this program? Is the audience's appreciation increased?
Review by panel, self study	Professional acceptance	How would professionals rate this program?
Quasi-legal procedures	Resolution	What are the arguments for and against the program?
Case studies, interviews, observations	Understanding diversity	What does the program look like to different people?

Figure 13.1
The evaluation process
Source: From *Evaluation Research* (p. 34) by E. A. Suchman, 1967, New York: Russell Sage Foundation. Reprinted by permission of the Russell Sage Foundation.

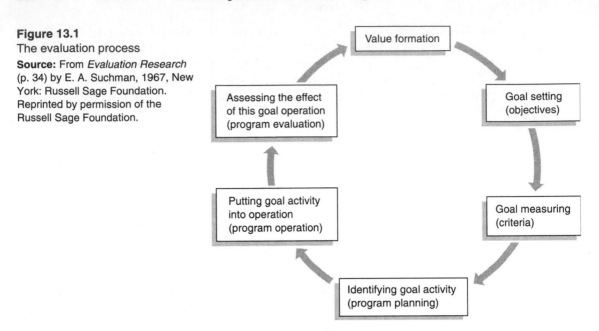

value; the goal is derived from this value, and objectives are set. The following steps include determining criteria to measure the goal, identifying the goal activity (program planning), and putting the goal activity into operation (program operation). The assessment step evaluates the extent to which the objectives have been met. Using this information, a judgment is made about the goal activity, which leads back to the initial value. At this point the value may be changed, reaffirmed, or reassessed.

Washington (1987, pp. 373–74) has identified five steps in measuring goal attainment. These steps include:

1. Specification of the goal to be measured.
2. Specification of the sequential set of performances that, if observed, would indicate that the goal has been achieved.
3. Identification of the performances that are critical to the achievement of the goal.
4. Description of the "indicator behavior" of each performance episode.
5. Collective testing to find whether each "indicator behavior" is associated with each other.

Within the general goal statement is the outcome behavior of the individual. The goal should be operationally defined—that is, it should consist of measurable objectives—and those objectives most critical in achieving the goal should be identified. An indicator of a performance episode refers to a measurable, observable behavior, based on normative criteria. Measurement should be standardized in order to compare outcomes from one behavior to another. (See Chapter 5 for a discussion of writing goals and objectives.)

A strength of the behavioral objective model is its objectivity. The values of the evaluator do not interfere with the outcome of the evaluation. Another strength is that the goal is predetermined: the evaluation is based on whether or not the goal was met, not on whether it was appropriate. The goal can be expressed as measurable objectives, making it easier to determine whether the goal was met.

A possible limitation of this model is how the goal is set, since the outcome of the evaluation is determined by the specification of the goal. The goal reflects the values or interests of the funding source, program staff, or consumers. Who sets the goal is an important factor, and consideration must be given to whose interests the goal represents.

Another limitation of this model is that only those items included in the objectives are evaluated. There may be other very positive outcomes of a program, but they will not be identified or evaluated because they were not included in the objectives. An example would be to include only behavior change in the objectives of a program; any other positive changes, such as in attitudes or knowledge, would be overlooked in the evaluation.

Goal-Free Model

The **goal-free model** of evaluation was developed in response to the limitations of the goal-attainment model. Scriven (1973), who developed the goal-free model, believed that evaluation should not be based on goals in order to enable the evaluator to remain unbiased. The evaluator must search for all outcomes, including unintended positive or negative side effects. Thus, the evaluator does not base the evaluation on reaching goals and remains unaware of the program goals.

Ideally, the evaluator suspends judgment concerning what the program is intended to accomplish and focuses on what actually happens. However, Popham (1988) sees this approach as oriented toward the output of the program and as a judgmental approach, since the evaluator is required to present a judgment regarding the program to the decision makers.

The techniques that the evaluator uses include examining pre-intervention test results, reading expert reviews, visiting program sites, reviewing the literature, examining similar programs, interviewing staff and clients, and examining materials. The techniques are generally qualitative methods, but quantitative methods can also be used.

The goal-free model is not often used in evaluation. It is difficult for evaluators to determine what to evaluate when program objectives are not to be used. One concern is that evaluators will substitute their own goals, since there is a lack of clear methodology as to how to approach the model. The goal-free evaluation model may be most useful in combination with other models.

On the other hand, this model has certain advantages. One is that it offers a bias-free approach. Another advantage is that this model avoids classifying side effects and unanticipated effects as being of secondary interest, since these may be crucial to setting new priorities in a program. A classic example of this model was an evaluation of an educational program for coronary care patients. The results of the evaluation indicated no increase in knowledge, which was the program goal. However, an unanticipated side effect was reduction in patients' anxiety during exercise. Without the use of goal-free evaluation, this benefit of the program might not have been discovered.

The main differences between the goal-attainment and goal-free models are presented in Table 13.2. The types of questions asked in each model reflect the difference in focus of the evaluation.

Decision-Making Model

According to Stufflebeam (1971), the developer of the **decision-making model**, there are three steps to the evaluation process: delineating (focusing of information), obtaining (collecting, organizing, and analyzing information), and providing (synthesizing information so it will be useful). The decision maker, usually a manager or administrator, wants and needs information to help answer relevant questions regarding a program.

The four types of evaluation in this model include context, input, process, and product (CIPP), with each providing information to the decision maker. Context evaluation describes the conditions in the environment, identifies unmet needs and unused opportunities, and determines why these occur. The purpose of input evaluation is to determine how to use resources to meet program goals. Process evaluation provides feedback to those responsible for program implementation. The purpose of product evaluation is to measure and interpret attainments during and after the program (Stufflebeam, 1971). It is the decision maker, not the evaluator, who uses this information to determine the worth of the program.

The main advantage to this type of model is the increased likelihood that the information will actually be used by the decision makers. The information most relevant to them will be obtained by this type of evaluation. The advantage for the evaluator is that the evaluation is focused, with criteria already determined. A limitation of the decision-making model is that the amount of input from administrators may reduce the objectivity of the evaluation.

Table 13.2
Comparison of the goal-attainment and goal-free models

Goal-attainment model	Goal-free model
Have the objectives been reached?	What is the outcome of the program?
Has the program met the needs of the target population?	Who has been reached by the program?
How can the objectives be reached?	How is the program operating?
Are the needs of the program administrators and funding source being met?	What has been provided?

Systems Analysis Model

The **systems analysis model** is based upon efficiency—determining which are the most effective programs. It focuses on the organization, determining whether appropriate resources are devoted to goal activities (and to nongoal activities, such as staff training or maintenance of the system). The measurement of general goals is central to this model, but it does not focus on the achievement of a specific goal. This is due to the recognition that organizations function at different levels with various goals at each level.

Economic evaluations, such as cost-benefit and cost-effectiveness analyses, are typical strategies used in the systems analysis model. **Cost-benefit analysis** looks at how resources can best be used. It will yield the dollar benefit received from the dollars invested in the program. **Cost-effectiveness analysis** is used to quantify the effects of a program in monetary terms. Cost-effectiveness analysis is more appropriate for health promotion programs than cost-benefit analysis, because a dollar value does not have to be placed on the outcomes of the program. Instead, a cost-effectiveness analysis will indicate how much it costs to produce a certain effect. For example, based on the cost of a program, the effect of years of life saved, number of smokers who stop smoking, or morbidity or mortality rates can be determined. A thorough explanation of both cost-benefit and cost-effectiveness analysis is presented in Appendix N in an article written by McKenzie (1986).

Two advantages of the systems analysis model are that the findings are objective and that the findings can convince decision makers that a program is effective in improving health status. A disadvantage, however, is that this is only one part of the data to be considered when making program decisions: information from program participants is not included. The fate of a program should not be based on cost-benefit or cost-effectiveness analysis alone.

Naturalistic Models

Models that focus more on qualitative data, using fewer constraints, are classified as less scientific and more naturalistic. An example of a **naturalistic model** is the responsive model, developed by Stake (1983). Compared to previous models, Stake's is much more attentive to the concerns of the individuals for whom the evaluation is being conducted, than to those of program planners or administrators. Responsive evaluation focuses on program activities rather than on goals or outcomes, looks at audience requirements for information, and considers the perspective of the participants in determining success or failure. The evaluator uses techniques such as observations and narratives about the program, validating the findings with participants and staff members. Much of this type of evaluation is informal, even the communication of the findings (Stake, 1983).

This evaluation model is best used when the main aim is to understand the program and there is a greater concern for the program stakeholders. Its characteristics of less structure and scientific base, informal communication and reporting, and less attention to program objectives may be a drawback for those who want a more formal, objective type of evaluation.

☐ SUMMARY

Several models have been presented in this chapter that could serve as a framework for an evaluation. No one model is useful in all situations. Therefore, we recommend that the evaluator select a model or parts of models to structure the evaluation based on the needs of the stakeholders involved with each program.

☐ QUESTIONS

1. Why is a model used in evaluation?
2. List the eight major evaluation approaches in the taxonomy by House (1980). Discuss the major audiences, the points on which the model assumes consensus, methodology, outcome, and some of the evaluation questions that could be answered.
3. Why is it difficult to categorize evaluation models, and how could the classification by Popham (1988) be used?
4. What are the major features of the behavioral objective, goal-free, decision-making, systems analysis, and naturalistic models? What are the strengths and limitations of each of these models?
5. What is the difference between cost-benefit analysis and cost-effectiveness analysis? Which is more appropriate for use in health promotion programs?

☐ ACTIVITIES

1. Develop your own model to evaluate a stress management program, using parts of the models presented in this chapter. Include information on your target group, the audience for your evaluation, and the questions you would like answered.
2. Look at an evaluation of a health promotion program that has been conducted in your community. Identify the evaluation model(s) it most closely follows. Discuss your view with the program evaluator.
3. Talk with a program administrator or other decision makers about their view of evaluation; discuss the advantages and disadvantages of the major models from their perspective. For example, who should make the decision about how the evaluation results are used? What are the questions they would like answered? Conduct the same activity using program participants instead of administrators. How does the view of the participants differ from the view of administrators?
4. Identify which model or models you would use in developing an evaluation for a program you are planning. Provide a rationale for your decision.

14

Evaluation Design

After reading this chapter and answering the questions at the end, you should be able to:

❑ Compare and contrast quantitative and qualitative approaches to evaluation.

❑ Differentiate among experimental, control, and comparison groups.

❑ Compare and contrast the major types of evaluation design.

❑ Explain the various types of validity.

❑ Identify the threats to internal and external validity and explain how evaluation design can increase control.

❑ Define reliability and explain why it is important in measurement and evaluation.

❑ List some considerations in selecting an evaluation design.

☐ KEY TERMS

blind

comparison group

concurrent validity

construct validity

content validity

control group

criterion-based validity

deductive

double blind

experimental design

experimental group

external validity

generalizability

inductive

internal consistency

internal validity

interrater reliability

measurement

nonexperimental design

posttest

predictive validity

pretest

qualitative approach

quantitative approach

quasi-experimental design

reliability

stability reliability

triple blind

validity

An evaluation design is used to organize the evaluation and to provide for planned, systematic data collection, analysis, and reporting. An evaluation helps furnish answers to properly formulated questions. A well-planned evaluation helps ensure that the conclusions drawn about the program will be as accurate as possible. The evaluation design is developed during the early stages of program planning and has program goals and objectives as its focus. As mentioned earlier, program planners must give consideration to the audience and/or stakeholders who will read the results of the evaluation; the design must produce information that will answer their evaluation questions.

QUANTITATIVE AND QUALITATIVE APPROACHES

A decision that must be made early in the evaluation design is whether to use a quantitative approach, a qualitative approach, or both. The **quantitative approach** is **deductive** in nature (applying a generally accepted principle to an individual case), so that the evaluation produces hard data, such as counts, ratings, scores, or classifications. Examples of quantitative data would be the number of participants in a stress management program, the ratings on a participant satisfaction survey, and the pretest scores on a nutrition knowledge test. This approach is suited to programs that are well defined and compares outcomes of programs with those of other groups or the general population. It is the method most often used in evaluation designs.

The **qualitative approach** is an **inductive** method (individual cases are studied to formulate a general principle) and produces soft data, such as descriptions. The methods most often used to collect qualitative data are interviews, case studies, focus groups, and observations. This is a good method to use for programs that emphasize individual outcomes or in cases where other descriptive information from participants is needed.

Patton (1988) offers a checklist to determine whether qualitative data might be appropriate in a particular program evaluation. Collecting qualitative data may be a good strategy if there is a need to describe individual outcomes, to understand the dynamics and process of the programs, to obtain in-depth information on certain clients or sites, or to focus on the diversity of program clients or sites; it is also helpful in gathering information to improve the program during formative evaluation.

Rather than choose one approach, it may be advantageous to combine quantitative and qualitative methods. For example, combining ratings or scores of program participants with interviews of a few selected participants can strengthen the evaluation. Supplementing the hard data with anecdotal information further describes the results.

EXPERIMENTAL AND CONTROL GROUPS

The group of individuals participating in the program that is to be evaluated is known, as in other types of research studies, as the **experimental group**. The evaluation is designed to determine what effects the program has on these individuals. To make sure that the effects are caused by the program and not by some other factor, a **control group** should be used. The control group should be as similar to the experimental group as possible, but the members of this group do not receive the program (intervention or treatment) that is to be evaluated.

Without the use of a properly selected control group, the apparent effect of the program could actually be due to a variety of factors, such as differences in participants' educational background, environment, or experience. By using a control group, the evaluator can show that the results or outcomes are due to the program and not to those other variables. In an ideal situation, participants should be randomly selected, then randomly assigned to one of two groups, and finally it should be randomly determined which group would become the experimental group and which the control group. Theoretically, this would evenly distribute the variables of the participants. This technique increases the credibility of the evaluation by controlling for extraneous events and factors.

It is not always possible or ethical to assign participants to a control group, especially if doing so would mean that they would be denied a necessary program or service. For example, a health promotion program could be designed for individuals with hypertension. Individuals diagnosed with hypertension could be referred by a physician into a health promotion class focused on reducing the risk factors associated with this disease. Denying some individuals access to the program in order to form a control group would clearly be unethical.

One way to deal with this problem is to provide the control group with an alternative program, or to offer the regular program to the group at a later time (if a delay is not potentially harmful). Another alternative is to compare two programs: offer an innovative program to some participants, and continue the conventional program for others. Wagner and Guild (1989) see the advantage of this strategy as providing service to all participants (which fulfills a moral obligation) and still providing a comparison to assess the effectiveness of the innovative program.

Since the main purpose of social programs is to help clients, the client's viewpoint should be the primary one. It is important to keep this in mind when considering ethical issues in the use of control groups. Conner (1980) identifies four underlying premises for the use of control groups in social program evaluation: (1) all individuals have a right to status quo services; (2) all individuals involved in the evaluation are informed about the purpose of the study and the use of a control group; (3) individuals have a right to new services, and random selection gives everyone a chance to participate; and (4) individuals should not be subjected to ineffective or harmful programs. The ethical issues that must be considered involve the potential denial of a service and allocation of scarce resources. When randomization is not feasible, planners should consider an equitable process of providing services for individuals while maintaining control over the evaluation design.

When participants cannot be randomly assigned to an experimental or control group, a nonequivalent control group may be selected. This is known as a **comparison group**. It is important to find a group that is as similar as possible to the experimental group, such as two classrooms of students with similar characteristics or residents in two comparable cities. Factors to consider include participants' age, gender, education, location, socioeconomic status, and experience, as well as any other variable that might have an impact on program results.

EVALUATION DESIGNS

Measurements can be collected in three main ways: after the program; both before and after the program; and several times before, during, and after the program. **Measurement** is defined by Green and Lewis (1986) as the method or procedure of assigning numbers to objects, events, and people. How such information is obtained will be discussed in Chapter 15.

Table 14.1 presents evaluation designs commonly used in health promotion. In the table, the letter M refers to measurement, such as surveys, tests, interviews, observations, or other methods of gaining information. Measurement before the program begins is known as the **pretest**, and measurement after the completion of the program is known as the **posttest**. The letter P represents the program; the relative positions of the two letters in the table indicate when measurements are made in relation to when the program is provided. The table also shows which groups receive the program and when participants are randomly assigned to groups [(R)].

Table 14.1
Evaluation designs

I. Experimental design								
1. Pretest-posttest design								
Experimental group		(R)	M		P	M		
Control group		(R)	M			M		
2. Posttest-only design								
Experimental group		(R)			P	M		
Control group		(R)				M		
3. Time series design								
Experimental group	(R)	M	M	M	P	M	M	M
Control group	(R)	M	M	M		M	M	M
II. Quasi-experimental design								
1. Pretest-posttest design								
Experimental group			M		P	M		
Comparison group			M			M		
2. Time series design								
Experimental group		M	M	M	P	M	M	M
Comparison group	M	M	M			M	M	M
III. Nonexperimental design								
1. Pretest-posttest design								
Experimental group			M		P	M		
2. Time series design								
Experimental group		M	M	M	P	M	M	M

Key: (R) = Random assignment
    M = Measurement
    P = Program

Windsor, Baranowski, Clark, and Cutter (1984) differentiate among three types of evaluation designs: experimental, quasi-experimental, and nonexperimental. **Experimental design** offers the greatest control over the various factors that may influence the results. It involves random assignment to experimental and control groups with measurement of both groups. It produces the most interpretable and defensible evidence of effectiveness. **Quasi-experimental design** results in interpretable and supportive evidence of program effectiveness, but usually cannot control for all factors that affect the validity of the results. There is no random assignment to the groups, and comparisons are made on experimental and comparison groups. **Nonexperimental design,** without the use of a comparison or control group, has little control over the factors that affect the validity of the results.

The most powerful design is the experimental design in which participants are randomly assigned to the experimental and control groups. The difference between I.1 and I.2 in Table 14.1 is the use of a pretest to measure the participants before the program begins. Use of a pretest would help assure that the groups are similar. Random assignment should equally distribute any of the variables (such as age, gender, and race) between the different groups. Potential disadvantages of the experimental design are that it requires a relatively large group of participants and that the intervention may be delayed for those in the control group.

A design more commonly found in evaluations of health promotion programs is the quasi-experimental pretest-posttest design using a comparison group (II.1 in Table 14.1). This design is often used when a control group cannot be formed by random assignment. In such a case, a comparison group (a nonequivalent control group) is identified, and both groups are measured before and after the program. For example, a program on fire safety for two fifth-grade classrooms could be evaluated by using a pre/post knowledge test. Two fifth-grade classrooms not receiving the program could serve as the comparison group. Similar pretest scores between the comparison and experimental groups would indicate that the groups were equal at the beginning of the program. However, without random assignment, it would be impossible to be sure that other variables (a unit on fire safety in a 4-H group, distribution of smoke detectors, information from parents) did not influence the results.

Sometimes participants cannot be assigned to a control group and no comparison group can be identified. In such cases, a nonexperimental pretest-posttest design (III.1 in Table 14.1) can be used, but the results are of limited significance since changes could be due to the program or to some other event. An example of this type of nonexperimental design would be the incidence of safety belt use after a community program on that topic. An increase in use might mean that the program successfully motivated individuals to use safety belts; however, it could also reveal the impact of increased enforcement of the mandatory safety belt law, of a traffic fatality in the community, or a safety article in the local newspaper.

A time series evaluation design (I.3, II.2, III.2 in Table 14.1) can be used to examine differences in program effects over time. Random assignment to groups (I.3) offers the most control over factors influencing the validity of the results. The use of a comparison group (II.2) offers some control; without a control group or comparison group (III.2), it is possible to determine changes in the participants over time, but one cannot be sure that the changes were due to the program.

In the time series design, several measurements are taken over time both before and after the program is implemented. This process helps to identify other factors that may account for a change between the pretest and posttest measurements and is especially appropriate for measuring delayed effects of a program. A time series design could be used in a weight loss program to indicate the amount of weight loss over time and the ability to maintain a desired weight.

When more than one experimental group is part of the evaluation, these can be included in the designs we have discussed. This design could be used to

Table 14.2
Staggered treatment design

Experimental group 1	(R)	P	M		M		M		M
Experimental group 2	(R)		M	P	M		M		M
Experimental group 3	(R)				M	P	M		M
Experimental group 4	(R)							P	M

Key: (R) = Random assignment
    M = Measurement
    P = Program

evaluate several types of programs, for example, to compare the effect of lectures, workshop, and self-study. Measurements could be collected from all groups at the same points in time, and programs could occur simultaneously.

Another design that may be used is the staggered treatment design (Table 14.2). It is used to determine the effects of a program over time by including several measurements after the end of the program. It also indicates the effects of testing, since not all groups in this design receive a pretest. The staggered treatment design can also be used in quasi-experimental and nonexperimental designs, although with the limitations of not using a control group or comparison group.

VALIDITY

When designing an evaluation, the planners must ensure that it measures what it is intended to measure. This refers to the **validity** of the measurement—whether it is correctly measuring the concepts under investigation. Using a valid instrument increases the chance that planners are measuring what they want to measure, thus ruling out other possible explanations for the results. We will discuss several types of validity.

Content Validity

The first type of validity, **content validity**, is based on the measurement reflecting the area(s) of information—that is, the items on the instrument come from each content area measured. A review of the literature is a good means of establishing content validity since current information about the topic is used to develop the instrument. For example, when planning an evaluation of a risk reduction program for cardiovascular disease, the program planner can conduct a review of the literature or consult a jury of experts in the area of cardiovascular risk reduction in order to ensure that all major risk factors, such as smoking, exercise, and diet, are included on a questionnaire.

Criterion-Based Validity

Criterion-based validity is determined by established criteria and looks at the degree of relationship between two measures of the same phenomenon. If the two measurements are focused on the present, such as scores on a knowledge test about AIDS and current grade point average, the type of criterion validity is known as **concurrent validity.** If the measurement used will be correlated with a future measurement of the same phenomenon, as with the use of standardized test scores to predict future college success, the criterion validity is known as **predictive validity**.

Construct Validity

Another type of validity is **construct validity**. This deals with psychological constructs, such as self-esteem, self-efficacy, or locus of control, which are difficult to define but have characteristics that are recognized. Individuals with high levels of the trait (as determined by experts) are given the instrument. If they receive high scores on the instrument, it is determined to have high construct validity—that is, it is measuring the construct as intended.

INTERNAL VALIDITY

The **internal validity** of evaluation is the degree to which the program caused the change that was measured. Many factors can threaten internal validity, either singly or in combination, making it difficult to determine if the outcome was brought about by the program or some other cause. Cook and Campbell (1979) have identified some of the threats to internal validity, which we summarize here.

History occurs when an event happens between the pretest and posttest and is not part of the health promotion program. An example of history as a threat to internal validity is having a national antismoking campaign coincide with a local smoking cessation program.

Maturation occurs when the participants in the program may show pretest-to-posttest differences due to growing older, wiser, or stronger. For example, in tests of muscular strength in an exercise program for junior high students, an increase in strength could be the result of muscular development and not the effect of the program.

Testing occurs when the participants become familiar with the test format due to repeated testing. This is why it is helpful to use a different form of the same test for pretest and posttest comparisons.

Instrumentation occurs when there is a change in the measuring between pretest and posttest, such as the observers becoming more familiar with or skilled in the use of the testing format over time.

Statistical regression is when extremely high or low scores (which are not necessarily accurate) on the pretest are closer to the mean or average scores on the posttest.

Selection reflects differences in the experimental and comparison groups generally due to lack of randomization. Selection can also interact with other threats to validity, such as history, maturation, or instrumentation, which may appear to be program effects.

Mortality refers to participants who drop out of the program between the pretest and posttest. For example, if most of the participants who drop out of a weight loss program are those with the least (or the most) weight to lose, the group composition is different at the posttest.

Diffusion or imitation of treatments results when participants in the control group interact and learn from the experimental group. Students randomly assigned to an innovative drug prevention program in their school (experimental group) may discuss the program with students who are not in the program (control group), biasing the results.

Compensatory equalization of treatments occurs when the program or services are not available to the control group and there is an unwillingness to tolerate the inequality. For instance, the control group from the previous example (students not enrolled in the innovative drug prevention program) may complain since they are not able to participate.

Compensatory rivalry is when the control group is seen as the underdog and is motivated to work harder.

Resentful demoralization of respondents receiving less desirable treatments occurs among participants receiving the less desirable treatments compared to other groups, and the resentment may affect the outcome. For example, an evaluation to compare two different smoking cessation programs may assign one group (control) to the regular smoking cessation program and another group (experimental) to the regular program plus an exercise class. If the participants in the control group become aware that they are not receiving the additional exercise class, they may resent the omission, and this may be reflected in their smoking behavior and attitude toward the regular program.

The major way in which threats to internal validity can be controlled is through randomization. By random selection of participants, random assignment to groups, and random assignment of types of treatment or no treatment to groups, any differences between pretest and posttest can be interpreted as a result of the program. When random assignment to groups is not possible and quasi-experimental designs are used, the evaluator must make all threats to internal validity explicit and then rule them out one by one.

EXTERNAL VALIDITY

The other type of validity that should be considered is **external validity**, or the extent to which the program can be expected to produce similar effects in other populations. This is also known as **generalizability**. The more a program is tailored to a particular population, the greater the threat to external validity, and the less likely it is that the program can be generalized to another group.

As with internal validity, several factors can threaten external validity. They are sometimes known as reactive effects, since they cause individuals to react in a certain way. We list here several types of threats to external validity.

Social desirability occurs when the individual gives a particular response to try to please or impress the evaluator. An example would be a child who tells the teacher she brushes her teeth every day, regardless of her actual behavior.

Expectancy effect is when attitudes projected onto individuals cause them to act in a certain way. For example, in a drug abuse treatment program, the facilitator may feel that a certain individual will not benefit from the treatment; projecting this attitude may cause the individual to behave in self-defeating ways.

Hawthorne effect refers to a behavior change because of the special status of those being tested. This effect was first identified in an evaluation of lighting conditions at an electric plant; workers increased their productivity when the level of lighting was raised, as well as when it was lowered. The change in behavior seemed to be due to the attention given to them during the evaluation process.

Placebo effect causes a change in behavior due to the participants' belief in the treatment.

Cook and Campbell (1979) discuss the threats to external validity in terms of statistical interaction effects. These include interaction of selection and treatment (the findings from a program requiring a large time commitment may not be generalizable to individuals who do not have much free time); interaction of setting and treatment (evaluation results from a program conducted on campus may not be generalizable to the worksite); and interaction of history and treatment (results from a program conducted on a historically significant day may not be generalizable to other days).

Conducting the program several times in a variety of settings, with a variety of participants, can reduce the threats to external validity. Threats to external validity can also be counteracted by making a greater effort to treat all subjects identically. In a **blind** study, the participants do not know what group (control or type of experimental group) they are in. In a **double blind** study, the type of group participants are in is not known by either the participants or the program planners. In a **triple blind** study, this information is not available to the participants, planners, or evaluators.

It is important to select an evaluation design that provides both internal and external validity. This may be difficult since lowering the threat to one type of validity may increase the threat to the other. For example, tighter evaluation controls make it more difficult to generalize the results to other situations. There must be enough control over the evaluation to allow evaluators to interpret the findings while sufficient flexibility in the program is maintained to permit the results to be generalized to similar settings.

RELIABILITY

When designing a measurement for evaluation, planners should consider both the validity and the reliability of the instrument. While validity refers to the ability to measure what one wants to measure, **reliability** refers to consistency in the measurement process. A reliable instrument gives the same (or nearly the same) result every time. However, no instrument will ever provide perfect accuracy in measurement. Green and Lewis (1986) illustrate the theory of reliability with an equation, where total score (obtained score) equals the true score (unobservable) plus an error score. The total score represents the individual's score obtained on the measuring instrument. The true score represents the score for the same individual if all conditions and the measuring instrument were perfect. An error score must be included since conditions are never perfect in the real world.

Several methods of determining reliability are available. **Internal consistency** refers to the intercorrelations among the individual items on the instrument, that is, whether all items on the instrument are measuring part of the total area. This can be done by logically examining the instrument to ensure that the items reflect what is to be measured and that the level of difficulty of all items is the same. Statistical methods can also be used to determine internal consistency by correlating the items on the test with the total score.

Stability reliability, or test-retest reliability, examines whether the results would be the same if the instrument were administered to the same person at a later date. The length of time between test and retest may vary from hours to weeks to years. A maximum amount of time should be allowed so individuals are not answering on the basis of remembering responses they made on the first test, but it should not be so long that other events could occur in the intervening time to influence their responses. To avoid the problems of retesting, parallel forms of the test can be administered to the participants and the results can be correlated.

Interrater reliability focuses on the consistency between test administrators. This comes into play when information is collected by observing or rating, or in other situations that could be affected by human error. It is measured as an agreement or correlation between the raters, as in the consistency of measurement between observers when measuring the amount of time preschool children spend in active play.

SELECTING AN EVALUATION DESIGN

When planning an evaluation, careful consideration should be given to the evaluation design since the design is critical to the outcome of the evaluation. There are few perfect evaluation designs because no situation is ideal and there are always constraining factors, such as limited resources. Planners should give much thought to selecting the best design for each situation. The following questions may be helpful in the selection of a design:

❑   How much time do you have to conduct the evaluation?

❑   What financial resources are available?

❑   How many participants can be included in the evaluation?

❑   Are you more interested in qualitative or quantitative data?

❑   Do you have data analysis skills or access to computers and statistical consultants?

❑   In what ways can validity be increased?

❑   Is it important to be able to generalize your findings to other populations?

❑   Are the stakeholders concerned with validity and reliability?

❑   Do you have the ability to randomize participants into experimental and control groups?

❑   Do you have access to a comparison group?

Dignan (1986) presents four steps in choosing an evaluation design. The first step is to orient oneself to the situation. The evaluator must identify resources (time, personnel), constraints, and hidden agendas (unspoken goals). During this step, the evaluator must determine what is to be expected from the program and what can be observed.

The second step involves defining the problem—determining what is to be evaluated. During this step, definitions are needed for independent variables (what the sponsors think makes the difference), dependent variables (what will show the difference), and confounding variables (what the evaluator thinks could explain additional differences).

The third step involves making a decision about the design, that is, whether to use a qualitative or quantitative design or both. The fourth step includes choosing how to measure the dependent variable, deciding how to collect the data and how the data will be analyzed, and determining how the results will be reported. These four steps are outlined in Figure 14.1.

Figure 14.1
Steps in selecting an evaluation design

Source: From *Measurements and Evaluation of Health Education* (p. 93) by M. B. Dignan, 1986, Springfield, IL: Charles C. Thomas, Publisher. Reprinted by permission of Charles C. Thomas, Publisher.

SUMMARY

During the program-planning stages, careful consideration should be given to the design of the evaluation. This will help to ensure that the evaluation is focused on the goals and objectives of the program and answers the questions of the individuals reading the results. Planners should consider ways to increase the accuracy of the evaluation, by focusing on assignment of participants to groups and on the validity and reliability of the measurement.

QUESTIONS

1. When would a quantitative approach be used in evaluation? A qualitative approach? How could the approaches be combined?

2. What are the advantages of using a control group? What types of evaluation design do not use control groups? What is the difference between a control group and a comparison group?

3. What are the strengths and weaknesses of the various evaluation designs?

4. What is the difference between validity and reliability? Between internal validity and external validity? Why are validity and reliability so important in evaluation design?

5. What are some considerations in the selection of an evaluation design presented in this chapter? What considerations can you add to this list?

ACTIVITIES

1. If you were hired to evaluate a safety belt program in a community, what evaluation design would you use and why? Assume you have all the resources you need to conduct the evaluation.

2. Explain what evaluation design you would use in evaluating the difference between two teaching techniques. Why would you choose this design?

3. Develop an evaluation design for a program you are planning. Explain why you chose this design, and list the strengths and weaknesses of the design.

15

Data Collection

After reading this chapter and answering the questions at the end, you should be able to:

❑   Describe the four main methods of data collection.

❑   Define *bias* in data collection and discuss how it can be reduced.

❑   Discuss the advantages and disadvantages of data collection from self-report (written surveys, telephone interviews, and face-to-face interviews), direct observation, existing records, and meetings.

❑   Describe how a sample can be obtained from a population.

❑   Differentiate between probability and nonprobability samples.

❑   Describe how a pilot test is used.

KEY TERMS

anonymous

bias

census

confidential

direct observation

nonprobability sample

pilot test

probability sample

random-digit dialing

randomization

respondents

response rate

sample

sampling

self-report

simple random sample

stratified random sample

survey population

systematic sample

A s discussed in Chapter 14, an evaluation should be designed so as to obtain specific information about the program. It is then necessary to collect data to be analyzed. Many methods of data collection can be used, depending upon the purpose of the evaluation, the informational needs of the audience, and practical constraints such as time and cost. Methods of data collection have been referred to in Chapter 4 in the discussion of needs assessment. The techniques used to collect the data in both cases are the same; the difference lies in how the information is used. In needs assessment, the data are used to determine initial need for the program; in an evaluation, the information collected is used to make decisions about the program or to determine the value of the program.

An extremely important aspect of data collection is consistency. All participants must be treated in the same manner in order to reduce the possibility of error that will affect the final results. Another consideration is the number of people who are willing to participate when asked, which is referred to as the **response rate**. More accurate results are gained when the response rate is high.

The response rate is usually higher when the responses are anonymous or confidential. **Anonymous** refers to data collected without requiring the person's name, Social Security number, or other identifying information. **Confidential** data may include information that would serve to identify the respondent, but this information is not released without the person's permission.

In this chapter, we present four main methods of data collection: self-report, direct observation, existing records, and meetings. We include information on how to select a sample to survey, how to conduct pilot tests, and how to reduce bias in data collection.

Bias is defined as the difference between the score obtained and the true score. Windsor and colleagues (1984) describe ways in which bias can occur in data collection: for example, when participants change behavior because they are being tested, when certain characteristics of the interviewer influence a response, and when participants answer questions in a particular way regardless of the questions. Using techniques to reduce bias during data collection helps increase the accuracy of the results.

METHODS OF DATA COLLECTION

Self-Report

Written questionnaires, telephone interviews, and face-to-face interviews are methods of collecting data from **respondents,** that is, the individuals who supply this information. In **self-report**, each respondent is asked to recall and report accurate information; inaccurate information may lead to bias in the data collected. The results are influenced by the person's ability to remember information ("When was your last visit to the dentist?") and report it honestly ("Do you floss your teeth daily?"). Offering anonymity is helpful in gaining honest answers from respondents.

Another possible bias in self-report is the desire to please the interviewer or to give a socially acceptable answer. If information is requested about a smoking cessation program, the respondent may want to give the "right" answer ("Yes, I quit smoking"). This bias may also work in reverse: a respondent may not like one aspect of a program and may give negative responses to all questions to emphasize displeasure. For example, a respondent may indicate that the time the class was offered was not convenient, the materials were not useful, and the location was not suitable, in order to downgrade the program because he feels that the instructor was ineffective. Skilled interviewing techniques can aid evaluators in obtaining correct information.

Questions Used in Self-Report

The presentation, wording, and sequence of questions in self-report questionnaires and interviews can be critical in gaining the necessary information. The questionnaire or interview should begin by explaining the purpose of the study and why the individual's responses are important. A cover letter should accompany a mailed questionnaire, explaining the need for the information and including very clear directions for supplying it. The name, address, and telephone number of the evaluator or another contact person can also be included in case the respondent needs additional information to complete the questionnaire. A stamped, addressed envelope should be enclosed. Udinsky, Osterlind, and Lynch (1981) have developed guidelines for writing a cover letter, which are presented in Table 15.1.

Table 15.1
Guidelines for a cover letter

1. This letter should contain a clear, brief, yet adequate statement of the purpose and value of the questionnaire.

2. It should be addressed to the respondent specifically.

3. It should provide good reason for the respondent to reply.

4. It should involve the respondent in a constructive and appealing way.

5. The respondent's professional responsibility, intellectual curiosity, personal worth, etc., are typical of response appeals.

6. The letter should establish a reasonable, but firm, return date.

7. An offer to send the respondent a report of the findings is often effective, though it carries with it the ethical responsibility to honor such a pledge.

8. The use of a letterhead, signature, and organizational endorsements lends prestige and official status to the letter.

9. The letter should guarantee anonymity and confidentiality.

10. Each letter should be signed individually by the researcher.

11. The researcher should include a stamped, self-addressed envelope for the return of the instrument.

Source: From *Evaluation Resource Handbook: Gathering, Analyzing, Reporting Data* (p. 120), by B. F. Udinsky, S. J. Osterlind, and S. W. Lynch, 1981, San Diego, CA: EdITS Publishers. Reprinted by permission of EdITS Publishers.

With telephone or face-to-face interviews, the interviewer can give information about the study and explain the need for information from the individual contacted. This introduction can be followed by general questions to put the respondent at ease or to develop a rapport between the interviewer and the respondent.

After several general questions come the questions of interest. Any questions that deal with sensitive topics should be posed at the end of the questionnaire or interview. Answers to questions about drug use, sexuality, or even demographic information such as income level are more readily answered when the respondents understand the need for the information, are assured of confidentiality or anonymity, and feel comfortable with the interviewer or the questionnaire. If the respondent ends the interview or does not complete the survey when asked sensitive questions, the other information collected can still be used; this is another advantage of putting these questions at the end.

The actual questions should be clear and unbiased. It is important to avoid questions with a specific direction ("How have you enjoyed the class?") that would guide the respondent's answer. Two-part (double-barreled) questions should also be avoided ("Do you brush and floss your teeth?"). Another problem with question design occurs when the question assumes knowledge that individuals may not have or includes terminology that they may not understand ("What cardiovascular benefits do you feel you gain from aerobic exercise?").

The way in which evaluation questions are worded is extremely important in gaining the needed information. The result of a poorly worded question was evident to one health promotion planner who was planning a smoking cessation program for employees. When asked, "Do you feel we need a smoking cessation program?" most employees said yes. The planner realized later that he should also have asked the question, "Would you attend a smoking cessation program?" since very few employees participated.

If possible, evaluators should use standardized questionnaires. This requires gaining permission from the author if the document is not in the public domain. (Documents in the public domain can be freely used without requesting permission.) The advantages to using questionnaires that have been developed by experts include increased credibility, lower cost, less planning time needed, and more documentation of validity and reliability. The major disadvantage—one that prevents the use of standardized questionnaires in many cases—is that all the items used to evaluate one program may not be relevant or appropriate to evaluate a similar program. Adaptations may be needed so that the questionnaire will fit with program objectives or the local target population.

When designing a questionnaire to collect self-reported data, evaluators can use several types of questions. The most structured or closed types of questions have yes-no or multiple-choice responses, and are most often used for knowledge questions. These types of responses are the easiest to tabulate but do not allow the individual to elaborate on the answers. They may also force a person into a choice because of the limited number of responses to each question. An "other" category, with space to list the exact nature of the "other" response, may serve to give the respondent another option. However, giving the respondents an opportunity to provide their own answers on multiple-choice questions makes it more difficult to categorize responses when the data are analyzed, thus reducing one of the main benefits of such questions. One way to ensure that the most common responses to questions are included in the multiple choices is to involve several individuals (especially those in the target population) in the formation of the instrument.

Attitude questions generally use less structured forms. Scales, such as Likert or semantic differentials, are often used, with the respondent choosing a response along a continuum, generally ranging from a five- to a seven-point scale. For example, responses to the statement, "I feel that it is important to limit my use of salt," might be rated on a seven-point scale ranging from "strongly agree" to "strongly disagree" (see examples in Table 15.2).

Unstructured or open-ended questions, such as essay, short-answer questions, journals, or logs, may be used to gain descriptive information about a program, but are generally not used when collecting quantitative data. Such responses are often difficult to summarize or to code for analysis. Table 15.2 provides examples of structured and unstructured types of questions.

Self-report, while widely used in evaluating health promotion programs, has limitations. To maximize the usefulness of self-report, Baranowski (1985, pp. 181–82) has developed eight steps to increasing the accuracy of this method of data collection. These steps include:

1.   Select measures that clearly reflect program outcomes.
2.   Select measures that have been designed to anticipate response problems and that have been validated.

Table 15.2
Examples of self-report questions

Structured

I. Dichotomy

    1. What is your gender?

        a. Female   b. Male

    2. A risk factor for heart disease is sedentary lifestyle.

        a. True   b. False

II. Multiple Choice

    1. The leading cause of death in the U.S. for adults is

        a. Cancer   b. Heart disease

        c. Injuries   d. AIDS

    2. What type of computer do you use?

        a. IBM   b. Apple

        c. Radio Shack   d. Other (please specify) _____

Less Structured (But Still Closed)

I. Likert

1. Women should be able to have an abortion if they choose to do so.	Strongly agree	Agree	Neutral	Disagree	Strongly disagree
2. I feel I can exercise regardless of weather conditions.	Strongly agree	Agree	Neutral	Disagree	Strongly disagree

II. Semantic Differentials

    1. Smokeless tobacco is   Good __ __ __ __ __ Bad

    2. When taking a test, I feel   Nervous __ __ __ __ __ Calm

III. Rank Order

    1. Put the following values in order, from most important in your life to least important: Health, Love, Emotional Security, Friendship, Financial Security

Unstructured (Open)

I. Completion

    1. I like to exercise because . . .

    2. The type of foods I generally eat are . . .

II. Short-answer

    1. List five advantages to conducting a worksite health promotion program.

    2. Describe the correct way to lift a heavy object to avoid straining your back.

III. Essay

    1. Explain the difference between aerobic and anaerobic exercise. Include examples of each type of exercise and discuss the importance of each in total fitness.

3. Conduct a pilot study with the target population.

4. Anticipate and correct major sources of unreliability.

5. Employ quality control procedures to detect other sources of error.

6. Employ multiple methods.

7. Use multiple measures.

8. Use experimental and control groups with random assignment to control for biases in self report.

By following these steps, evaluators can enhance the accuracy of self-report, making this a more effective method of data collection.

Written Questionnaires

Probably the most often used method of collecting self-reported data is the written questionnaire. It has several advantages, notably the ability to reach a large number of respondents in a short period of time, even if there is a large geographic area to be covered. This method offers low cost with minimum staff time needed. However, it often has the lowest response rate.

With a written questionnaire, each individual receives the same questions and instructions in the same format, so that the possibility of response bias is lessened. The corresponding disadvantage, however, is the inability to clarify any questions or confusion on the part of the respondent.

As mentioned, the response rate for mailed questionnaires tends to be low, but there are several ways to overcome this problem. One way is to include with the questionnaire a postcard that identifies the person in some way (such as by name or identification number). The individual is asked to return the questionnaire in the envelope provided and to send the postcard back separately. Anonymity is thus maintained, but the evaluator knows who returned a questionnaire. The evaluator can then send a follow-up mailing (including a letter indicating the importance of a response and another copy of the questionnaire with a return envelope) to the individuals who did not return a postcard from the first mailing. This step should increase the response rate.

Another way to overcome the drawback of a low response rate from a mailed questionnaire is to use this method for a homogeneous group, that is, one composed of similar individuals. The problem of underrepresentation of certain types of individuals may still occur, but if the group is homogeneous in, for example, age or health behaviors the likelihood that the missing data will be different from the data collected is much less.

The appearance of the questionnaire is extremely important. It should be attractive, easy to read, and offer ample space for the respondent's answers. It should also be easy to understand and complete, since written questionnaires provide no opportunity to clarify a point while the respondent is completing the questionnaire. All mailed questionnaires should be accompanied by a cover letter, as previously discussed.

Short questionnaires that do not take a long time to complete and questionnaires that clearly explain the need for the information are more likely to be returned. Evaluators should give thought to designing a questionnaire that is as easy to complete and return as possible.

Telephone Interviews

Compared to mailed surveys or face-to-face interviews, the telephone interview offers a relatively easy method of collecting self-reported data at a moderate cost. The evaluator must choose a way of selecting individuals to participate in this type of data collection; this method will reach only those individuals who have access to a telephone. One possibility is to call a randomly selected group of people who have completed a health promotion program. Another method is to select telephone numbers at random from a telephone directory, for example, a local telephone book, student directory, church directory, or employee directory. This method will not reach all the population since some people have unlisted telephone numbers. One way to overcome this problem is a method known as **random-digit dialing**, in which telephone number combinations are chosen at random. This method would include businesses as well as residences, and nonworking as well as valid numbers, making it more time-consuming. The numbers may be obtained from a table of random numbers or generated by a computer. The advantage of random-digit dialing is that it includes all the survey population with a telephone in the area, including people with unlisted numbers. Drawbacks to this method include some people's resistance to answer questions over the telephone or resentment in being interrupted with an unwanted call. Those conducting the interviews may also have difficulty reaching individuals due to unanswered phones or answering machines.

Telephone interviewing requires trained interviewers; without proper training and use of a standardized questionnaire, the interviewer may not be consistent during the interview. Explaining a question or offering additional information can cause a respondent to change an initial response, thus creating a chance for interviewer bias. The interviewer does have the opportunity to clarify questions, which is an advantage over the written questionnaire, but does not have the advantage of visual cues that the face-to-face interview offers.

Face-to-Face Interviews

At times it is advantageous to administer the instrument to the respondents in an interview setting. This method is time-consuming, since it may require not only time for the actual interview but also travel time to the interview site and/or waiting time between interviews. As with telephone interviews, the interviewer must be carefully trained to conduct the interview in an unbiased manner. It is important to explain the need for the information in order to conduct the evaluation and to accurately record the responses. Methods of probing, or eliciting additional information about an individual's responses, are used in the face-to-face interview, and the interviewer must be skilled at this technique.

This method of self-report allows the interviewer to develop rapport with the respondent. The flexibility of this method, along with the availability of visual cues, has the advantage of gaining more complete evaluation data from respondents. Smaller numbers of respondents are included in this method, but the rate of participation is generally high. It is important to establish and follow procedures for selecting the respondents. There are also several disadvantages to the face-to-face interview. It is more expensive, requiring more staff time and training of interviewers. Variations in the interviews, as well as differences between interviewers, may influence the results.

Direct Observation

Direct observation can be used to obtain information regarding the behavior of participants in a program. For example, evaluators might observe students in the cafeteria to gain information about actual food choices and consumption. This method is somewhat time-consuming, but it seldom encounters the problem of people refusing to participate in the evaluation, resulting in a high response rate.

Observation is generally more accurate than self-report, but the presence of the observer may alter the behavior of the people being observed. For example, having someone observe smoking behavior may cause smokers to smoke less out of self-consciousness due to being under observation, and not as a result of the program. Observers must be unobtrusive; conspicuous note taking or recording behavior may bias the evaluation.

Differences among observers may also bias the results, since different observers may not observe and report behaviors in the same manner. Some behaviors, such as safety belt use, are very easy to observe accurately. Others, such as degree of tension, are more difficult to observe. This method of data collection requires a clear definition of the exact behavior to observe and how to record it, in order to avoid subjective observations. Observer bias can be reduced by providing training and by determining interrater reliability (see Chapter 14 for a discussion of interrater reliability). If the observers are skilled, observation can provide accurate evaluation data at a moderate cost.

Indirect methods can also be used to determine whether a behavior has occurred. Examples of indirect methods include measuring weight loss and monitoring blood pressure. These measures can be used to verify self-reports when observations of the actual changes in behavior cannot be observed.

Existing Records

Using existing records may be an efficient way to obtain the necessary information for evaluation without the need for additional data collection. The advantages include low cost, minimum staff needed, and ease in randomization. The disadvantages to using this method of data collection include difficulty in gaining access to necessary records and the possible lack of availability of all the information needed for program evaluation.

Examples of the use of existing records include checking physician records to monitor blood pressure and cholesterol levels of participants in an exercise program, reviewing insurance usage of employees enrolled in an employee health promotion program, and comparing the academic records of students engaging in an after-school weight loss program. In these situations, as with all evaluations using existing records, the cooperation of the agencies that hold the records is essential. At times, agencies may be willing to collect additional information to aid in the evaluation of a health promotion program. Keepers of records are concerned about confidentiality and the release of private information. Evaluators can deal with this by getting permission from all participants in the evaluation to use their records or by using only anonymous data.

Meetings

Meetings are a good source of information for process evaluation. For example, if a fitness program is being evaluated, the evaluators, staff, and some participants may meet early in the planning and implementation stages to discuss the status of the program. Focus groups or community forums are other examples of engaging potential program participants in discussions to gain insight for program planning (see Chapter 4 for a discussion of the use of focus groups and community forums in needs assessment).

The meeting structure can be flexible to avoid limiting the scope of the information gained. The cost of this form of evaluation is minimal. Possible biases may occur, however, when meetings are used as a source of evaluation data. Those involved may give "socially acceptable" responses to questions rather than discussing actual concerns. There also may be limited input if relatively few participants are included, or if one or two participants dominate the discussion.

Summarized in Table 15.3 are the advantages and disadvantages of the various methods of data collection. As discussed in Chapter 14, it may be beneficial to combine methods of data collection as well as to incorporate quantitative and qualitative data.

SAMPLING

Once a method of collecting the data has been chosen, evaluators should consider how to select the group of individuals who will be included. Depending on the size of the population, they may want to collect data from all participants (**census**) or from only some of the participants (**sample**). Evaluators must exercise care in selecting the sample: the sample should be representative of the total target group included in the program, and the selection procedure should be unbiased.

Figure 15.1 illustrates the relationship between groups of individuals. All individuals, unspecified by time or place, constitute the universe. Within the universe is a population of individuals specified by time or place. Within this population is a **survey population**, composed of all individuals who can be contacted. For example, all individuals who have participated in an aerobic fitness class through a local hospital constitute a population. Those participating in the past year may become the survey population, since most of them can still be contacted.

Table 15.3
Methods of data collection

Method	Advantages	Disadvantages
Self report		
Written questionnaire	Large outreach	Possible low response rate
	No interviewer bias	Possible unrepresentation
	Convenient	No clarification of questions
	Low cost	Need homogeneous group if response is low
	Minimum staff time required	
	Easy to administer	
	Quick	
	Standardized	
Telephone interview	Moderate cost	Possible problem of representation
	Relatively easy to administer	Possible interviewer bias
	Good response rate	Requires trained interviewers
Face-to-face interview	High response rate	Expensive
	Flexibility	Requires trained interviewers
	Gain in-depth data	Possible interviewer bias
	Develop rapport	Limits sample size
		Time-consuming
Observation	Accurate behavioral data	Requires trained observers
	Can be unobtrusive	May bias behavior
	Moderate cost	Possible observer bias
		May be time-consuming
Existing records	Low cost	May need agency cooperation
	Easy to randomize	Certain data may be unavailable
	Avoid data collection	
	Minimum staff needed	
Meetings	Good for formative evaluation	Possible result bias
	Low cost	Limited input from participants
	Flexible	

A survey population may still be too large to include in its entirety. For this reason, a sample is chosen from the survey population, a process called **sampling**. These are the individuals who will be included in the evaluation. Using a sample rather than an entire survey population helps contain costs of an evaluation. For example, using a sample reduces the amount of staff time needed to conduct interviews, the cost of postage for written questionnaires, and the time and cost of travel to conduct observations.

Figure 15.1
Relationship of groups of
individuals

How the sample is chosen is critical to the result of the evaluation: does the information gained from the sample reflect the knowledge, attitudes, and behaviors of the population? According to Green and Lewis (1986), the sampling bias is the difference between the sampling estimate and the actual population value. The sampling bias can be controlled by controlling the sampling procedure, that is, how the sample is chosen. The ability to generalize the results to the population is greater when the sampling bias is reduced.

Probability Sample

Increasing the chance that the sample is representative of the population is achieved by **randomization**. This assures that each person in the survey population has a known probability of being selected, thus creating a **probability sample**. A **simple random sample** can be obtained by taking a list of all participants and choosing the sample by following a list of random numbers, giving each individual an equal chance of being selected. A **systematic sample** also uses a list of participants and takes every Nth person beginning with a randomly selected individual.

If it is important that certain groups should all be represented in a sample, a **stratified random sample** can be obtained. For example, if representatives from all age groups are needed, a predetermined number from each age group would be randomly chosen. The predetermined number is based upon representation. For example, if the evaluator is selecting 100 out of a population of 1,000 college students (1 in 10), it may be important to ensure that all class ranks are represented. If 400 of the students are freshmen, 300 sophomores, 200 juniors, and 100 seniors, then the representative sample would contain 1 in 10 of each of those subgroups: 40 freshmen, 30 sophomores, 20 juniors, and 10 seniors. Within each class rank, the appropriate number of students would be randomly selected.

Nonprobability Sample

There are times when a probability sample cannot be obtained. In such cases, evaluators can take **nonprobability samples**, samples in which all individuals in the survey population did not have a known probability of being selected to participate in the evaluation. Nonprobability samples have limitations in the extent to which the results can be generalized to the total survey population. Bias may also occur since those who are not included in the sample may differ in some way from those who are included. For example, including only the individuals who complete a health promotion program may bias the results; the findings might be different if all participants, including those who attended but did not complete the program, were surveyed.

Nonprobability samples can be used when evaluators are unable to identify or contact all those in the survey population. These samples can also be used when resources are limited and a probability sample is too costly or time-consuming. It is important that evaluators understand the limitations of this type of sample when reporting the results.

Sample Size

How many individuals to include in the sample is difficult to determine. Green and Lewis (1986) give guidelines for determining the sample size, with the objective being to obtain the highest level of precision for a given cost. *Precision* refers to how accurately the sample values reflect the actual values in the population. Another consideration is variability in the survey population; the greater the differences among the survey population, the larger the sample size needed.

Additional guidelines refer to the sampling method selected, with stratified random sampling offering the greatest level of precision for a given cost. The cost of the evaluation is also a consideration in determining whether a desired sample size is affordable. Evaluators can choose actual numbers of participants with the help of statistics textbooks, giving consideration to statistical power and level of statistical significance.

PILOT TEST

Once a method of data collection has been selected and the instrument developed, a trial run of the instrument, data collection procedures, and analyses can be conducted. This is known as a **pilot test**, or piloting. A very small sample of individuals can be selected to participate in the pilot test. If possible, this sample should be representative of the survey population. Controls are applied to simulate the testing situation, and data are collected. After the interview has been completed, the survey filled out, the observation conducted, or another method of data collection has been carried out, a follow-up interview may be held to gain information about the method of data collection.

In survey research, the instrument could be reviewed by colleagues, by potential users of the data, and by a sample of program participants. Stacy (1987) offers guidelines on this review process. The person reviewing the instrument is asked to complete a short questionnaire. For example, the colleague would answer questions on the appropriateness of the title, the introductory statement explaining the purpose of the study, the directions, the grouping of the questions, and the length of the questionnaire. The individuals in the sample population are questioned on the directions, the title, the appropriateness of the questions (unclear, too personal), length of the instrument, purpose of the study, and method for returning the questionnaire. The potential users of the data could review the instrument with regard to how well the questions reflect the topic being studied, whether the questions are consistent with current knowledge of the topic, and whether questions should be added or deleted. Information collected from this process can then be used to revise the questionnaire.

The purpose of the pilot test is to refine the method of data collection on the basis of comments from those reviewing the instrument and suggestions from the respondents. Any problems in the data collection process should be evident in the pilot test, such as ambiguous questions, difficulty with code sheets, and misunderstood directions. The data collected in the pilot test should be statistically analyzed or compiled to make sure that there is no difficulty with this step in the evaluation process. Revising the data collection process using the information gained from the pilot test helps ensure that the actual data collection will proceed smoothly.

SUMMARY

This chapter presented four main areas of data collection: self-report, direct observation, existing records, and meetings. Advantages and disadvantages of each method of data collection should be considered when selecting an appropriate method. Many steps can be taken to reduce bias, or error, in information gained, such as selecting a representative sample and conducting a pilot test.

QUESTIONS

1. What is bias in data collection? Name some ways in which it can be reduced.

2. Describe each method of data collection (self-report, direct observation, existing data, and meetings), and list two advantages and disadvantages of each.

3. When could standardized questions be used?

4. How does an evaluator determine who will participate in the data collection?

5. Describe three types of probability samples.

6. When, if ever, should nonprobability samples be used?

7. What is the purpose of a pilot test, and how is it conducted?

☐ ACTIVITIES

1. Construct a three-page written questionnaire on a health promotion topic of your choice that could be administered to a group of college students.

2. Conduct a pilot test of your written questionnaire on 10 of your friends, colleagues, or classmates. After the pilot test, identify any flaws you see in the questionnaire or data collection process.

3. Assume that you are charged with the responsibility of collecting data from all the students on your campus who have enrolled in a jogging course. Assume also that this group of students is too large to collect data from everyone. Explain how you would obtain a representative sample from this population.

4. Visit a survey research center on your campus or in your community. Ask about the methods of data collection, and if possible arrange to observe a face-to-face or telephone interview. Write a two-page paper describing your reaction to this experience.

16
Data Analysis and Reporting

After reading this chapter and answering the questions at the end, you should be able to:

❑   Differentiate between descriptive and inferential statistics.

❑   List types of descriptive and inferential statistics and explain how they could be used in an evaluation.

❑   Explain the difference between the null hypothesis and alternative hypothesis in significance testing.

❑   Define *level of significance, Type I error,* and *Type II error.*

❑   Define *independent variable* and *dependent variable.*

❑   Describe how statistical results can be interpreted.

❑   Describe the format for the evaluation report, guidelines for presenting data, and ways to enhance the report.

❑   Discuss ways to increase the utilization of the evaluation findings.

KEY TERMS

alpha level

alternative hypothesis

analysis of variance (ANOVA)

chi square

correlation

dependent variable

descriptive data analysis

independent variable

inferential data analysis

level of significance

mean

measures of central tendency

measures of spread or variation

median

mode

null hypothesis

practical significance

program significance

statistical significance

Type I error

Type II error

variables

L ike all other aspects of evaluation, the types of data analysis to be used in the evaluation should be determined in the program-planning stage. Basically, the analysis determines whether the outcome was different than what was expected. The evaluator then draws conclusions and prepares reports and/or presentations. The types of analysis to be used and how the information is presented are determined by the evaluation questions and the needs of the stakeholders.

In this chapter, we describe different types of analyses commonly used in evaluating health promotion programs. To present them in detail or to include all possible techniques is beyond the scope of this text. Readers needing more information are referred to statistics textbooks, research methods and statistics courses, or statistical consultants.

Evaluations that suffer from major methodological problems are not likely to inspire confidence. A common problem is inadequate documentation of methods, results, and data analysis. The evaluation itself should be well designed; the report should contain a complete description of the program, objective interpretation of facts, information about the research design and statistical analysis, and a discussion of features of the study that may have influenced the findings. In order to add accurate findings to the knowledge base of the profession, appropriate evaluation standards should be adopted to serve as guidelines for reporting and reviewing evaluation research (Moskowitz, 1989).

ORGANIZATION OF DATA

Once evaluators have collected the data, they must compile and analyze the information collected in order to interpret the findings. The data must be cleaned, reduced, coded, and pulled into a usable form. Information from surveys and observation sheets, for example, must be coded and entered into the computer to be compiled and analyzed. This is done with both quantitative and qualitative data. With qualitative data, a coding system is used to assign numerical values to various responses.

TYPES OF ANALYSES

Statistical analysis techniques can be used to describe data, generate hypotheses, or test hypotheses. Techniques that summarize and describe characteristics of a group or make comparisons of characteristics between groups are known as descriptive statistics. Inferential statistics is used to make generalizations or inferences about a population based on findings from a sample.

Variables are characteristics, such as age, level of knowledge, or type of educational program. **Independent variables** are controlled by the evaluator; an example is the type of fitness program chosen (high impact aerobics or stretching and toning). This choice results in an outcome, known as the **dependent variable.** Examples of dependent variables include scores on an alcohol knowledge test, fitness level, or attitude toward safety.

The choice of a type of analysis is based on the evaluation questions. For some types of evaluation, descriptive data are all that is needed, and techniques are chosen to determine frequencies or relationships between variables. Other evaluation questions focus on testing a hypothesis about relationships between variables, and in such cases more elaborate statistical techniques are needed. Table 16.1 lists the types of evaluation questions that can be answered by using descriptive or inferential statistics.

Descriptive Data Analysis

Descriptive data analysis is used to describe, classify, and summarize data. Summary counts (frequencies) are totals, and are the easiest type of data to collect and report. Summary counts could be used in formative evaluation, to count the number of participants in blood pressure screening programs at various sites.

Table 16.1
Types of evaluation questions answered using descriptive or inferential statistics

Descriptive statistics	Inferential statistics
What was the average score on the cholesterol knowledge test?	Is there a difference in smoking behavior between the individuals in the experimental and control groups after the healthy lifestyle program?
How similar are students' attitudes toward the drinking and driving prevention workshop?	Is peer education, classroom instruction, or media presentations more effective in increasing knowledge about the effects of drug abuse?
How many participants at the worksite attended the healthy lifesyle presentation?	
What is the relationship between participation in the corporate fitness program and in the number of sick days taken during the past year?	Do students' attitudes about bicycle helmets differ in rural and urban settings?

The information would assist the program planners in publicizing sites with low attendance or adding additional personnel to busy sites. Other examples of frequencies, or summary counts, are the number of participants in a workshop, those who scored over 80% on a knowledge posttest, or number of individuals wearing a safety belt.

Measures of central tendency are other forms of descriptive statistics. The **mean** is the arithmetic average of all the scores. The **median** is the midpoint of all the scores, dividing scores ranked by size into equal halves. The **mode** is the score that occurs most frequently. These are all useful in describing the results, and reporting all three measures of central tendency will be especially helpful if extreme scores are found.

Measure of spread or variation refers to how spread out the scores are. Range is the difference between the highest and lowest scores. For example, if the high score is 100 and the low score is 60, the range is 40. **Measures of spread or variation**, such as range, standard deviation, or variance, can be used to determine whether scores from groups are similar or spread apart.

Measures of relationship, or **correlation**, are used to establish a relationship between variables. Correlation is expressed as a value between +1 (positive correlation) and -1 (negative correlation), with 0 indicating no relationship between the variables. Correlation between variables only indicates a relationship; this technique does not establish cause and effect. An example of the use of correlation would be to determine the relationship between safety belt use and age of the driver. If older people were found to wear their safety belts more often than young people, that would constitute a positive correlation between age and belt use. If younger people wore their safety belts more often, it would be a negative correlation. If age made no difference in who wore the belts more often, the correlation would be 0.

Inferential Data Analysis

Inferential data analysis uses statistical tests to draw tentative conclusions about the relationship between variables; conclusions are drawn in the form of probability statements, not absolute proof. The evaluation question is stated in the form of hypotheses. The **null hypothesis** holds that there is no observed difference between the variables. The **alternative hypothesis** says that there is a difference between the variables. For example, a null hypothesis states that there is no difference between the experimental and control groups in knowledge about cancer risk factors. The alternative hypothesis states that there is a difference.

Statistical tests are used to determine whether the null hypothesis can be rejected (meaning that a relationship between the variables probably does exist) or whether it should be retained (indicating that any apparent relationship between variables is due to chance). There is the possibility that the null hypothesis can be rejected when it is, in fact, true: this is known as a **Type I error**. There is also the possibility of failing to reject the null hypothesis when it is, in fact, not true: this is a **Type II error**. The probability of making a Type I error is reflected in the alpha level. The **alpha level**, or **level of significance**, is established before the statistical tests are run and is generally set at .05 or .01. This indicates that the decision to reject the null hypothesis is incorrect 5% (or 1%) of the time; that is, there is a 5% probability (or 1% probability) that the outcome occurred by chance alone.

When a smaller alpha level is used (.01 or .001), the possibility of making a Type I error is reduced; at the same time, however, the possibility of a Type II error increases. An example of a Type I error is the adoption of a new program due to higher scores on a knowledge test, when in reality increases in knowledge occurred by chance and the new program is not more effective than the existing program. An example of a Type II error is not adopting the new program when it is, in reality, more effective.

Analysis of variance (ANOVA) is a statistical test used to compare the difference in means of two or more groups. It does not prove that there is a difference between groups; it only allows the evaluator to reject or retain the null hypothesis, then make inferences about the population.

The **chi square** is a statistical technique to test hypotheses about frequencies in various categories. This technique uses categories that can be distinguished from one another but are not hierarchical. This type of analysis could be used to analyze attitudes toward the use of bicycle helmets (strongly agree, agree, neutral, disagree, and strongly disagree) between children in three different grade levels.

Other types of statistical techniques may be used to test hypotheses or describe data. The method should be chosen during the evaluation planning process and should be in place well before data are collected.

INTERPRETING THE RESULTS

Once the results of the analyses are available, evaluators must interpret them to answer the evaluation questions. Utilization-focused evaluation suggests having a session with the stakeholders to simulate interpreting the results of the data. The purpose of this session is to check on the evaluation design, train the stakeholders to interpret data, help stakeholders set realistic expectations, and build a commitment to use the findings, or else reveal the lack of commitment (Patton, 1986).

Evaluators should seek input from the leaders of the group affected by the program to assist in the interpretation of the results and to develop recommendations. They should present the facts in a logical order, allowing for questions about the possible relationships among the findings. Various courses of action can then be discussed (Solomon, 1987).

Standards of acceptability can be established in the program-planning stage. These standards can be modified after a session with stakeholders, during instrument development, or before data collection. The role of evaluators as decision makers may vary in the different evaluation models. Even if evaluators are responsible for making decisions and recommendations, they should still seek input from stakeholders.

The interpretation of the results must distinguish between **program significance (practical significance)** and **statistical significance**. Programmatic significance measures the meaningfulness of an observation, like validity. Statistical significance is determined by data analysis. It is possible—especially when a large number of people are included in the data collection—to have statistically significant results that indicate gains in performance but are not meaningful in terms of program goals. Statistical significance is similar to reliability in that they are both measures of precision. It is important to consider whether statistical significance justifies the development, implementation, and costs of a program (Fink and Kosecoff, 1978).

EVALUATION REPORTING

The results and interpretation of the data analyses, as well as a description of the evaluation process, are incorporated into the final report to be presented to the stakeholders. The report itself generally follows the format of a research report, including an introduction, methodology, results, conclusions, and discussion.

The number and type of reports needed are determined at the beginning of the evaluation based on the needs of the stakeholders. For a formative evaluation, reports are needed early and may be provided on a weekly or monthly basis. The formative evaluations may be formal or informal, ranging from scheduled presentations to informal telephone calls. They must be submitted on time in order to provide immediate feedback so that program modifications can be made. Generally, a report is submitted at the end of an evaluation and may be written and/or oral.

Evaluators must be able to communicate to all audiences when presenting the results of the evaluation. The reaction of each audience—participants, media, administrators, funding source—must be anticipated in order to prepare the necessary information. In some cases, technical information must be included; in other cases, anecdotal information may be appropriate. The evaluator must fit the report to the audience and also prepare for a negative response if the results of the evaluation are not favorable. This involves looking critically at the results and developing responses to anticipated reactions.

The format for communicating the evaluation results may include several methods, such as a technical report, journal article, news release, meeting, presentation, press conference, letter, or workshop. Generally, more than one method is selected in order to meet the needs of all stakeholders. For example, following an innovative worksite health promotion program, the evaluator might prepare a news release for the community, a letter to all staff who participated, a technical report for the funding source, and an executive summary for the administrators.

Designing the Written Report

As previously mentioned, the evaluation report follows a similar format to that used in a research report. The evaluation report generally includes the following sections:

❑ *Abstract or executive summary.* This is a summary of the total evaluation, including goals and objectives, methods, results, conclusions, and recommendations. It is a concise presentation of the evaluation, since it may be the only portion of the report that some of the stakeholders may read. Most abstracts/executive summaries range in length from 150 to 600 words.

❑ *Introduction.* This section of the report includes a complete description of the program and the evaluation. Goals and objectives of the program are listed, as are the evaluation questions to be answered.

❑ *Methods/procedures.* The methods/procedures section of the report includes information on the evaluation design, the target groups, the instruments used, and how the data were collected and analyzed.

❑   *Results.* This section is the main part of the report. It includes the findings from the evaluation, summarizing and simplifying the data and presenting them in a clear, concise format. Data are presented for every evaluation question.

❑   *Conclusions/recommendations.* This section uses the findings (presented in the previous section) to answer the evaluation questions. The results are interpreted to determine significance and explanations. Judgments and recommendations are included in this section; they may have been made by the evaluator and/or the administrator, depending on the evaluation model used.

Table 16.2 summarizes what is included in the evaluation report.

Table 16.2
What to include in the evaluation report

Abstract/executive summary	Overview of the program and evaluation
	General results, conclusions, and recommendation
Introduction	Purpose of the evaluation
	Program and participant description (including staff, materials, activities, procedures, etc.)
	Goals and objectives
	Evaluation questions
Methods/procedures	Design of the evaluation
	Target population
	Instrument
	Sampling procedures
	Data collection procedures
	Pilot study results
	Validity and reliability
	Limitations
	Data analyses procedures
Results	Description of findings from data analyses
	Answers to evaluation questions
	Address any special concerns
	Explanation of findings
	Charts and graphs of findings
Conclusions/recommendations	Interpretation of results
	Conclusions about program effectiveness
	Program recommendations
	Determining if additional information is needed

Presenting Data

The data that have been collected and analyzed are presented in the evaluation report. Graphs and tables may be used to illustrate certain findings, and these are often a central portion of the results section. The narrative should not repeat what is shown in the graphs and tables but should expand and enhance this information. If many tables are included, the main ones can be placed in the text of the report and the rest relegated to an appendix. Table 16.3 lists guidelines to follow when presenting data in the evaluation report and/or presentation.

How and When to Present the Report

Evaluators must consider carefully the logistics of presenting the evaluation findings. They should discuss this with the decision makers involved in the eval-

Table 16.3
Guidelines for presenting data

1. Use graphic methods of presenting numerical data whenever possible.

2. Build the results and discussion section of the evaluation report—and perhaps other sections as well—around tables and figures. Prepare the tables and graphs first; then write text to explain them.

3. Make each table and figure self-explanatory. Use a clear, complete title, a key, label, footnotes, and so forth.

4. Discuss in the text the major information to be found in each table and figure.

5. Play with, and consider using, as many graphs as you have the time and ingenuity to prepare. Not only do they communicate clearly to your audiences, they also help you to see what is happening.

6. Since graphs tend to convey fewer details than numerical tables, consider providing both tables and graphs for the same data, where appropriate.

7. If you have used a mixed evaluation design with both quantitative and qualitative data collection procedures, use the direct quotations and descriptions from the qualitative results to add depth and clarity to information reported graphically.

8. When presenting complicated graphs to a live audience, give some instruction about how to read the graph and a few sample interpretations of simpler versions, then present the real data.

9. When a complete draft of the report has been completed, ask yourself the following questions:

    a. Do the figure titles give a comprehensive description of the figures? Could someone leafing through the report understand the graphs?

    b. Are both axes of every graph clearly labeled with a name?

    c. Is the interval size marked on all axes of graphs?

    d. Is the number of cases on which each summary statistic has been based indicated in each table or on each graph?

    e. Are the tables and figures labeled and numbered throughout the report?

    f. If the report is a lengthy one, does it include a list of tables and figures at the front following the table of contents?

Source: From *How to Communicate Evaluation Findings* (pp. 75–76) by L. L. Morris, C. T. Fitz-Gibbon, and M. E. Freeman, 1987, Newbury Park, CA: Sage Publications, Inc. Reprinted by permission of Sage Publications, Inc.

uation. An evaluator may be in the position of presenting negative results, encountering distrust among staff members, or submitting a report that will never be read. We offer several suggestions for enhancing the evaluation report:

❑   Give key decision makers advance information on the findings; this increases the likelihood that the information will actually be used and prevents the decision makers from learning about the results from the media or another source.

❑   Maintain anonymity of individuals, institutions, and organizations; use sensitivity to avoid judging or labeling people in negative ways; maintain confidentiality of the final report according to the wishes of the administrators; maintain objectivity throughout the report (Windsor et al., 1984).

❑   Choose ways to report the evaluation findings so as to meet the needs of the stakeholders, and include information that is relevant to each group.

INCREASING UTILIZATION OF THE RESULTS

Far too often, an evaluation will be conducted and a report submitted to the decision makers, but the recommendations will not be implemented. This occurs due to a variety of reasons. Decision makers may not use findings because they are conducting the evaluation only to fulfill the requirements of the funding source, to serve their own self-interest, or to gain recognition for a successful program. Even decision makers who plan to use the evaluation results in their health promotion program may find that they are unable to state the evaluation question or that the final report contains language and concepts that are unfamiliar to them. Weiss (1984) sees the need to improve the quality both of evaluation research and of modes of disseminating the findings. Weiss (1984) developed the following guidelines to increase the chances that evaluation results will actually be used.

1.   Plan the study with program stakeholders in mind and involve them in the planning process.

2.   Continue to gather information about the program after the planning stage; a change in the program should result in a change in the evaluation.

3.   Focus the evaluation on conditions about the program which the decision makers can change.

4.   Write reports in a clear, simple manner and submit them on time. Use graphs and charts within the text and include complicated statistical information in an appendix.

5.   Base whether to make recommendations or not on how specific and clear cut the data are, how much is known about the program, whether differences between programs are obvious. A joint interpretation between evaluator and decision maker may be best.

6.   Disseminate the results to all stakeholders, using a variety of methods.

7. Integrate evaluation findings with other research and evaluation about the program area.

8. Provide high quality research.

SUMMARY

Evaluation questions developed in the early program-planning stages can be answered once the data have been analyzed. Descriptive statistics can be used to summarize or describe the data, and inferential statistics can be used to generate or test hypotheses. Evaluators then interpret the findings and present the results to the stakeholders, via a formal or informal report.

QUESTIONS

1. What are some common problems with evaluations, and how can these problems be reduced or overcome?

2. What are some types of descriptive statistics used in evaluation? When would these be used?

3. How are inferential statistics used in evaluation?

4. Explain the concepts of hypothesis testing, level of significance, Type I error, and Type II error.

5. What is the role of evaluators and decision makers in interpreting the results and making recommendations?

6. What is the difference between statistical significance and program significance?

7. What information is included in the written evaluation report? How is the information modified for various audiences?

8. What are some guidelines for presenting data in an evaluation report?

9. How can the evaluation report be enhanced?

10. How can the evaluator increase the likelihood of utilization of the evaluation findings?

ACTIVITIES

1. Obtain an actual report from a program evaluation. Look for the type of statistical test used, the level of significance, the independent and dependent variables, the interpretation of the findings, recommendations, and format for the report.

2. Discuss evaluation with a decision maker from a health agency. Find out what types of evaluation have been conducted, who has conducted them,

what the findings have been, whether the findings were implemented, and how the information was reported.

3. Compare an evaluation report with a research report. What are the similarities and differences? How could you improve the report?

4. Using data that you have generated or data presented by your instructor, create one table and one graph.

Appendixes

Appendix A   Responsibilities and Competencies for Entry-Level Health Educators   254

Appendix B   Health Style: A Self-Test   260

Appendix C   Model Alcohol Policy   267

Appendix D   Indiana Bell Telephone Company Safety Belt Policy 269

Appendix E   Model Ordinance Eliminating Smoking in Workplaces and Enclosed Public Places   270

Appendix F   Sample Letter for Letter-Writing Campaign   275

Appendix G   Examples of PSAs from the Indiana State Department of Health   277

Appendix H   Code of Practice for Smoking Cessation Programs 280

Appendix I   How to Select the Right Vendor for Your Company's Health Promotion Program   282

Appendix J   Health Behavior Contract   287

Appendix K   Example of an Informed Consent Form for a Cholesterol Screening Program   288

Appendix L   Sample Medical Clearance Form   289

Appendix M   Society for Public Health Education Code of Ethics 290

Appendix N   Cost-Benefit and Cost-Effectiveness as a Part of the Evaluation of Health Promotion Programs   292

RESPONSIBILITY I: ASSESSING INDIVIDUAL AND COMMUNITY NEEDS FOR HEALTH EDUCATION

Competency A

Obtain health-related data about social and cultural environments, growth and development factors, needs, and interests.

Sub-Competencies

1.   Select valid sources of information about health needs and interests.
2.   Utilize computerized sources of health-related information.
3.   Employ or develop appropriate data-gathering instruments.
4.   Apply survey techniques to acquire health data.

Competency B

Distinguish between behaviors that foster, and those that hinder, well-being.

Sub-Competencies

1.   Investigate physical, social, emotional, and intellectual factors influencing health behaviors.
2.   Identify behaviors that tend to promote or compromise health.
3.   Recognize the role of learning and affective experience in shaping patterns of health behavior.

Competency C

Infer needs for health education on the basis of obtained data.

Sub-Competencies

1.   Analyze needs assessment data.
2.   Determine priority areas of need for health education.

RESPONSIBILITY II: PLANNING EFFECTIVE HEALTH EDUCATION PROGRAMS

Competency A

Recruit community organizations, resource people, and potential participants for support and assistance in program planning.

Sub-Competencies

1.   Communicate need for the program to those who will be involved.
2.   Obtain commitments from personnel and decision makers who will be involved in the program.
3.   Seek ideas and opinions of those who will affect, or be affected by, the program.
4.   Incorporate feasible ideas and recommendations into the planning process.

Competency B

Develop a logical scope and sequence plan for a health education program.

Sub-Competencies

1.   Determine the range of health information requisite to a given program of instruction.
2.   Organize the subject areas comprising the scope of a program in logical sequence.

Competency C

Formulate appropriate and measurable program objectives.

Sub-Competencies

1.   Infer educational objectives facilitative of achievement of specified competencies.
2.   Develop a framework of broadly stated, operational objectives relevant to a proposed health education program.

Competency D

Design educational programs consistent with specified program objectives.

Sub-Competencies

1.   Match proposed learning activities with those implicit in the stated objectives.
2.   Formulate a wide variety of alternative educational methods.
3.   Select strategies best suited to implementation of educational objectives in a given setting.
4.   Plan a sequence of learning opportunities building upon, and reinforcing mastery of, preceding objectives.

RESPONSIBILITY III: IMPLEMENTING HEALTH EDUCATION PROGRAMS

Competency A

Exhibit competence in carrying out planned educational programs.

Sub-Competencies

1.   Employ a wide range of educational methods and techniques.
2.   Apply individual or group process methods as appropriate to given learning situations.
3.   Utilize instructional equipment and other instructional media effectively.
4.   Select methods that best facilitate practice of program objectives.

Competency B

Infer enabling objectives as needed to implement instructional programs in specified settings.

Sub-Competencies

1.   Pretest learners to ascertain present abilities and knowledge relative to proposed program objectives.
2.   Develop subordinate measurable objectives as needed for instruction.

Competency C

Select methods and media best suited to implement program plans for specific learners.

Sub-Competencies

1.   Analyze learner characteristics, legal aspects, feasibility, and other considerations influencing choices among methods.
2.   Evaluate the efficacy of alternative methods and techniques capable of facilitating program objectives.
3.   Determine the availability of information, personnel, time, and equipment needed to implement the program for a given audience.

Competency D

Monitor educational programs, adjusting objectives and activities as necessary.

Sub-Competencies

1.   Compare actual program activities with the stated objectives.
2.   Assess the relevance of existing program objectives to current needs.
3.   Revise program activities and objectives as necessitated by changes in learner needs.
4.   Appraise applicability of resources and materials relative to given educational objectives.

RESPONSIBILITY IV: EVALUATING EFFECTIVENESS OF HEALTH EDUCATION PROGRAMS

Competency A

Develop plans to assess achievement of program objectives.

Sub-Competencies

1.   Determine standards of performance to be applied as criteria of effectiveness.
2.   Establish a realistic scope of evaluation efforts.
3.   Develop an inventory of existing valid and reliable tests and survey instruments.
4.   Select appropriate methods for evaluating program effectiveness.

Competency B

Carry out evaluation plans.

Sub-Competencies

1.   Facilitate administration of the tests and activities specified in the plan.
2.   Utilize data-collecting methods appropriate to the objectives.
3.   Analyze resulting evaluation data.

Competency C

Interpret results of program evaluation.

Sub-Competencies

1.   Apply criteria of effectiveness to obtained results of a program.
2.   Translate evaluation results into terms easily understood by others.
3.   Report effectiveness of educational programs in achieving proposed objectives.

Competency D

Infer implications from findings for future program planning.

Sub-Competencies

1.   Explore possible explanations for important evaluation findings.
2.   Recommend strategies for implementing results of evaluation.

RESPONSIBILITY V: COORDINATING PROVISION OF HEALTH EDUCATION SERVICES

Competency A

Develop a plan for coordinating health education services.

Sub-Competencies

1.   Determine the extent of available health education services.
2.   Match health education services to proposed program activities.
3.   Identify gaps and overlaps in the provision of collaborative health services.

Competency B

Facilitate cooperation between and among levels of program personnel.

Sub-Competencies

1.   Promote cooperation and feedback among personnel related to the program.
2.   Apply various methods of conflict reduction as needed.
3.   Analyze the role of health educator as liaison between program staff and outside groups and organizations.

Competency C

Formulate practical modes of collaboration among health agencies and organizations.

Sub-Competencies

1.   Stimulate development of cooperation among personnel responsible for community health education program.
2.   Suggest approaches for integrating health education within existing health programs.
3.   Develop plans for promoting collaborative efforts among health agencies and organizations with mutual interests.

Competency D

Organize in-service training programs for teachers, volunteers, and other interested personnel.

Sub-Competencies

1. Plan an operational, competency-oriented training program.
2. Utilize instructional resources that meet a variety of in-service training needs.
3. Demonstrate a wide range of strategies for conducting in-service training programs.

RESPONSIBILITY VI: ACTING AS A RESOURCE PERSON IN HEALTH EDUCATION

Competency A

Utilize computerized health information retrieval systems effectively.

Sub-Competencies

1. Match an information need with the appropriate retrieval system.
2. Access principal on-line and other database health information resources.

Competency B

Establish effective consultative relationships with those requesting assistance in solving health-related problems.

Sub-Competencies

1. Analyze parameters of effective consultative relationships.
2. Describe special skills and abilities needed by health educators for consultation activities.
3. Formulate a plan for providing consultation to other health professionals.
4. Explain the process of marketing health education consultative services.

Competency C

Interpret and respond to requests for health information.

Sub-Competencies

1. Analyze general processes for identifying the information needed to satisfy a request.
2. Employ a wide range of approaches in referring requesters to valid sources of health information.

Competency D

Select effective educational resource materials for dissemination.

Sub-Competencies

1. Assemble educational material of value to the health of individuals and community groups.
2. Evaluate the worth and applicability of resource materials for given audiences.

3.   Apply various processes in the acquisition of resource materials.

4.   Compare different methods for distributing educational materials.

RESPONSIBILITY VII: COMMUNICATING HEALTH AND HEALTH EDUCATION NEEDS, CONCERNS, AND RESOURCES

Competency A

Interpret concepts, purposes, and theories of health education.

Sub-Competencies

1.   Evaluate the state of the art of health education.

2.   Analyze the foundations of the discipline of health education.

3.   Describe major responsibilities of the health educator in the practice of health education.

Competency B

Predict the impact of societal value systems on health education programs.

Sub-Competencies

1.   Investigate social forces causing opposing viewpoints regarding health education needs and concerns.

2.   Employ a wide range of strategies for dealing with controversial health issues.

Competency C

Select a variety of communication methods and techniques in providing health information.

Sub-Competencies

1.   Utilize a wide range of techniques for communicating health and health education information.

2.   Demonstrate proficiency in communicating health information and health education needs.

Competency D

Foster communication between health care providers and consumers.

Sub-Competencies

1.   Interpret the significance and implications of health care providers' messages to consumers.

2.   Act as liaison between consumer groups and individuals and health care provider organizations.

Source: Reprinted from *A Framework for the Development of Competency-Based Curricula for Entry-Level Health Educators* by the National Task Force on the Preparation and Practice of Health Educators, Inc., with permission of the National Commission for Health Education Credentialing, Inc., copyright 1985.

U.S. DEPARTMENT OF HEALTH AND HUMAN SERVICES • Public Health Service

Source: *Healthstyle: A Self-Test* by U.S. Department of Health and Human Services (USDHHS), n.d., DHHS Publication No. (PHS) 81-50155, Washington, DC: U.S. Government Printing Office.

How This Booklet Can Help You

All of us want good health. But, many of us do not know how to be as healthy as possible. Good health is not a matter of luck or fate. You have to work at it.

Good health depends on a combination of things . . . the environment in which you live and work . . . the personal traits you have inherited . . . the care you receive from doctors and hospitals . . . and the personal behaviors or habits that you perform daily, usually without much thought. All of these work together to affect your health. Many of us rely too much on doctors to keep us healthy, and we often fail to see the importance of actions we can take ourselves to look and feel healthy. You may be surprised to know that by taking action individually and collectively, you can begin to change parts of your world which may be harmful to your health.

Every day you are exposed to potential risks to good health. Pollution in the air you breathe and unsafe highways are two examples. These are risks that you, as an individual, can't do much about. Improving the quality of the environment usually requires the effort of concerned citizens working together for a healthier community.

There are, however, risks that you can control: risks stemming from your personal behaviors and habits. These behaviors are known as your lifestyle. Health experts now describe lifestyle as one of the most important factors affecting health. In fact, it is estimated that as many as seven of the ten leading causes of death in the United States could be reduced through common sense changes in lifestyle.

That's what the brief test contained in this booklet is all about. The few minutes you take to complete it may actually help you add years to your life! How? Well to start, it will enable you to identify aspects of your present lifestyle that are risky to your health. Then it will encourage you to take steps to eliminate or minimize the risks you identify. All in all, it will help you begin to change your present lifestyle into a new HEALTHSTYLE. If you do, it's possible that you may feel better, look better, and live longer too.

Before You Take the Test

This is not a pass-fail test. Its purpose is simply to tell you how well you are doing to stay healthy. The behaviors covered in the test are recommended for most Americans. Some of them may not apply to persons with certain chronic diseases or handicaps. Such persons may require special instructions from their physician or other health professional.

You will find that the test has six sections: smoking, alcohol and drugs, nutrition, exercise and fitness, stress control, and safety. Complete one section at a time by circling the number corresponding to the answer that best describes your behavior (2 for "Almost Always", 1 for "Sometimes", and 0 for "Almost Never"). Then add the numbers you have circled to determine your score for that section. Write the score on the line provided at the end of each section. The highest score you can get for each section is 10.

A Test for Better Health

Cigarette Smoking

	Almost Always	Sometimes	Almost Never

If you never smoke, enter a score of 10 for this section and go to the next section on *Alcohol and Drugs*.

	Almost Always	Sometimes	Almost Never
1. I avoid smoking cigarettes.	2	1	0
2. I smoke only low tar and nicotine cigarettes *or* I smoke a pipe or cigars.	2	1	0

Smoking Score: _____

Alcohol and Drugs

	Almost Always	Sometimes	Almost Never
1. I avoid drinking alcoholic beverages *or* I drink no more than 1 or 2 drinks a day.	4	1	0
2. I avoid using alcohol or other drugs (especially illegal drugs) as a way of handling stressful situations or the problems in my life.	2	1	0
3. I am careful not to drink alcohol when taking certain medicines (for example, medicine for sleeping, pain, colds, and allergies), or when pregnant.	2	1	0
4. I read and follow the label directions when using prescribed and over-the-counter drugs.	2	1	0

Alcohol and Drugs Score: _____

Eating Habits

	Almost Always	Sometimes	Almost Never
1. I eat a variety of foods each day, such as fruits and vegetables, whole grain breads and cereals, lean meats, dairy products, dry peas and beans, and nuts and seeds.	4	1	0
2. I limit the amount of fat, saturated fat, and cholesterol I eat (including fat on meats, eggs, butter, cream, shortenings, and organ meats such as liver).	2	1	0
3. I limit the amount of salt I eat by cooking with only small amounts, not adding salt at the table, and avoiding salty snacks.	2	1	0
4. I avoid eating too much sugar (especially frequent snacks of sticky candy or soft drinks).	2	1	0

Eating Habits Score: _____

Exercise/Fitness

	Almost Always	Sometimes	Almost Never
1. I maintain a desired weight, avoiding overweight and underweight.	3	1	0
2. I do vigorous exercises for 15-30 minutes at least 3 times a week (examples include running, swimming, brisk walking).	3	1	0
3. I do exercises that enhance my muscle tone for 15-30 minutes at least 3 times a week (examples include yoga and calisthenics).	2	1	0
4. I use part of my leisure time participating in individual, family, or team activities that increase my level of fitness (such as gardening, bowling, golf, and baseball).	2	1	0

Exercise/Fitness Score: _____

Stress Control

	Almost Always	Sometimes	Almost Never
1. I have a job or do other work that I enjoy.	2	1	0
2. I find it easy to relax and express my feelings freely.	2	1	0
3. I recognize early, and prepare for, events or situations likely to be stressful for me.	2	1	0
4. I have close friends, relatives, or others whom I can talk to about personal matters and call on for help when needed.	2	1	0
5. I participate in group activities (such as church and community organizations) or hobbies that I enjoy.	2	1	0

Stress Control Score: _____

Safety

	Almost Always	Sometimes	Almost Never
1. I wear a seat belt while riding in a car.	2	1	0
2. I avoid driving while under the influence of alcohol and other drugs.	2	1	0
3. I obey traffic rules and the speed limit when driving.	2	1	0
4. I am careful when using potentially harmful products or substances (such as household cleaners, poisons, and electrical devices).	2	1	0
5. I avoid smoking in bed.	2	1	0

Safety Score: _____

Your HEALTHSTYLE Scores

After you have figured your scores for each of the six sections, circle the number in each column that matches your score for that section of the test.

Remember, there is no total score for this test. Consider each section separately. You are trying to identify aspects of your lifestyle that you can improve in order to be healthier and to reduce the risk of illness. So let's see what your scores reveal.

What Your Scores Mean to YOU

Scores of 9 and 10

Excellent! Your answers show that you are aware of the importance of this area to your health. More importantly, you are putting your knowledge to work for you by practicing good health habits. As long as you continue to do so, this area should not pose a serious health risk. It's likely that you are setting an example for your family and friends to follow. Since you got a very high score on this part of the test, you may want to consider other areas where your scores indicate room for improvement.

Scores of 6 to 8

Your health practices in this area are good, but there is room for improvement. Look again at the items you answered with a "Sometimes" or "Almost Never". What changes can you make to improve your score? Even a small change can often help you achieve better health.

Scores of 3 to 5

Your health risks are showing! Would you like more information about the risks you are facing and about why it is important for you to change these behaviors. Perhaps you need help in deciding how to successfully make the changes you desire. In either case, help is available. See the last page of this booklet.

Scores of 0 to 2

Obviously, you were concerned enough about your health to take the test, but your answers show that you may be taking serious and unnecessary risks with your health. Perhaps you are not aware of the risks and what to do about them. You can easily get the information and help you need to improve, if you wish. A source of contact appears on the last page. The next step is up to you.

YOU Can Start Right Now!

In the test you just completed were numerous suggestions to help you reduce your risk of disease and premature death. Here are some of the most significant:

 Avoid cigarettes. Cigarette smoking is the single most important preventable cause of illness and early death. It is especially risky for pregnant women and their unborn babies. Persons who stop smoking reduce their risk of getting heart disease and cancer. So if you're a cigarette smoker, think twice about lighting that next cigarette. If you choose to continue smoking, try decreasing the number of cigarettes you smoke and switching to a low tar and nicotine brand.

 Follow sensible drinking habits. Alcohol produces changes in mood and behavior. Most people who drink are able to control their intake of alcohol and to avoid undesired, and often harmful, effects. Heavy, regular use of alcohol can lead to cirrhosis of the liver, a leading cause of death. Also, statistics clearly show that mixing drinking and driving is often the cause of fatal or crippling accidents. So if you drink, do it wisely and in moderation.

 Use care in taking drugs. Today's greater use of drugs—both legal and illegal— is one of our most serious health risks. Even some drugs prescribed by your doctor can be dangerous if taken when drinking alcohol or before driving. Excessive or continued use of tranquilizers (or "pep pills")can cause physical and mental problems. Using or experimenting with illicit drugs such as marijuana, heroin, cocaine, and PCP may lead to a number of damaging effects or even death.

Eat sensibly. Overweight individuals are at greater risk for diabetes, gall bladder disease, and high blood pressure. So it makes good sense to maintain proper weight. But good eating habits also mean holding down the amount of fat (especially saturated fat), cholesterol, sugar and salt in your diet. If you must snack, try nibbling on fresh fruits and vegetables. You'll feel better—and look better, too.

Exercise regularly. Almost everyone can benefit from exercise—and there's some form of exercise almost everyone can do. (If you have any doubt, check first with your doctor.) Usually, as little as 15-30 minutes of vigorous exercise three times a week will help you have a healthier heart, eliminate excess weight, tone up sagging muscles, and sleep better. Think how much difference all these improvements could make in the way you feel!

Learn to handle stress. Stress is a normal part of living; everyone faces it to some degree. The causes of stress can be good or bad, desirable or undesirable (such as a promotion on the job or the loss of a spouse). Properly handled, stress need not be a problem. But unhealthy responses to stress—such as driving too fast or erratically, drinking too much, or prolonged anger or grief—can cause a variety of physical and mental problems. Even on a very busy day, find a few minutes to slow down and relax. Talking over a problem with someone you trust can often help you find a satisfactory solution. Learn to distinguish between things that are "worth fighting about" and things that are less important.

Be safety conscious. Think "safety first" at home, at work, at school, at play, and on the highway. Buckle seat belts and obey traffic rules. Keep poisons and weapons out of the reach of children, and keep emergency numbers by your telephone. When the unexpected happens, you'll be prepared.

Where Do You Go From Here?

Start by asking yourself a few frank questions: *Am I really doing all I can to be as healthy as possible? What steps can I take to feel better? Am I willing to begin now?* If you scored low in one or more sections of the test, decide what changes you want to make for improvement. You might pick that aspect of your lifestyle where you feel you have the best chance for success and tackle that one first. Once you have improved your score there, go on to other areas.

If you already have tried to change your health habits (to stop smoking or exercise regularly, for example) don't be discouraged if you haven't yet succeeded. The difficulty you have encountered may be due to influences you've never really thought about—such as advertising—or to a lack of support and encouragement. Understanding these influences is an important step toward changing the way they affect you.

There's Help Available. In addition to personal actions you can take on your own, there are community programs and groups (such as the YMCA or the local chapter of the American Heart Association) that can assist you and your family to make the changes you want to make. If you want to know more about these groups or about health risks contact your local health department. There's a lot you can do to stay healthy or to improve your health—and there are organizations that can help you. Start a new HEALTHSTYLE today!

☆ U.S. Government Printing Office: O-1981-344-829

INTER-ASSOCIATION TASK FORCE

MODEL CAMPUS ALCOHOL POLICY GUIDELINES

The Task Force recommends that a comprehensive campus policy on alcohol include a summary of state and city laws covering each of the following areas:

1.   Drinking Age Laws pertaining to the possession, consumption, and sale of alcoholic beverages as well as penalties for violation of such laws.

2.   Regulations of Sale Laws with special emphasis on Alcohol Beverage Control (ABC) Board's requirements for special permits or licenses by groups that charge admission or dues for events involving alcoholic beverages.

3.   Open Container Laws governed by city or county ordinances or state statutes concerning the consumption of alcoholic beverages in outdoor areas or automobiles.

4.   Other Laws pertinent to the jurisdiction (such as dram shop or implied consent laws).

College Regulations

In addition to legal responsibilities, The Task Force recommends that the following regulations be instituted as part of an alcohol policy on campus:

1.   Locations where alcoholic beverages are permitted to be possessed, served, and consumed by persons of legal drinking age on the campus should be visibly marked. A specific listing of such places (e.g., in private rooms, designated common areas of residence halls, college unions, etc.) helps clarify questions that students, faculty, or staff might have about where alcoholic beverages are permitted on campus.

2.   Locations where alcoholic beverages are permitted to be sold as opposed to merely served on campus (e.g., faculty lounge, college union, pub, etc.) should be delineated clearly.

3.   Guidelines should be established regarding public and private social events that involve alcoholic beverages within the institution's jurisdiction. An event that is open to the public (i.e., where admission is charged or public announcement is made) should be registered with the appropriate campus office before the event. Such events should be conducted within the following guidelines:

  a.   If the function includes the sale of alcoholic beverages, a permit should be obtained from the appropriate state office or ABC Board.

  b.   Individuals sponsoring the event should implement precautionary measures to ensure that alcoholic beverages are not accessible or served to persons under the legal drinking age or to persons who appear intoxicated.

  c.   At social functions where alcoholic beverages are provided by the sponsoring organization, direct access should be limited to a person(s) designated as the server(s).

  d.   Consumption of alcoholic beverages should be permitted only within the approved area designated for the event.

  e.   Nonalcoholic beverages must be available at the same place as the alcoholic beverages and featured as prominently as the alcoholic beverages.

f.   A reasonable portion of the budget for the event shall be designated for the purchase of food items.

g.   No social event shall include any form of "drinking contest" in its activities or promotion.

h.   Advertisements for any university event at which alcoholic beverages are served shall mention the availability of nonalcoholic beverages as prominently as alcohol. Alcohol should not be used as an inducement to participate in a campus event.

i.   Promotional materials including advertising for any university event shall not make reference to the amount of alcoholic beverages (such as number of beer kegs) available.

j.   Institutionally approved security personnel shall be present at all times during the event.

4.   A specific statement concerning the use or nonuse of alcoholic beverages at membership recruitment functions (e.g., fraternity/sorority rush, departmental clubs, and special interest groups) should be an integral part of a comprehensive campus alcohol policy.

5.   A specific statement concerning the use or nonuse of alcoholic beverages in athletic facilities or at athletic events should be included as part of a comprehensive campus alcohol policy. Such a statement should apply equally to students, faculty, staff, alumni, and others attending the event.

6.   Guidelines for any marketing, advertising, or promotion of alcoholic beverages on campus or at campus events involving alcohol should be stated as part of a comprehensive campus alcohol policy.

7.   Procedures for adjudicating violations of the alcohol policy should be articulated. Such procedures should include an explicit statement of sanctions.

Source: *Alcohol programs and policies on campus: NASPA monograph #7* ed. S. Sherwood, 1987, Washington, DC: National Association of Student Personnel Administrators. Reprinted by permission of National Association of Student Personnel Administrators.

Indiana Bell Telephone Company, Incorporated

Safety Practice 14
Effective December 15, 1982

Seat Belt Policy

It is the policy of Indiana Bell Telephone Company that all occupants of Company vehicles will wear seat belts when the vehicle is in motion. Likewise, occupants of leased or privately-owned vehicles being operated at Company expenses are required to abide by the above-stated policy.

Violations of this policy may result in disciplinary action up to and including dismissal.

Source: Indiana Bell Telephone Company, Inc., Indianapolis, IN. Reprinted by permission of Indiana Bell Telephone Company, Inc.

SEC. 1000. TITLE

This article shall be known as the Smoking Pollution Control Ordinance.

SEC. 1001. FINDINGS AND PURPOSE

The City Council does hereby find that:

Numerous studies have found that tobacco smoke is a major contributor to indoor air pollution, and that breathing secondhand smoke is a cause of disease, including lung cancer, in nonsmokers. At special risk are elderly people, individuals with cardiovascular disease, and individuals with impaired respiratory function, including asthmatics and those with obstructive airway disease; and

Health hazards induced by breathing second-hand smoke include lung cancer, heart disease, respiratory infection, decreased respiratory function, bronchoconstriction, and broncho-spasm.

Accordingly, the City Council finds and declares that the purposes of this ordinance are (1) to protect the public health and welfare by prohibiting smoking in public places and places of employment; and (2) to guarantee the right of nonsmokers to breathe smoke-free air, and to recognize that the need to breathe smoke-free air shall have priority over the desire to smoke.

SEC. 1002. DEFINITIONS

The following words and phrases, whenever used in this article, shall be construed as defined in this section:

1.   "Bar" means an area which is devoted to the serving of alcoholic beverages for consumption by guests on the premises and in which the serving of food is only incidental to the consumption of such beverages. Although a restaurant may contain a bar, the term "bar" shall not include the restaurant dining area.

2.   "Business" means any sole proprietorship, partnership, joint venture, corporation or other business entity formed for profit-making purposes, including retail establishments where goods or services are sold as well as professional corporations and other entities where legal, medical, dental, engineering, architectural or other professional services are delivered.

3.   "Employee" means any person who is employed by any employer in the consideration for direct or indirect monetary wages or profit, and any person who volunteers his or her services for a non-profit entity.

4.   "Employer" means any person, partnership, corporation, including a municipal corporation, or non-profit entity, who employs the services of one or more individual persons.

5.   "Enclosed Area" means all space between a floor and ceiling which is enclosed on all sides by solid walls or windows (exclusive of door or passage ways) which extend from the floor to the ceiling, including all space therein screened by partitions which do not extend to the ceiling or are not solid, "office landscaping" or similar structures.

6.   "Place of Employment" means any enclosed area under the control of a public or private employer which employees normally frequent during the course of employment, including, but not limited to, work areas, employee lounges and restrooms, conference and class rooms, employee cafeterias and hallways. A private residence is not a "place of employment" unless it is used as a child care or health care facility.

7.   "Public Place" means any enclosed area to which the public is invited or in which the public is permitted, including but not limited to, banks, educational facilities, health facilities, laundromats, public transportation facilities, reception areas, restaurants, retail food production and marketing establishments, retail service establishments, retail stores, theatres and waiting rooms. A private residence is not a "public place."

8.   "Restaurant" means any coffee shop, cafeteria, sandwich stand, private and public school cafeteria, and any other eating establishment which gives or offers for sale food to the public, guests, or employees, as well as kitchens in which food is prepared on the premises for serving elsewhere, including catering facilities, except that the term "restaurant" shall not include a cocktail lounge or tavern if said cocktail lounge is a "bar" as defined in Section 1002(1).

9.   "Retail Tobacco Store" means a retail store utilized primarily for the sale of tobacco products and accessories and in which the sale of other products is merely incidental.

10.   "Service Line" means any indoor line at which one (1) or more persons are waiting for or receiving service of any kind, whether or not such service involves the exchange of money.

11.   "Smoking" means inhaling, exhaling, burning or carrying any lighted cigar, cigarette, weed, plant or other combustible substance in any manner or in any form.

12.   "Sports Arena" means sports pavilions, gymnasiums, health spas, boxing arenas, swimming pools, roller and ice rinks, bowling alleys and other similar places where members of the general public assemble either to engage in physical exercise, participate in athletic competition, or witness sports events.

SEC. 1003. APPLICATION OF ARTICLE TO CITY-OWNED FACILITIES

All enclosed facilities owned by the City of _____ shall be subject to the provisions of this article.

SEC. 1004. PROHIBITION OF SMOKING IN PUBLIC PLACES

A.   Smoking shall be prohibited in all enclosed public places within the City of _____ , including, but not limited to, the following places, and with the following exceptions:

1.   Elevators

2.   Buses, taxicabs, and other means of public transit under the authority of the City of _____ , and ticket, boarding, and waiting areas of public transit depots.

3.   Restrooms.

4.   Service lines.

5.   Retail stores.

6.   All areas available to and customarily used by the general public in all businesses and non-profit entities patronized by the public, including but not limited to, attorneys' offices and other offices, banks, laundromats, hotels and motels.

7.   Restaurants.

8. Public areas of aquariums, galleries, libraries and museums when open to the public.

9. Any facility which is primarily used for exhibiting any motion picture, stage, drama, lecture, musical recital or other similar performance, except when smoking is part of a stage production.

10. Sports arenas and convention halls.

11. Every room, chamber, place of meeting or public assembly, including school buildings under the control of any board, council, commission, committee, including joint committees, or agencies of the City or any political subdivision of the State during such time as a public meeting is in progress, to the extent such place is subject to the jurisdiction of the city.

12. Waiting rooms, hallways, wards and semiprivate rooms of health facilities, including, but not limited to, hospitals, clinics, physical therapy facilities, doctors' offices, and dentists' offices.

13. Lobbies, hallways, and other common areas in apartment buildings, condominiums, retirement facilities, nursing homes, and other multiple-unit residential facilities.

14. Lobbies, hallways, and other common areas in multiple-unit commercial facilities.

15. Polling places.

B. Notwithstanding any other provision of this section, any owner, operator, manager or other person who controls any establishment or facility may declare that entire establishment or facility as a nonsmoking establishment.

SEC. 1005. REGULATION OF SMOKING IN PLACES OF EMPLOYMENT

A. It shall be the responsibility of employers to provide a smoke-free workplace for all employees, but employers are not required to incur any expense to make structural or other physical modifications.

B. Within 90 days of the effective date of this article, each employer having an enclosed place of employment located within the city shall adopt, implement, make known and maintain a written smoking policy which shall contain the following requirements:

Smoking shall be prohibited in all enclosed facilities within a place of employment without exception. This includes common work areas, auditoriums, classrooms, conference and meeting rooms, private offices, elevators, hallways, medical facilities, cafeterias, employee lounges, stairs, restrooms, vehicles, and all other enclosed facilities.

C. The smoking policy shall be communicated to all employees within three (3) weeks of its adoption.

D. All employers shall supply a written copy of the smoking policy upon request to any existing or prospective employee.

SEC. 1006. WHERE SMOKING IS NOT REGULATED

A. Notwithstanding any other provision of this article to the contrary, the following areas shall not be subject to the smoking restrictions of this article:

1.   Bars.

2.   Private residences, except when used as a child care or health care facility.

3.   Retail tobacco stores.

4.   Restaurants, hotel and motel conference or meeting rooms and public and private assembly rooms while these places are being used for private functions.

B.   Notwithstanding any other provision of this section, any owner, operator, manager or other person who controls any establishment described in this section may declare that entire establishment as a nonsmoking establishment.

SEC. 1007. POSTING OF SIGNS

A.   "No Smoking" signs or the international "No Smoking" symbol (consisting of a pictorial representation of a burning cigarette enclosed in a red circle with a red bar across it) shall be clearly, sufficiently and conspicuously posted in every building or other place where smoking is regulated by this article, by the owner, operator, manager or other person having control of such building or other place.

B.   Every restaurant shall have posted at every entrance a conspicuous sign clearly stating that smoking is prohibited.

SEC. 1008. ENFORCEMENT

A.   Enforcement of this article shall be implemented by the Department of Health [or the City Manager].

B.   Any citizen who desires to register a complaint under this chapter may initiate enforcement with the Department of Health [or the City Manager].

C.   The Fire Department or the Health Department shall require, while an establishment is undergoing otherwise mandated inspections, a "self-certification" from the owner, manager, operator or other person having control of such establishment that all requirements of this article have been complied with.

D.   Any owner, manager, operator or employee of any establishment regulated by this article may inform persons violating this article of the appropriate provisions thereof.

E.   Notwithstanding any other provision of this article, a private citizen may bring legal action to enforce this article.

SEC. 1009. VIOLATIONS AND PENALTIES

A.   It shall be unlawful for any person who owns, manages, operates or otherwise controls the use of any premises subject to regulation under this article to fail to comply with any of its provisions.

B.   It shall be unlawful for any person to smoke in any area where smoking is prohibited by the provisions of this article.

C.   Any person who violates any provision of this article shall be guilty of an infraction, punishable by:

1.   A fine not exceeding one hundred dollars ($100) for a first violation.

2.   A fine not exceeding two hundred dollars ($200) for a second violation of this article within one (1) year.

3.   A fine not exceeding five hundred dollars ($500) for each additional violation of this article within one (1) year.

SEC. 1010. NONRETALIATION

No person or employer shall discharge, refuse to hire or in any manner retaliate against any employee or applicant for employment because such employee or applicant exercises any right to a smoke-free environment afforded by this article.

SEC. 1011. PUBLIC EDUCATION

The Department of Health [or City Manager] shall engage in a continuing program to explain and clarify the purposes and requirements of this ordinance to citizens affected by it, and to guide owners, operators and managers in their compliance with it. Such program may include publication of a brochure for affected businesses and individuals explaining the provisions of this ordinance.

SEC. 1012. OTHER APPLICABLE LAWS

This article shall not be interpreted or construed to permit smoking where it is otherwise restricted by other applicable laws.

SEC. 1013. SEVERABILITY

If any provision, clause, sentence or paragraph of this article or the application thereof to any person or circumstances shall be held invalid, such invalidity shall not affect the other provisions of this article which can be given effect without the invalid provision or application, and to this end the provisions of this article are declared to be severable.

SEC. 1014. EFFECTIVE DATE

This article shall be effective thirty (30) days from and after the date of its adoption, and shall be reviewed within one year of its effective date.

Source: Americans for Nonsmokers' Rights, Berkeley, CA. Reprinted by permission of Americans for Nonsmokers' Rights.

AMERICAN PUBLIC HEALTH ASSOCIATION
1015 Fifteenth Street, N.W., Washington, D.C. 20005   •   (202) 789-5600

"HEALTH CARE FOR ALL"

ACTION ALERT

August 6, 1990

Dear Colleague:

Over the past year I have visited many states and talked to thousands of public health professionals about the need for a national health program in our country. I have been both encouraged and impressed with the number of individuals who are willing to work together to help us achieve this goal. As you know, APHA is working with Representative Henry Waxman (D-CA) to introduce "Health Care For All", a Sense of the Congress resolution outlining broad policy goals based on public health principles for a national health program in the United States.

You can help us gather cosponsors by writing to Representative Sharp and asking that he become an original cosponsor of the "HEALTH CARE FOR ALL" resolution. Additionally, you may wish to set up a meeting in your Representative's district office at which time you can discuss the need for a national health program and request that he cosponsor the resolution.

We all know that the United States health care system is in crisis. A growing number of Americans — now estimated at 37 million people — have neither private health insurance nor coverage by government programs. An additional 20 million persons have inadequate health care coverage.

The United States spends more than $600 billion a year on health care, constituting over 11 percent of our Gross National Product. Our per capita expenditure is about $2,300. These expenditures are larger than that of any other nation. Despite these costs the health status of Americans is clearly worse than that of many other nations which spend less than the U.S.

There is a growing recognition of the multitude of problems we face in the health care field. Increasingly, Congress is being asked to examine alternative ways to adjust our health care system. The "Health Care For All" resolution addresses these issues by expressing public health principles that

118th APHA ANNUAL MEETING • NEW YORK, NY • SEPT 30–OCT 4, 1990

Source: American Public Health Association, Washington, DC. Reprinted by permission of American Public Health Association and Myron Allukian, Jr.

should guide us as we examine and evaluate proposals to improve our nation's health care system.

Please join in this effort of APHA for the "HEALTH CARE FOR ALL" resolution. Write your Representative today and/or set up a meeting and help call attention to the need for a cost efficient system that will provide access to quality health care for every man, woman, and child in America.

Ask your Representative to cosponsor this resolution! We need your help! Enclosed is a copy of the "Health Care For All" resolution. Thank you for your assistance.

Very truly yours,

Myron Allukian Jr., DDS, MPH
President

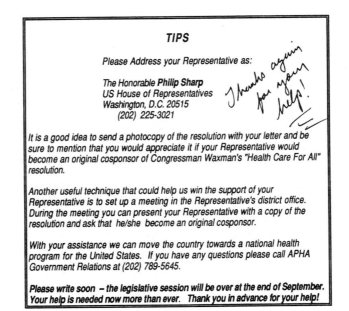

TIPS

Please Address your Representative as:

The Honorable **Philip Sharp**
US House of Representatives
Washington, D.C. 20515
(202) 225-3021

Thanks again for your help!

It is a good idea to send a photocopy of the resolution with your letter and be sure to mention that you would appreciate it if your Representative would become an original cosponsor of Congressman Waxman's "Health Care For All" resolution.

Another useful technique that could help us win the support of your Representative is to set up a meeting in the Representative's district office. During the meeting you can present your Representative with a copy of the resolution and ask that he/she become an original cosponsor.

With your assistance we can move the country towards a national health program for the United States. If you have any questions please call APHA Government Relations at (202) 789-5645.

Please write soon – the legislative session will be over at the end of September. Your help is needed now more than ever. Thank you in advance for your help!

Mammograms for Mother's Day
Indiana State Board of Health
Television Public Service Announcement

Video	Audio/Narration
Susan Bayh (wife of Gov. Evan Bayh)	I'm Susan Bayh, and this is my mother. My husband lost his mother to breast cancer.
Carolyn Breshears Susan's Mom	And there's a history of breast cancer in our family.
Susan	Today there is no reason why any woman should die from breast cancer.
B-roll of exam	A mammogram x-ray can detect breast cancer 2 years before you can feel it through self-exam. Almost all breast cancers can be successfully treated if caught early.
Susan & Mom	So this year, give your Mom something really special. . . give her a mammogram.
Squeeze box with font	We'll give you this special card to go along with it.

For information call Indiana's
American Cancer Society
1-800-ACS-2345

Total Tape Time :30   Begin airdates 4/18/91   End 5/9/91

Source: Indiana State Department of Health, Indianapolis. Reprinted by permission of the Indiana State Department of Health.

Ryan White "For Teens Only" PSA #1
Choices

Produced by the Indiana State Board of Health   :30
For air 10/2/90 – 9/31/91

Video	Audio
Ryan up full on camera	You know there's 3 ways to get aids.
	Sex, needles and ignorance.
	It's the last one that gets most people today.
	I didn't have a choice. You do. Don't be afraid to ask questions.
	You can get confidential answers by calling the AIDS Hotline.
Lower third key over Elton:	(Elton John singing to end)
Indiana AIDS Hotline 1-800-848-AIDS	"Skyline Pigeon fly, to all the dreams he left so very far behind."
	(piano under to end)

TTT – :30

Please note we put :04 pad at the end for those who need a little extra time.
You can cut out at your discretion. It won't affect the PSA.

Baby Bottle Tooth Decay
Indiana State Board of Health
Childhood Dental Health PSA Feb. 1990 :30

Video	**Audio**
Mom puts child down	Bedtime bottles could be dangerous to your child's health. If your child has a bedtime bottle habit—break that habit now.
Closeup pouring milk into bottle	When sweetened liquids, juices or milk stay on their teeth all night long, or naptime your child's teeth can go from
Good teeth wipe to bad teeth	this – to this – before you know it.
Cee'Ann in dental chair	Find out how you can prevent this painful tooth decay and break the
Get kid to throw down his bottle	bottle habit.
Squeeze box and font Phone #	Call the Indiana State Board of Health Dental Division at (317) 633-8418.

PREAMBLE

The national organizations listed below have developed and subscribe to the following Code of Practice for group programs of smoking cessation. They, thereby, have agreed that all such programs conducted under their aegis will comply with this code of self-regulation. The Code of Practice is intended to provide assurance and protection to individuals seeking assistance in smoking cessation. It is not intended either to endorse or to interfere with the methodology or content of any program or eliminate its unique features. The Code will be reviewed annually by the subscribing organizations.

I. CRITERIA OF SUCCESS

Complete cessation, and continued abstinence from smoking for one year, should be the primary criteria of success. A uniform approach to the determination of rates of success is set forth in *Standards for the Evaluation of Group Smoking Cessation Programs*.

II. DISCLOSURE

Program participants should be given an accurate description of the services rendered including a general explanation of the treatment approach, time and costs involved and qualifications of leaders or facilitators.

Introductory sessions or some other method of informing participants of the major facts about the program, including any possible physiological risks involved, should be provided. Participants with relevant medical problems should be referred to their family physicians.

III. CONTINUITY/AVAILABILITY

Maintenance programs or other services should be available to participants (or past participants who require continued help).

Each program should have some provision for furnishing information, counseling or referral to the participants who do not respond to its approach.

IV. TRAINING OF LEADERS

Only adequately trained and experienced individuals should be allowed to lead groups.

A written protocol for training and written criteria for evaluation of leaders should be on file in each organization.

V. PROGRAM UNIFORMITY

Programs identified with a particular organization should be similar, unless otherwise noted.

Each organization should plan for quality control and standardization of its approved program models.

VI. RECORD KEEPING

Adequate records of all participants should be maintained in accordance with the standards set forth in *Standards for the Evaluation of Group Smoking Cessation Programs*.

VII. EVALUATION

All national organizations should carry out evaluation of their own programs on at least an annual basis in accordance with *Standards for the Evaluation of Group Smoking Cessation Programs*.

Reports of these annual evaluations should be made to the Peer Review Committee on National Smoking Cessation Programs. In addition, organizations should participate in peer-reviewed evaluation as requested by this body.

VIII. ADVERTISING, PROMOTION AND PUBLIC RELATIONS

No quantitative claims of success should be made in advertising.

No guarantees of success should be made.

Statistics cited to the press should be referenced to peer-reviewed evaluation conducted in accordance with *Standards for the Evaluation of Group Smoking Cessation Programs* and must include results both at the end of treatment and after one year.

IX. HUMAN DIGNITY

All programs should respect the human dignity of their participants.

There should be no discrimination in admission to or treatment in programs on the basis of race, religion, color or sex.

All records should be confidential and lists of names should not be sold to outside groups without the approval of the participants.

American Cancer Society
American Health Foundation
American Heart Association
American Lung Association
Five-Day Plan to Stop Smoking
SmokEnders

Source: American Cancer Society, Atlanta, GA. Reprinted by permission of the American Cancer Society.

How to Select the Right Vendor for Your Company's Health Promotion Program

JOHN H. HARRIS, III, M.ED.
JAMES F. MCKENZIE, PH.D., M.P.H.
WILLIAM B. ZUTI, PH.D.

The development of interest by employers in health promotion programs for their employees has been paralleled by a growth of vendors interested in selling health promotion services to these employers. A checklist indicating the particular services offered and the methods by which they will be provided and at what costs can help the employer make the decision for the most suitable and efficient service.

There has been a tremendous growth during the past 15 years in the number of corporate employers who have begun offering employee health promotion programs (EHPPs) (1). Many of the early programs were begun because of the intuitive projection that improved employee lifestyle would not only improve the health of the individual employees but also have an impact on the health care programs of the company. However, much of the recent growth has come about because of the relatively recent empirical data indicating that EHPPs can be cost-effective and can have a significant effect on employee health, absenteeism, morale and productivity. Additionally, the data have indicated that EHPPs may help a company increase its own image and its ability to recruit new personnel and decrease employee turnover (2–9).

With the growth of EHPPs in the business community there has come a parallel growth in the number of organizations (vendors) who are interested in selling health promotion services (products) to the companies. It is not uncommon to find hospitals, health clubs, YMCAs/YWCAs, voluntary health agencies (i.e., American Lung Association, American Red Cross, etc.), health departments, other community organizations and for-profit health promotion companies trying to market their services. Just like any service, some of what these vendors are marketing is good, while some is not. Unless your company employs trained health promotion professionals who can identify the difference in these services, a good salesperson can make the poor services appear comparable, if not better, than the good ones. Because of the newness of the EHPPs there are few guidelines (10) to help companies select appropriate vendors. Thus, in order to help those companies who do not employ trained health promotion professionals and those who have hired one with limited experience, a checklist for evaluating health promotion vendors has been developed.

The Instrument

The checklist comprises 50 yes-no type questions. It includes several questions that are "common sense" or basic "good business" questions. However, it has been our experience that unless a company specifically asks the questions of the vendor, the vendor may not provide information and thus a company must make a decision to buy or not to buy based upon insufficient and/or perhaps inaccurate data.

The checklist is divided into six sections. The first section deals with the initial meeting with the vendor. Basically this portion of the checklist presents questions which ask: "How well prepared was the vendor for the meeting?"

Direct correspondence to:
John H. Harris, III
Manager, Health Enhancement
Owens-Illinois, Inc.
One Seagate
Toledo, OH 43666

The second and third portions of the checklist pose questions that ask about the quality of the service being marketed. These include questions such as: "How effective is it?" "How does it compare to services being marketed by other vendors?" and "What are the qualifications of those who will actually provide the service?"

Section four of the checklist presents a series of questions that examine how the vendor will deliver and service the product. You want to work with a vendor who will provide excellent service when the agreement has been signed. The fifth section of the checklist provides questions that can be used in determining an appropriate cost for the product. The last portion of the checklist includes several general questions that deal with image, contracts and legal concerns.

It should be noted that the checklist has not been standardized and there is no set score that will assure that a vendor will be a good supplier of health promotion services. When using the checklist, those responsible for EHPPs should be very skeptical of those vendors who have a large number of checks in the "no" column of the instrument. At the same time, it will probably be difficult to find a vendor that will receive all "yes" responses. Although final decisions are usually made on a subjective basis, one should feel more confident when using the services of a vendor with a large number of "yes" responses. And finally, it should be pointed out that some areas of the country are better supplied with vendors than others, and thus all ratings would be relative to the geographic locations.

References

1. Fielding JE, Breslow L. Health promotion programs sponsored by California employers. *Am J Public Health* 73:538–542, 1983.
2. Erfurt JC, Foote A. Cost-effectiveness of work-site blood pressure control programs. *J Occup Med* 26:892–900, 1984.
3. Fielding JE. Effectiveness of employee health improvement programs. *J Occup Med* 24:907–916, 1982.
4. Fielding JE. Health promotion and disease prevention at the worksite. *Annu Rev Public Health* xx:237–265, 1984.
5. Gibbs JO, Mulvaney D, Henes C, Reed RW. Work-site health promotion: five-year trend in employee health care costs. *J Occup Med* 27:826–830, 1985.
6. Kristein MM. The economics of health promotion at the worksite. *Health Educ Q* 9 (special suppl):27–36, 1982.
7. Rogers PJ, Eaton EK, Bruhn JG. Is health promotion cost effective? *Prev Med* 10:324–339, 1981.
8. Schwartz RM, Rollins PL. Measuring the cost benefit of wellness strategies. *Business Health* 2(10):24–26, 1985.
9. Stason WG. Measuring the "payoff" of worksite health strategies. *Business Health* 1(4):19–22, 1984.
10. Zuti WB. Weighting—and minimizing—the risks of joint venturing. *Promoting Health* January–February, 4–5, 1985.
11. Kelly KE. Building a successful health promotion program. *Business Health* 3(March):44–45, 1986.
12. Opatz JP. *A Primer of Health Promotion: Creating Healthy Organizational Cultures.* Oryn Publications, Inc., Washington, DC, 1985.
13. Kelly KE. Separate yourself from the crowd. *Optimal Health* 2(March/April):30–32, 34, 1986.

Source: "How to Select the Right Vendor for Your Company's Health Promotion Program" by J. H. Harris, J. F. McKenzie, and W. B. Zuti, 1986, *Fitness in Business*, 1(October), pp. 53–56. Reprinted by permission of Association for Fitness in Business, a resource for health promotion professionals.

Checklist for selecting health promotion vendors

Code: Yes—Yes, the vendor does/did this.   **NA**—Not applicable
No —No, the vendor does not/did not do this.   **NS**—Not sure

	Yes	No	NA/NS	Comments
1. Initial experience with vendor				
A. Did the vendor present a good professional image?				
B. Did the vendor do his/her homework on your company prior to the initial meeting?				
C. Is the vendor's philosophy of health promtion consistent with that of your company's philosophy (11)?				
D. Can the vendor explain why his/her product is appropriate for your company?				
E. Did the vendor appear responsive to your company's needs?				
F. Did the vendor explain how his/her product can meet the needs of your company (11)?				
G. Was the vendor willing to listen to you or was he/she too busy trying to sell his/her product?				
H. Is the vendor willing to make a presentation to your company's management?				
I. Did the vendor demonstrate his/her organization's expertise with regard to the product?				
J. Did the vendor provide you with a reference list of other customers (12)?				
K. Did the vendor leave written materials that summarize his/her product?				
2. Product quality				
A. Did the vendor provide an overview of the product content?				
B. Can the vendor provide careful documentation of product effectiveness?				
C. Does the vendor have evaluative data to back up the product?				
D. Does the vendor have data to compare sucess rates of the product to those of his/her competitors?				
E. Can the vendor provide data which shows the adequacy of his/her products with a population similar to yours (12)?				
F. Can the vendor provide several different products (health promotion activities) or does he/she just specialize in one area?				

	Yes	No	NA/NS	Comments

2. Product quality, *continued*

G. Did the vendor explain the types of interventions (behavior modification, aversive techniques, etc.) that are used with the product?

H. Will the vendor "customize" the product to meet the needs of your company?

I. Can the vendor offer a variety of interventions (i.e. different approaches to smoking cessation) from which you can choose to best meet the needs of your employees (13)?

J. Can the vendor offer a product which can meet special needs of your employees (e.g. reading levels, various levels of health status, etc.) (13)?

K. When appropriate, does the vendor provide written instructional materials to accompany the product?

L. If written informational materials are provided, are they written clearly and presented in an attractive way?

3. Individuals who provide the service

A. What type of education and training do the staff and/or instructors have.?

B. Are the instructors certified by a professional and/ or health organization?

C. Are the instructors required to update their training periodically?

D. Are the instructor-to-participant ratios reasonable?

4. Product delivery and service

A. Can the vendor put in writing the actual services that will be provided?

B. If a written presentation of services is made, does it spell out the responsibilities of both parties?

C. Is the vendor willing to market the product inside your company?

D. Does purchase of the product include an evaluation?

E. Can the vendor appropriately serve the size of your company's population?

F. Can the vendor provide the product at all sites desired?

G. Can the vendor provide the product at the time desired?

	Yes	No	NA/NS	Comments
4. Product delivery and service, *continued*				
H. Are the length of the product sessions appropriate for your work day?				
I. Does the vendor provide you with the name of one of their employees who can act as a trouble-shooter?				
J. Can the vendor also provide other products/services to other departments (units) (i.e., the safety division, health policy, etc.) in your company?				
K. Has the vendor been in business for at least five years (10)?				
L. Is the vendor's company well managed and financially sound (10)?				
M. Does the vendor enjoy a good reputation in the community (10)?				
5. Product cost				
A. Is the cost of the product competitive with the cost of other vendors?				
B. Does the vendor provide written bids for the product?				
C. Does the cost per unit go down when the number of participants increase?				
D. Does the cost per unit go down if additional products are purchased from the same vendor?				
E. Does the vendor offer corporate discounts?				
6. General concerns				
A. Does the vendor carry adequate liability insurance?				
B. Does the vendor put in writing a "statement of reasonable expectations" for the product (13)?				
C. Is the vendor willing to sign a contract?				
D. If you buy the product of this vendor, will it improve the image of your company in the community?				
E. If you buy the product of this vendor, will it improve the image of your company with the employees?				

Being of sound mind and in need of health behavior change, I (insert name of person wanting to make the change) do hereby commit myself to the following health behavior change for the next eight weeks. This contract with (insert the name of the other person who is entering into this contract) shall be in effect from (insert starting date) to (insert ending date) . For completing this contract I will be rewarded/reinforced with (insert reward or reinforcer) . This reward/reinforcer will be received when I (insert desired behavior) . If I do not successfully fulfill this contract I will (insert what will happen if person is not successful) .

A.   The behavior I plan to change is:

_____

_____

B.   The reason I want to change this behavior is because:

_____

_____

C.   I have set the following objectives for myself. (Reminder: objectives must be measurable so you will know if you have reached them. For example, choose practicing relaxation techniques once a day, 5 times per week as an objective rather than indicating stress reduction as a goal.)

  1. _____

  2. _____

  3. _____

D.   To meet these goals I will (provide a description of your daily/weekly activity):

_____

_____

E.   To carry out my plan I am going to solicit the help of (names of friends, family, roomate, or significant others and how they will help:)

_____

_____

F.   I expect to receive the following benefits from this activity:

_____

_____

Your signature: _____ Date: _____

Facilitator's signature: _____ Date: _____

I hereby grant permission to the Institute for Health Promotion personnel to perform a cholesterol screening on me. I am engaging in this screening voluntarily. I have been told that this screening is an analysis of total blood cholesterol and that my blood will be taken from a fingerstick blood sample by a trained employee. I understand that the results of this screening are considered to be preliminary in nature and in no way conclusive. Results of a blood cholesterol screening like this can be affected by a number of factors including, but not limited to, smoking, stress level, amount of exercise, hormone levels, foods eaten, heredity, and pregnancy. I also understand that my physician can perform a more complete blood lipid (fat) analysis for me, if I so desire.

Further, I have been told that all information related to this screening is considered confidential.

I have read the above statement and understand what it means. I have also had an opportunity to ask questions about the screening, and all my questions have been answered to my satisfaction.

_____   _____   _____

Participant's Signature   Date   Signature of Witness

To ensure it meets with all related local and state laws, this form, or any others like it, should be submitted to legal counsel before use.

I hereby certify that ___(name of participant)___ has been examined and cleared by me to participate, with the noted restrictions, in the programs indicated below. This person should not be placed into any of the other programs until he/she has been cleared by me to do so.

☐ Vigorous exercise programs. This type of program would include all out effort for the development of cardiovascular endurance, muscular strength, and flexibility.
   Physician's comments: _____

   _____

   _____

☐ Moderate exercise program. This type of program is for those participants who would be unable to participate in the vigorous exercise program because of physical limitations. These programs should be modified as per my instructions.
   Physician's comments: _____

   _____

   _____

☐ Mild exercise program. This type of program is for those participants who would be unable to participate in the moderate exercise program because of physical limitations. These programs should be modified as per my instructions.
   Physician's comments: _____

   _____

   _____

_____   _____
Physician's signature   Date

SOPHE'S MAJOR GOALS

In 1975, the SOPHE Board of Trustees and the Society's Chapters collaborated on the development of major goals to be worked toward for the rest of the decade. Some of these goals are:

- To determine the relevance of national health legislation to SOPHE concerns

- To influence health policies and programs in which there should be an identifiable health education component

- To stimulate research in health education programs and methods, including evaluation

- To develop standards for the professional preparation and practice of health education

- To encourage high quality practice through professional development, continuing education, and training

- To assure that a mechanism for credentialing health educators exists and that it is properly used

- To increase career opportunities for health educators

- To maintain effective liaison with other organizations having allied interests in health education

- To improve communication with Chapters and members on critical issues that affect health education

- To provide guidance and support for Chapter development and expansion

SOPHE'S CODE OF ETHICS

To guide professional behaviors of its members toward highest standards, SOPHE adopted a Code of Ethics in 1976, and acknowledged the need for periodic review and improvement of the Code.

- I will accurately represent my capability, education, training, and experience, and will act within the boundaries of my professional competence

- I will maintain my competence at the highest level through continuing study, training, and research

- I will report research findings and practice activities honestly and without distortion

- I will not discriminate because of race, color, national origin, religion, age, sex, or socio-economic status in rendering service, employing, training, or promoting others

- I value the privacy, dignity, and worth of the individual, and will use skills consistent with these values

- I will observe the principle of informed consent with respect to individuals and groups served

- I will support change by choice, not by coercion

- I will foster an educational environment that nurtures individual growth and development

- If I become aware of unethical practices, I am accountable for taking appropriate action concerning these practices

Source: Society for Public Health Education, San Francisco, CA. Reprinted by permission of Society for Public Health Education.

WHAT IS SOPHE?

The Society for Public Health Education is a national professional service organization formed in 1950 to promote the health of all people by stimulating research, developing criteria for professional preparation, and elevating performance standards for the practice of health education. Cumulative efforts by its members have helped SOPHE achieve international recognition for its outstanding contributions to the improvement of individual and community health.

Affairs of the Society are guided by a Board of Trustees, which is composed of elected officers, at-large, and Chapter members. The Board determines organizational direction, develops policies, and sets the framework for achievement by its committees and the Society's Chapters. More than 80 percent of the members belong to local Chapters.

SOPHE's membership extends health educational principles and practice into many settings: The community . . . colleges and universities . . . the home . . . hospitals and other health care facilities . . . official, professional, and voluntary health agencies and organizations . . . schools . . . and the workplace. The Society derives its strength from the united efforts of its members, who include: Administrators . . . behavioral scientists . . . community health educators . . . consumers . . . dentists . . . faculty . . . health planners . . . mental health educators . . . nurses . . . physicians . . . school health educators . . . teachers . . . and volunteers.

WHAT SOPHE MEMBERSHIP OFFERS YOU

One-year subscription to *Health Education Quarterly,* SOPHE's scholarly journal

National health legislation information/action network activities

Annual Membership Directory

Chapter affiliation for regular contact and idea exchange with colleagues

Discount prices on SOPHE publication

Opportunities to achieve professional identity and recognition through service on SOPHE committees and task forces

SOPHE *News & Views,* the Society's newsletter

Long-term professional development and continuing education activities

Opportunities to influence standards for professional preparation and práctice

SOPHE Annual Report

Opportunities to know other members who are active at local, state, national, and international levels

Reduced registration fees for SOPHE'S annual meeting, held each fall in conjunction with the annual meeting of the American Public Health Association

SOPHE membership benefits and services are designed to help you fulfill your health education responsibilities and increase your professional competence.

Cost-Benefit and Cost-Effectiveness as a Part of the Evaluation of Health Promotional Programs

James F. McKenzie, Ph.D., M.P.H.,
Beta Gamma Chapter

Abstract
Economic evaluation should be a component of program evaluation. To encourage and help with this process, definitions of common economic terms, a review of the literature, steps for conducting an economic evaluation, and the use of economic evaluation, with health promotion program is presented.

Introduction

The idea of promoting good health practices is not new in the United States. However, it is only in recent years that the concept of health promotion has grown in popularity and that the number of health promotion programs has flourished. The growth has occurred because of the ". . . increasing evidence of an association between patterns of lifestyle and health status of individuals and population groups, and associations between environmental and workplace hazards and the health and well-being of communities and workers" (Work Group on Health Promotion/Disease Prevention, 1987).

Though the number of health promotion programs continues to increase, the evaluation of said programs lags behind. There are several reasons for this. First, many of the first generation health promotion programs were developed without regard to an appropriate plan of evaluation. Thus data were not and could not be collected. Second, because of the very nature of health promotion programs, that of being "in the field" and being geared toward the long-term outcome of "improved health," make them difficult to evaluate. Concerns such as evaluation expertise, confidentiality of participants, and resources of time, money and personnel, have proven to be stumbling blocks in collecting the needed data.

If health promotion programs are to prosper and grow, empirical evidence of their worth should be provided. This can only be done through appropriate evaluation of the programs; evaluation that pays considerable attention to problems of design and measurement, and that can be reproducible. Green (1979) stated that "Evaluation of a health promotion plan certifies its appropriateness and its effectiveness and ensures that the practitioner is accountable to the patient (consumer), the community, and the hospital administrator." Though Green's comments were directed toward hospital health promotion programs these same ideas can be transferred to any health promotion setting because all program planners need to be accountable to the consumer (Work Group on Health Promotion/Disease Prevention, 1987).

The question now is not whether or not health promotion programs should be evaluated but how should it be done?

James F. McKenzie is Associate Professor in the Health Education Division, School of HPER, Bowling Green State University, Bowling Green, Ohio 43403. The author wishes to gratefully acknowledge the help of Bonnie McKenzie in the preparation of this manuscript.

Green (1979) has defined three different levels of evaluation—process, impact and outcome. Process evaluation deals with the professional practice of those presenting the health promotion program. Impact evaluation is concerned with the immediate difference that the health promotion program has on the knowledge, attitude, behavior and environment. Outcome evaluation focuses on long-term concerns such as morbidity, mortality and years of survival following the health promotion program. There are many strategies for evaluating health promotion programs within each of these levels and they have been thoroughly covered in the works of Windsor, Baranowski, Clark, and Cutter (1984) and Green and Lewis (1986). However, there is one evaluation strategy that these authors have addressed that merits further discussion because of the importance being placed on it in today's practice: the economic evaluation of health promotion programs. In the business world the economic evaluation of a program is often referred to as the "bottom line."

In writing about corporate health promotion programs Fielding (1982, p. 85) has stated:

> Although current evidence suggests a very favorable return on investment for disease prevention and health promotion programs, much more information is needed to quantify costs and benefits and to suggest which models work best in different corporate settings. Therefore, it is imperative that all efforts include long-term evaluation of effects of programs on both direct and indirect costs.

The remaining portion of this paper will focus on the economic evaluation of health promotion programs. This refers to the cost-benefit and cost-effectiveness analysis (CBA and CEA, respectively) of the programs.

Definitions of CBA and CEA

Simply stated, CBA and CEA are formal analytical techniques used for comparing the negative and positive consequences of alternative uses of resources. They are not formulas for making decisions but rather they are tools to help individuals make decisions (Warner & Luce, 1982). More specifically, Green and Lewis (1986, p. 361) have defined cost-benefit as "a measure of the cost of an intervention relative to the benefits it yields, usually expressed as a ratio of dollars saved or gained for every dollar spent on the program," and cost-effectiveness as "a measure of the cost of an intervention relative to its impact, usually expressed in dollars per unit of effect." Common CEA measures may include years of life saved, days of morbidity and disability avoided, number of smokers who quit, and number of pounds lost.

Source: "Cost-Benefit and Cost-Effectiveness as a Part of the Evaluation of Health Promotion Programs" by J. F. McKenzie, 1986, *The Eta Sigma Gamman, 18*(2), pp. 10–16. Reprinted by permission of The Eta Sigma Gamman.

When first reading these definitions, they appear to be very much alike. The basic technical distinction between CBA and CEA lies in the process of valuing the desirable consequences of health promotion programs (Warner & Luce, 1982). CBA requires that all desirable consequences be expressed in monetary (dollar) terms. For many of the consequences this is a manageable task, but there are some desirable consequences that researchers have found most difficult to quantify in dollars—the value of human life may be the most notable. Several researchers (Rice, 1966; Cooper and Rice, 1976; Acton, 1976) have offered means of dealing with the problem.

More recently the difference between CBA and CEA seems to be fading. Warner and Luce have pointed out that as they have reviewed the literature on CBA and CEA, the two techniques are becoming more alike in the way analysts are applying the concepts. They have indicated that "recent sophisticated health care CEAs are incorporating some dollar-valued benefits into the cost side of the equation (as negative costs), and increasing recognition of the meaning of CBA in health care is bringing it closer to CEA. The human capital approach to measuring indirect benefits in CBA values livelihood, not life itself; thus a CBA is really a net dollar benefit for some nonmonetized health outcomes. The newer more sophisticated CEA seems to be a significant step forward in that it combines the best of both CBA and CEA" (Warner & Luce, 1982, p. 213).

The Popularity of CBA and CEA
The evaluation techniques of CEA and CBA are by no means new concepts, for they can be traced back hundreds of years. However, there has been a tremendous growth in their use and interest in the health professions in the past fifteen years. Much of this growth has paralleled the increase of health care costs during the same period of time. Many feel that this burgeoning interest of CEA and CBA in the health professions has resulted from health professionals seeking to identify and convey the meaning of cost-beneficial and cost-effective health care interventions. It is now quite common to find CBA and CEA citations on most all health care topics.

Review of Literature
As Warner and Hutton (1980) have pointed out, the contributions to the health care CBA and CEA literature have grown exponentially in recent years. Over the years the majority of the literature has dealt with medical interventions. Since this paper is focused on nonmedical interventions—health promotion activities—the medical intervention CBA and CEA literature is not reviewed here. However, it is well presented in Warner and Luce (1982).

The references to the nonmedical CBA and CEA literature are much more limited. The nonmedical literature falls into three major areas—public health measures (i.e., water fluoridation, food inspection, etc.), identification of health risks via screenings (for hypertension, cancer and other diseases) and personal health lifestyle (i.e., exercise, smoking, nutrition, stress, etc.). Public health measures have generally not been considered a part of health promotion activities.

And even though screenings have been a portion of a number of health promotion programs, it is the category of personal health lifestyle on which most health promotion programs are planned. It is this literature that is reviewed below.

A number of reviews of the CBA and CEA of health promotion type activities have been found in the literature (Fielding, 1982; Rogers, Eaton, & Bruhn, 1981; Scheffler, & Paringer, 1980; and Warner, 1979). These reviews report on basically two types of studies. One group includes studies that have calculated a CBA or CEA on a specific health problem in terms of what the costs and benefits would be for the entire United States if a health promotion program were implemented. One such paper is presented by Kristein (1977). In his paper, Kristein examines several different health concerns such as hypertension, cancer of the colon, heavy cigarette smoking, alcohol abuse and breast cancer. A summary of his heavy cigarette smoking calculations provides a good example of this approach. He calculated that the costs of heavy cigarette smoking were approximately $20.3 billion (in 1975 dollars). This includes the cost of hospital care, medical care, absenteeism, and premature deaths. If a smoking cessation program were implemented for the 22 million heavy smokers in the United States (a 1975 estimate) at $125 per person and there was a 25% success rate, Kristein estimated a cost-benefit ratio of 1.8 to 1.0. This means that for every dollar put into such a program a $1.80 could be saved. This type of CBA is useful in showing that smoking cessation programs can provide financial benefits, but the exactness of the figures must be put into perspective because of the lack of detail in the analysis.

The other major group of studies that appear in the reviews are those which report on the results of a CBA or CEA calculated on a specific health promotion activity offered by a specific organization. For example, Fielding (1982) has reviewed the results of a number of employee health promotion programs. His findings show that a number of different techniques have been used to calculate CBAs and CEAs, that calculations are based on a number of assumptions and thus the results are difficult to compare. In another paper Fielding (1984) offers the following example:

> Campbell's analysis of the savings attributable to their colorectal cancer screening programs hinges on assumptions regarding the number of cases of colorectal cancer that would have occurred in the absence of screening, and the direct and indirect costs associated with each case. It also assumes that all cases prevented were due to on-site screening rather than screening that occurred in another setting (e.g., doctor's office or HMO) at the encouragement of an outside health professional. While these estimates of savings due to health promotion measures are useful in showing the value companies themselves have placed in the savings, it is difficult to know if their assertions can be applied to other companies. (p. 259).

Further indication of the inconsistency in the way CBA and CEA for health promotion activities have been calculated was noted by Rogers et al. (1981, p. 333)—". . .carefully designed cost analyses have not been conducted so that various approaches can be compared as to the expense, as well as to short-term impact and long-term outcome." There is clearly a need for authors to describe in detail all the steps they follow in calculating their CBA or CEA so that other evaluators can use the same steps and thus be able to compare results.

The health promotion literature includes more reports of CBAs and CEAs on identification of health risks than in personal health lifestyle change, with the more reports dealing with hypertension screening programs than any other (Alderman, Madhavan, & Davis, 1983; Erfurt & Foote, 1984; Foote & Erfurt, 1977; Ruchlin & Alderman, 1980; and Ruchlin, Melcher, & Alderman, 1984). Only two recent reports on personal health lifestyle change could be found. One dealt with weight loss (Seidman, Sevelius & Ewald, 1984) and the other with smoking cessation (Weiss, Jurs, Lesage, & Iverson, 1984). Scheffler and Paringer (1980) have pointed out the need for empirical evidence of the economic soundness of other lifestyle change programs such as physical exercise and dietary changes.

Finally, there are many more reports using CEA than CBA in the health promotion literature. Only two reports of CBA (Alderman et al., 1983; and Weiss, et al., 1984) could be found. All others were CEAs. The reasons for this will become clear from subsequent discussion.

Calculating CBAs and CEAs
As suggested in preceding portions of this paper, the calculation of CBAs and CEAs for health promotion activities is no easy task. In most cases they will be difficult and in some cases impossible to calculate. However, if evaluations of health promotion activities are going to be complete, they should be attempted.

Though there are certain processes that must be included in calculating CBAs and CEAs, the exact steps one could use may vary. The important point to remember is that whatever steps are used, they should be reported accurately and in detail so others can replicate and compare results. The steps presented below are a combination of techniques suggested by a governmental agency and several different individuals (OTA, 1978; OTA, 1980; Rogers et al, 1981; Shepard & Thompson, 1979; and Warner & Luce, 1982).

Step 1: Defining the Problem
The initial step in calculating a CBA or CEA is defining the problem to be analyzed. The problem should be stated as clearly and explicitly as possible. Seemingly small differences in the definition of the problem could have a large impact on the calculated costs, benefits and effects. The statement of the problem should also clearly specify for whom the analysis is going to be calculated. For example, a cost-analysis of a health promotion program would differ greatly if it were being calculated from the employer's point of view as opposed to the costs, benefits and effects experienced by the employee.

Commonly defined problems for which health promotion programs are usually designed either deal with a specific health concern or an economic issue. An example of a problem that deals with a health concern might be to reduce the risk of cardiovascular disease in white collar employees, while a problem revolving around an economic issue may be to reduce the amount of money the company spends on health insurance claims per year. Both of these problems would be appropriate for calculating a CBA or CEA, however for the purposes of this paper, the cardiovascular disease problem will be used as an example through the remaining steps in the process.

Step 2: Specifying the Objectives
Closely related to defining the problem is setting one or more objectives against which programmatic alternatives are to be evaluated. If the defined problem is not readily measurable, further specification may help qualify it. For example, the problem of reducing cardiovascular disease in white collar employees is too broad to be readily quantified.

A possible specification of an appropriate objective would be to reduce the risk of cardiovascular disease in this employee group by getting 50% of the high risk employees in an appropriate exercise program. It is known that the high risk group includes individuals who have hypertension and are overweight. These individuals cost a company more money in medical care, accidents, etc. than individuals without them. Exercise has been shown to help both of these health concerns.

Step 3: Identifying Alternatives
To determine if a specific approach to a problem is cost-effective or cost-beneficial, it needs to be compared to other approaches that could also be used to achieve the stated objectives. Again using the problem of cardiovascular disease as an example, an alternative approach may be to reduce disease via a nutrition and weight control program as opposed to the exercise program.

When identifying alternatives for health promotion programs, it should be noted that the alternatives do not need to attack the problem using similar approaches. For example, if the problem is to reduce health costs due to cigarette smoking within an organization, one cost analysis may be completed on an educational smoking cessation approach. Another analysis of costs could be calculated on the alternative which mandates, via a company policy, that there be no smoking in the workplace.

It is helpful to keep the following concerns in mind when identifying appropriate alternatives: 1) select only alternatives that are believed to be potentially quite cost-effective, 2) select alternatives that offer variety in their approach, and 3) select alternatives that would be appropriate for comparison—do not select an alternative that is obviously an inappropriate approach for solving the problem (i.e., getting *every* employee to adopt a specific exercise program).

Step 4: Describing Production Relationships
The first three steps of this process set the conceptual

framework for calculating a CBA or CEA. When one describes the production relationships he/she is creating the technical framework for the quantitative assessment and comparison of costs and benefits of the alternatives. This may be the most important step in the CBA and CEA processes. To set up the technical framework the evaluator must identify the resources necessary to carry out the alternative, explain how the resources are combined, and then predict the outcome(s). As Warner and Luce (1982) have pointed out, this can be completed in several different ways ranging from a simple flow chart to a sophisticated, multi-equation computer simulation.

In the cardiovascular disease problem, the resources would include personnel time—of both the high risk employees participating in this program and the program leaders, educational materials (i.e. booklets, films, handouts, etc.), supplies (i.e. exercise clothing, laundry expenses, etc.), pre- and post-program exercise testings, pre-program medical examinations, fee for facility use, and any other pre-participant program expenses. The outcomes of the program may include 50% of the participants getting involved in a life-long exercise program, 50% reducing their weight, and 75% getting their blood pressure under control. These in turn may result in fewer health insurance claims because of reduced illness, less absenteeism, and fewer accidents thus increasing productivity. In the long run it is hoped these programs will decrease both morbidity and premature mortality.

As one can see from this example, this step can become quite involved. One may need to examine previous programs—either conducted in house or in another setting—or obtain the services of a technical consultant to try to adequately identify all resources and outcomes. However, the evaluator of the health promotion programs should be aware that even this additional work may not insure the identification of all health outcomes. It is because of this inability to identify specific health outcomes that the use of CBA with health promotion programs has been limited. If the health benefits of a program cannot be identified, then one cannot put a dollar value on them and thus the cost of the benefit cannot be analyzed. For example, what are the health benefits of a nutrition education program? Unless these benefits can be identified*, CBA would be an inappropriate cost analysis technique to use with health promotion programs.

On the other hand, CEA can be applied very well to some health promotion programs. For the outcomes of concern are not benefits but effects and with a CEA the evaluator is not required to put a dollar value on the effects. Thus when analyzing the nutrition education program one can identify effects such as the reduction of calorie intake or the reduction of serum fat levels without trying to identify the health benefit of such. It should be noted that these effects are immediate (i.e. reduction in calories) or intermediate (i.e. decrease in serum fat levels) outcomes only and not long-term (i.e. decreased pre-mature mortality) like some financiers of health promotion programs want to see.

*See the related literature section of this paper for examples of where evaluators have been able to apply CBA to health promotion programs.

Whether one is using CBA or CEA, the more completely the production relationships have been described, the easier it will be to complete steps 5 and 6 in the process—analyzing costs, benefits and effectiveness.

Step 5: Analyzing the Costs

Costs should be defined as those resources that one must give up to gain some benefit or effect (Warner & Luce, 1982). This would include not only those direct controllable costs but also overhead uncontrollable costs.

The cost of some resources may be obvious. Using the cardiovascular disease example, it may be very easy to determine that the cost of the educational materials because they can be purchased at a cost of Y per set. The cost of the group leader may be obvious, too, but how about the cost of the four volunteers who are helping conduct the program? Since the program could not be run without the four volunteers, this is a cost to the program. In this situation the economic concept of "opportunity cost" would be used. "The opportunity cost is its value in another use" (Warner & Luce, 1982, p. 77). So if these volunteers were not helping in this program how much would they be worth in another setting? It may be found that they would be worth $7.50 per hour working in a similar capacity at a local health agency. Therefore, their cost could be determined with this figure.

Since one of the major reasons for calculating CBAs and CEA is to be able to compare alternatives it is important that costs (and for that matter benefits and effects) of the different alternatives are calculated in a similar manner. For example, if one is comparing different cardiovascular exercise programs and both programs include the help of volunteers, the same opportunity costs should be used in determining the total cost of volunteers.

Step 6: Analyzing Benefits and Effectiveness

There are usually numerous desired outcomes (benefits) that result from health promotion programs. Some are obvious while others are much more difficult to identify. For this reason, it may help the evaluator to try to categorize the different outcomes. Warner and Luce (1982) have identified the following classification scheme for outcomes associated with health care activities: 1) Personal health benefits—improvements in health such as increased life expectancy, decreased morbidity and reduced disability; 2) Health care resource benefits—the saving of unused resources resulting from the implementation of an activity (for example an exercise program could reduce the resources put into cardiac surgery); 3) Other economic benefits—desired outcomes that are not identified as either health or health care benefits, such as work productivity; 4) Other social benefits—desired outcomes that have positive social effects like increased access to health services or compassion; and 5) Intermediate outcomes—benefits that occur prior to a final outcome. Because it is sometimes difficult to measure final outcomes, one often must use the intermediate outcome. For example, the long-term impact of an exercise program on one's health would be difficult to determine but one could measure the intermediate outcome of weight loss.

It should be noted that not all outcomes are benefits. The best example of this appears in screening programs when false positive outcomes appear. If such outcomes do exist they need to be treated as costs.

The measurement of benefits and effectiveness is very much like the measurement of costs in that some aspects are straightforward while others are very difficult. For example not all social benefits can be quantified, such as compassion. There is no standard unit of compassion on which one could attach a dollar value.

It is at this point in the calculations of CBA and CEA that the differences in the two analyses can be seen. The CEA ends with the measurement of effectiveness. No dollar value is placed on the outcomes. Thus, the number of lives saved, trips to the health clinic, or persons involved in the exercise program are all that are needed. However, in order to calculate a CBA, monetary units must be attached to each outcome. This is not too difficult when market prices are available. But they are not always available and the one area that has caused considerable discussion is trying to put a monetary label on the "value of life." Techniques that have been used include 1) human capital - value of being productively employed in the labor market plus direct benefit of health care resource savings, 2) willingness to pay—value that individuals place on reducing risks of death and illness, 3) court awards in civil cases—value of productive life and emotional costs, and 4) life insurance holdings—value of one's life insurance.

Step 7: Discounting
A necessary step in calculating an accurate CBA or CEA is that of discounting. Since the costs and benefits of some programs do not occur entirely in the present, for comparison purposes all future costs and monetary values of future benefits should be discounted to their present value. In other words, a dollar today is worth more to an individual than the promise of having the dollar tomorrow and more still than having the dollar the day after tomorrow. "The discount rate attempts to adjust for what a dollar invested today would earn in interest" (Collen & Goodman, 1985). "...Discounting is particularly important in the case of preventive activities since so many of the benefits occur well into the future. In addition, discounting helps to explain how 'postponing' illness costs can have the effect of 'containing them.' (Warner, 1979)

To carry out the discounting process one must first decide on a discount rate. The discount rate expresses the degree to which tomorrow's dollar loses value relative to today's dollar. Since there is little consensus on what discount rate should be used and because the particular discount rate chosen can have a substantial impact on the outcome of the analysis [In relative terms, low discount rates tend to favor projects whose benefits occur in the distant future (OTA, 1980)], CBAs and CEAs are usually calculated using several different rates usually ranging from 3-10%. This process of using several different rates is called sensitivity analysis.

For example, if one wanted to spend $1,000 today on an exercise program expecting to save $2,000 in medical costs in

five years, there would be a need to discount the benefit ($2,000) to its estimated present value. For the sake of the example the discount rate will be set at 5%. The present discounted value today of the net benefit would be $567 ($1,567-$1,000) and not $1,000 ($2,000-$1,000).

Both time (in years) and the discount rate have an impact on the discounted value. Tables 1 and 2 are presented to illustrate the effect of each. Table 1 shows how an expected $2,000 benefit decreases in value over time when the discount rate stays constant (5% in this example).

Table 1
Effect of Time on Discounted Value

Discount Rate	Time (in years)	Present Value of Cost	Present Value of Benefit	Present Value Of Net Benefit
.05	0	$1,000	$2,000	$1,000
.05	1	1,000	1,905	905
.05	2	1,000	1,814	814
.05	5	1,000	1,567	567
.05	10	1,000	1,228	228
.05	20	1,000	754	− 246

Table 2 illustrates how again a $2,000 benefit decreases in value as the discount rate increases and the time stays constant (5 years in this example).

Table 2
Effect of Discount Rate on Discounted Value

Discount Rate	Time (in years)	Present Value of Cost	Present Value of Benefit	Present Value of Net Benefit
0	5	$1,000	$2,000	$1,000
3	5	1,000	1,725	725
5	5	1,000	1,567	567
7	5	1,000	1,426	426
10	5	1,000	1,242	242
15	5	1,000	994	− 6

It is obvious from these tables that given a large enough discount rate and/or substantial number of years, the net benefit could be a negative number. Such a number would indicate that the costs would outweigh the benefits and the cost-benefits ratio would be less than one point zero (1.0) to 1.0. In other words, it would cost more than one dollar to get a dollar worth of benefit.

For those interested in other examples of the discounting process, see Collen and Goodman (1985) and Warner and Luce (1982).

Step 8: Analyzing Uncertainties
As has been demonstrated throughout this discussion of calculating a CBA or CEA, there will be times when the evaluator will be uncertain of some data that need to be included. In such cases there are several alternatives available to the evaluator. As with discounting, the evaluator could use a sensitivity analysis. For example, if the evaluator were figuring a CEA on a smoking cessation program and was not sure of the cost of an instructor for the program, he/she could make several different estimates of the cost. Each of these estimates

could then be "plugged into" the analysis to give the evaluator a range for the CEA.

Another approach to dealing with uncertainties would be to elicit the help of a group of experts in the field. Such a technique is called consensus development. With this technique a group of experts is brought together to listen to a presentation of uncertain areas. Following the presentation, the group is then isolated to discuss the presentation and to reach a consensus as to what should be used in place of the uncertain data.

Step 9: Interpreting the Results

Because of all the concerns noted in calculating a CBA or CEA, one needs to be careful in interpreting the results of an analysis. There are many assumptions and uncertainties that both the evaluator and/or the interpreter of the results could overlook. Thus, one needs to proceed with caution when reading the analysis reports.

Asssuming all steps have been carried out properly and appropriate CBA and CEA data have been calculated, the decision-maker must not forget that the economic evaluation is only one piece of the data needed to make decisions about programs. Most programs have important ethical, legal and/or societal issues that must be identified and discussed before final program decisions can be made.

Using CBAs and CEAs with Health Promotion Programs

The need for incorporating an economic component in the evaluation of a health promotion program should be obvious. The question that remains is, what specific technique would be most appropriate? In most situations the answer would be CEA. The reasons for using CEA as opposed to CBA with health promotion programs are: 1) the inability to determine and then measure all the effects of a program, and 2) the inability to put a monetary value on the measured effect. These inabilities of not being able to identify the effects and then in turn being able to determine the value (in dollars) of these effects are critical steps in the CBA process. Without them an evaluator could not calculate an accurate CBA. It would probably be a rare situation in which a CBA would be an appropriate technique to use in an evaluation of a health promotion program. Even if an evaluator were able to determine these values, there are some (Fielding, 1979; Kristein, 1983) who believe the cost-benefit ratio would not favor the health promotion programs. These individuals have indicated that there are several cost issues that evaluators to date have not considered when calculating a CBA. One of these issues revolves around the additional costs of human longevity. When an individual lives longer he/she is more likely to have incurred additional medical costs and an employee will have to pay pensions for a longer period of time.

Conclusion

Many of the early health promotion programs planned in this country were implemented on the premise that it was more economically sound to spend health care dollars on prevention activities than on curing disease..At the present time there is little empirical data to prove such economic evaluation - even though CBA and CEA have been used in many other areas of the health care system. As one looks to the future, it seems reasonable that if health promotion program planners are going to convince policy makers that such programs are an effective means of improving health status, then economic evaluation must be a part of the total evaluation process.

REFERENCES

Acton, J. (1976). Measuring the monetary value of lifesaving programs. *Law and Contemporary Problems, 40,* 46.

Alderman, M.H., Madhavan, S., & Davis, T. (1983). Reduction of cardiovascular disease events by worksite hypertension treatment. *Hypertension, 5* (supplement V). V138-V143.

Collen, M., & Goodman, C. (1985). Cost-effectiveness and cost-benefit analaysis. In Institute of Medicine, *Assessing Medical Technologies* (pp. 136-144, 160-164). Washington, D.C.: National Medical Press.

Cooper, B., & Rice, D. (1976). The economic cost of illness revisited. *Social Security Bulletin, 39,* 21.

Erfurt, J.C., & Foote, A. (1984). Cost-effectiveness of work-site blood pressure control programs. *Journal of Occupational Medicine, 26,* 892-900.

Fielding, J.E. (1982). Effectiveness of employee health improvement programs. *Journal of Occupational Medicine, 24,* 907-916.

Fielding, J.E., (1984). Health promotion and disease prevention at the worksite. In L. Breslow (Ed.), *Annual review in public health* (pp. 237-265). Palo Alto, California: Annual Reviews, Inc.

Fielding, J.E. (1979). Preventive medicine and the bottom line. *Journal of Occupational Medicine, 21,* 79-88.

Foote, A., & Erfurt, J.C. (1977). Controlling hypertension: A cost effective model. *Preventive Medicine, 6,* 319-343.

Green, L.W. (1979). How to evaluate health promotion. *Hospitals, 53,* 106-108.

Green, L.W., & Lewis, F.M. (1986). *Measurement and evaluation in health education and health promotion.* Palo Alto, California: Mayfield Publishing Company.

Kristein, M.M. (1977). Economic issues in prevention. *Preventive Medicine, 6,* 252-264.

Kristein, M.M. (1983). How much can business expect to profit from smoking cessation? *Preventive Medicine, 12,* 358-381.

Office of Technology Assessment, U.S. Congress. (1978). *Assessing the efficacy and safety of medical technologies.* Washington, D.C.: U.S. Government Printing Office.

Office of Technology Assessment, U.S. Congress. (1980). *The implications of cost-effectiveness analysis of medical technology/background paper #1: Methodological issues and literature review.* Washington, D.C.: U.S. Government Printing Office.

Rogers, P.J., Eaton, E.K. & Bruhn, J.G. (1981). Is health promotion cost effective? *Preventive Medicine, 10,* 324-339.

Rice, D. (1966). *Estimating the cost of illness.* U.S. Department of Health Education and Welfare, PHS, Health Economic Series No. 6.

Ruchlin, H.S., & Alderman, M.H. (1980). Cost of hypertension control at the workplace. *Journal of Occupational Medicine, 22,* 795-800.

Ruchlin, H.S., Melcher, L.A., & Alderman, M.H. (1984). A comparative economic analysis of work-related hypertension care programs. *Journal of Occupational Medicine, 26,* 45-49.

Scheffler, R.M., & Paringer, L. (1980). A review of the economic evidence on prevention. *Medical Care, 18,* 473-484.

Schwartz, R.M., & Rollins, P.L. (1985). Measuring the cost benefit of wellness strategies. *Business and Health, 2,* 10, 24-26.

Seidman, L.S., Sevelius, G.G., & Ewald, P. (1984). A cost-effective weight loss program at the worksite. *Journal of Occupational Medicine, 26,* 725-730.

Shepard, D.S., & Thompson, M.S. (1979). First principles of cost-effectiveness analysis in health. *Public Health Reports, 94,* 535-543.

Warner, K.E., & Hutton, R.C. (1980). Cost-benefit and cost-effective analysis in health care. *Medical Care, 18,* 1069-1084.

Warner, K.E., & Luce, B.R. (1982). *Cost-benefit and cost-effectiveness in health care: Principles, practice and potential.* Ann Arbor, Michigan: Health Administration Press.

Warner, K.E. (1979). The economic implications of preventive health care. *Social Science and Medicine, 13C*, 227-237.

Weiss, S.J., Jurs, S., Lesage, J.P., & Iverson, D.C. (1984). A cost-benefit analysis of a smoking cessation program. *Evaluation and Program Planning, 7*, 337-346.

Windsor, R.A., Baranowski, T., Clark, N., & Cutter, G. (1984). *Evaluation of health promotion and education programs.* Palo Alto, California: Mayfield Publishing Company.

Work Group on Health Promotion/Disease Prevention. (1987). Criteria for the development of health promotion and education programs. *American Journal of Public Health, 77*, 89-92.

References

Adcock, A. G., Nagy, S., & Adcock, A. S. (1990). Utilizing mass media to promote health education. *Health Education, 21*(1), 22–25.

Ad Hoc Work Group of the American Public Health Association. (1987). Criteria for the development of health promotion and education programs. *American Journal of Public Health, 77*(1), 89–92.

Ajzen, I. (1988). *Attitudes, personality, and behavior.* Chicago: Dorsey Press.

Alexy, B. J. (1985). Health risk appraisal: Reliability demonstrated. In *Proceedings of the 20th Meeting of the Society of Prospective Medicine.* Bethesda, MD: Society of Prospective Medicine.

Alinsky, S. D. (1971). *Rules for radicals: A pragmatic primer for realistic radicals.* New York: Random House.

American College of Sports Medicine. (1980). *Guidelines for graded exercise testing and exercise prescription* (2nd ed.). Philadelphia: Lea & Febiger.

American Public Health Association (1991). *Healthy communities 2000: Model standards - Guidelines for community attainment of the year 2000 national health objectives* (3rd ed.). Washington, DC: Author.

Amler, R. W., Moriarty, D. G., & Hutchins, E. B. (Eds.). (1988). *Healthier people: The Carter Center of Emory University health risk appraisal program guides and documentation.* Atlanta: The Carter Center of Emory University.

Anderson, D. M., & Portnoy, B. (1989). Diffusion of cancer education into the schools. *Journal of School Health, 59*(5), 214–217.

Archer, S. E., & Fleshman, R. P. (1985). *Community health nursing.* Monterey, CA: Wadsworth Health Sciences.

Archer, S. E., Kelly, C. D., & Bisch, S. A. (1984). *Implementing change in communities: A collaborative process.* St. Louis: C.V. Mosby.

Arkin, E. B. (1990). Opportunities for improving the nation's health through collaboration with the mass media. *Public Health Reports, 105*(3), 219–223.

Bandura, A. (1977a). Self-efficacy: Toward a unifying theory of behavioral change. *Psychological Review, 84*(2), 191–215.

Bandura, A. (1977b). *Social learning theory.* Englewood Cliffs, NJ: Prentice Hall.

Bandura, A. (1986). *Social foundations of thought and action*. Englewood Cliffs, NJ: Prentice Hall.

Baranowski, T. (1985). Methodologic issues in self-report of health behavior. *Journal of School Health, 55*(5), 179–182.

Bartlett, E. E., Windsor, R. A., Lowe, J. B., & Nelson, G. (1986). Guidelines for conducting smoking cessation programs. *Health Education, 17*(1), 31–37.

Basch, C. (1984). Research on disseminating and implementing health education programs in schools. *Health Education, 15*(4), 57–66; *Journal of School Health, 54*(6), 57–66.

Basch, C. E., & Sliepcevich, E. M. (1983). Innovators, innovations and implementation: A framework for curricular research in school health education. *Health Education, 14* (2), 20–24.

Bates, I. J., & Winder, A. E. (1984). *Introduction to health education*. Palo Alto, CA: Mayfield.

Becker, M. H., Drachman, R. H., & Kirscht, J. P. (1974). A new approach to explaining sick-role behavior in low income populations. *American Journal of Public Health, 64*(March), 205–216.

Becker, M. H., & Green, L. W. (1975). A family approach to compliance with medical treatment, a selective review of the literature. *International Journal of Health Education, 18*(3), 2–11.

Becker, M. H., & Maiman, L. (1983). Models of health-related behavior. In D. Mechanic (Ed.), *Handbook of health, health care and the health professions* (pp. 539–568). New York: Free Press.

Behrens, R. (1983). *Work-site health promotion: Some questions and answers to help you get started*. Washington, DC: Office of Disease Prevention and Health Promotion.

Bellicha, T., & McGrath, J. (1990). Mass media approaches to reducing cardiovascular disease risk. *Public Health Reports, 105*(3), 245–252.

Bensley. L. B. (1989). A review of the use of mass media and marketing in health education: A look at theory and practice. *Eta Sigma Gamman, 21*(1), 18–23.

Berkman, L. F., & Syme, S. L. (1979). Social networks, host resistance and mortality: A nine-year follow-up of Alameda County residents. *American Journal of Epidemiology, 109*(2), 186–204.

Best, J. A., & Milsum, J. H. (1978). HHA and the evaluation of lifestyle change programs: Methodological issues. In *Proceedings of the 13th Meeting of the Society of Prospective Medicine*. Bethesda, MD: Society of Prospective Medicine.

Blackburn, H. (1983). Research and demonstration projects in community cardiovascular disease prevention. *Journal of Public Health Policy, 4*(4), 398–421.

Blair, S. N., Collingwood, T. C., Reynolds, R., Smith, M., Hagen, R. D., & Sterling, C. L. (1984). Health promotion for educators: Impact on health behaviors, satisfaction, and general well-being. *American Journal of Public Health, 74*(2), 147–149.

Bloomquist, K. (1981). Physical fitness programs in industry: Applications of social learning theory. *Occupational Health Nursing, 29*(7), 30–33.

Bly, L., Jones, R. C., & Richardson, J. E. (1986). Impact of worksite health promotion on health care costs and utilization: Evaluation of Johnson & Johnson's live for life program. *Journal of the American Medical Association, 256*(23), 3235–3240.

Borg, W. R., & Gall, M. D. (1989). *Educational research: An introduction* (5th ed.). New York: Longman.

Bowne, D. W., Russell, M. L., Morgan, J. L., Optenberg, S. A., & Clarke, A. E. (1984). Reduced disability and health care costs in an industrial fitness program. *Journal of Occupational Medicine, 26*(1), 809–816.

Brager, G., Specht, H., & Torczyner, J. L. (1987). *Community organizing*. New York: Columbia University Press.

Braithwaite, R. L., Murphy, F., Lythcott, N., & Blumenthal, D. S. (1989). Community organization and development for health promotion within an urban black community: A conceptual model. *Health Education, 20*(5), 56–60.

Breckon, D. J., Harvey, J. R., & Lancaster, R. B. (1989). *Community health education: Settings, roles, and skills* (2nd ed.). Rockville, MD: Aspen Systems.

Chaplin, J. P., & Krawiec, T. S. (1979). *Systems and theories of psychology* (4th ed.). New York: Holt, Rinehart & Winston.

Checkoway, B. (1989). Community participation for health promotion: Prescription for public policy. *Wellness Perspectives: Research, Theory and Practice, 6*(1), 18–26.

Checkoway, B., & Van Til, J. (1978). What do we know about citizen participation? A selected review of research. In S. Langton (Ed.), *Citizen participation in America* (pp. 25–42). Lexington, MA: Lexington Books.

Chenoweth, D. H. (1987). *Planning health promotion at the worksite*. Indianapolis: Benchmark Press.

Chess, C., Salomone, K. L., & Sandman, P. M. (1991). Risk communication activities of state health agencies. *American Journal of Public Health, 81*(4), 489–491.

Cinelli, B., Rose-Colley, M., & Hayes, D. M. (1988). Health promotion efforts in Pennsylvania schools. *American Journal of Health Promotion, 2*(4), 36–44.

Clinton, J. (Ed.). (1988). *National guide to foundation funding in health*. New York: The Foundation Center.

Colletti, G., & Brownell, K. (1982). *The physical and emotional benefits of social support: Application to obesity, smoking and alcoholism*. In M. Eisler et al. (Eds.), *Progress in behavior modification* (vol. 13). New York: Academic Press.

Conner, R. F. (1980). Ethical issues in the use of control groups. In R. Perloff, & E. Perloff, (Eds.) *New Directions for Program Evaluation* (pp. 63-75), San Francisco: Jossey-Bass Inc., Publishers.

Connor, D. M. (1968). *Strategies for development*. Ottawa: Development Press.

Cook, T. D., & Campbell, D. T. (1979). *Quasi-experimentation: Design and analysis issues for field settings*. Boston: Houghton Mifflin.

Cooper, K. H. (1982). *The aerobics program for total well-being*. Toronto: Bantam Books.

Covello, V. T., & Allen, F. (1988, April). *Seven cardinal rules of risk communication*. Washington, DC: U.S. Environmental Protection Agency.

Covello, V. T., McCallum, D., & Pavlova, M. (1989). Principles and guidelines for improving risk communication. In V. T. Covello, D. McCallum, & M. Pavlova (Eds.), *Effective risk communication: The role and responsibility of government and nongovernment organizations* (pp. 3–18). New York: Plenum.

Cox, M., Shephard, R. J., & Corey, P. (1981). Influence of an employee fitness programme upon fitness, productivity and absenteeism. *Ergonomics, 24*(10), 795–806.

Cummings, C., Gordon, J. R., & Marlatt, G. A. (1980). Relapse: Prevention and prediction. In W. R. Miller (Ed.), *Addictive behaviors* (pp. 291–322). Oxford, U. K.: Pergamon Press.

Cummings, K., Becker, M. H., & Maile, M. (1980). Bringing the models together in an empirical approach to combining variables used to explain health actions. *Journal of Behavioral Medicine, 3*(2), 123–145.

Dennison, D. (1984). Activated health education: The development and refinement of an intervention model. *Health Values, 8*(2), 18–24.

DiBlase, D. (1985). Small businesses lead into wellness. *Business Insurance,* (December 2), 16.

DiClemente, C. C., & Prochaska, J. O. (1982). Self-change and therapy change of smoking behavior: A comparison of processes of change in cessation and maintenance. *Addictive Behaviors, 7*(2), 133–142.

Dignan, M. B. (1986). *Measurement and evaluation of health education.* Springfield, IL: Charles C. Thomas.

Dignan, M. B., & Carr, P. A. (1987). *Program planning for health education and health promotion.* Philadelphia: Lea & Febiger.

Directory of research grants 1991. (1991). Phoenix, AZ: Oryx Press.

Dishman, R. K. (Ed.). (1988). *Exercise adherence: Its impact on public health.* Champaign, IL: Human Kinetics.

Dishman, R. K., Sallis, J. F., & Orenstein, D. R. (1985). The determinants of physical activity and exercise. *Public Health Reports, 100*(2), 158–171.

Dunbar, J. M., Marshall, G. D., & Howell, M. F. (1979). Behavioral strategies for improving compliance. In R. B. Haynes, D. W. Taylor, & D. L. Sackett (Eds.), *Compliance in health care* (pp. 174–190). Baltimore: Johns Hopkins University Press.

Elias, W. S., & Dunton, S. (1981). Effect of reliability on risk factor estimation by a health hazard appraisal. In *Proceedings of the 16th Meeting of the Society of Prospective Medicine.* Bethesda, MD: Society of Prospective Medicine.

Emont, S. L., & Cummings, K. M. (1989). Adoption of smoking policies by automobile dealerships. *Public Health Reports, 104* (5), 509–514.

Erfurt, J. C., Foote, A., Heirich, M. A., & Gregg, W. (1990). Improving participation in worksite wellness: Comparing health education classes, a menu approach, and follow-up counseling. *American Journal of Health Promotion, 4*(4), 270–278.

Erickson, A. C., McKenna, J. W., & Romano, R. M. (1990). Past lessons and new uses of the mass media in reducing tobacco consumption. *Public Health Reports, 105*(3), 239–244.

Feldman, R. H. L. (1983). Strategies for improving compliance with health promotion programs in industry. *Health Education, 14*(4), 21–25.

Fennell, R., & Beyrer, M. K. (1989). AIDS: Some ethical considerations for the health educator. *Journal of American College Health, 38*(November), 145–147.

Fink, A., & Kosecoff, J. (1978). *An evaluation primer.* Washington, DC: Capitol Publications.

Fishbein, M., & Ajzen, I. (1975). *Belief, attitude, intention and behavior: An introduction to theory and research.* Reading, MA: Addison-Wesley.

Forster, J., Jeffery, R., Sullivan, S., & Snell, M. (1985). A worksite weight control program using financial incentives collected through payroll deduction. *Journal of Occupational Medicine, 27*(11), 804–808.

Frederiksen, L. (1984). Using incentives in worksite wellness. *Corporate Commentary, 1*(2), 51–57.

Freimuth, V. S., & Mettger, W. (1990). Is there a hard-to-reach audience? *Public Health Reports, 105*(3), 232–238.

Freire, P. (1973). *Education: The practice of freedom.* London: Writer's and Reader's Publishing.

Freire, P. (1974). *Pedagogy of the oppressed.* New York: Seabury Press.

Gilmore, G., Campbell, M. D., & Becker, B. L. (1989). *Needs assessment strategies for health education and health promotion.* Indianapolis: Benchmark Press.

Green, L. W. (1989, March). *The health promotion program of the Henry J. Kaiser Family Foundation*. Paper presented at a public lecture at Mankato State University, Mankato, MN.

Green, L. W. (1990). The revival of community and the public obligation of academic health centers. In R. E. Bulger and S. J. Reiser (Eds.), *Integrity in institutions: Humane environments for teaching* (pp. 163–178). Iowa City: University of Iowa Press.

Green, L. W., & Kreuter, M. W. (1991). *Health promotion planning: An educational and environmental approach* (2nd ed.). Mountain View, CA: Mayfield.

Green, L. W., Kreuter, M. W., Deeds, S. G., & Partridge, K. B. (1980). *Health education planning: A diagnostic approach*. Palo Alto, CA: Mayfield.

Green, L. W., & Lewis, F. M. (1986). *Measurement and evaluation in health education and health promotion*. Palo Alto, CA: Mayfield.

Greenberg, J. (1978). Health education as freeing. *Health Education, 9*(2), 20–21.

Hall, C. L. (1943). *Principles of behavior*. New York: Appleton-Century-Crofts.

Harris, J. H., McKenzie, J. F., & Zuti, W. B. (1986). How to select the right vendor for your company's health promotion program. *Fitness in Business, 1*(October), pp. 53–56.

Health Insurance Association of America. (1983). *Your guide to wellness at the worksite*. Pamphlet issued by the Public Relations Division of the Health Insurance Association of America, Washington, DC.

Healthy people: The surgeon general's report on health promotion and disease prevention. (1979). (Publication No. 79-55071). Washington, DC: Department of Health, Education, and Welfare (Public Health Service).

Hempel, C. (1977). Formulation and formation of scientific theories. In F. Suppe (Ed.), *The structure of scientific theories* (2nd ed.) (pp. 244–265). Urbana: University of Illinois Press.

Horman, S. (1989). The role of social support on health throughout the lifestyle. *Health Education, 20*(4), 18–21.

Horne, W. M. (1975). Effects of a physical activity program on middle-aged, sedentary corporation executives. *American Industrial Hygiene Journal*, (March), 241–245.

Hosokawa, M. C. (1984). Insurance incentives for health promotion. *Health Education, 15*(6), 9–12.

House, E. R. (1980). *Evaluating with validity*. Beverly Hills, CA: Sage.

Hunt, W. A., Barnett, L. W., & Branch, L. G. (1971). Relapse rates in addiction programs. *Journal of Clinical Psychology, 27*(4), 455–456.

IOX Assessment Associates. (1988). Program evaluation handbooks for health promotion and health education. Los Angeles: Author.

Jacobsen, D., Eggen, P., & Kauchak, D. (1989). *Methods for teaching: A skills approach* (3rd ed.). Columbus, OH: Merrill, an imprint of Macmillan Publishing Company.

Janz, N. K., & Becker, M. H. (1984). The health belief model: A decade later. *Health Education Quarterly, 11*(1), 1–47.

Jason, L. A., Jayaraj, S., Blitz, C. C., Michaels, M. H., & Klett, L. E. (1990). Incentives and competition in a worksite smoking cessation intervention. *American Journal of Public Health, 80*(2), 205–206.

Jessor, R., Graves, T. D., Hanson, R. C., & Jessor, S. L. (1968). *Society, personality, and deviant behavior: A study of tri ethnic community*. New York: Holt, Rinehart & Winston.

Jessor, R., & Jessor, S. L. (1977). *Problem behavior and psychosocial development: A longitudinal study of youth*. New York: Academic Press.

Joint Committee on Health Education Terminology. (1991). Report of the 1990 joint committee on health education terminology. *Journal of Health Education, 22*(2), 97–108.

Kaplan, B., & Cassel, J. (1977). Social support and health. *Medical Care, 15*(5), 47–58.

Kendall, R. (1984). Rewarding safety excellence. *Occupational Hazards,* (March), 45–50.

Kickbusch, I. (1989). Healthy cities: A working project and a growing movement. *Health Promotion, 4*(2), 77–82.

Kolbe, L. J., & Iverson, D. C. (1981). Implementing comprehensive health education: Educational innovations and social change. *Health Education Quarterly, 8*(1), 57–80.

Kotler, P., & Andreasen, A. R. (1987). *Strategic marketing for nonprofit organizations* (3rd ed.). Englewood Cliffs, NJ: Prentice-Hall.

Kotler, P., & Andreasen, A. R. (1991). *Strategic marketing for nonprofit organizations* (4th ed.). Englewood Cliffs, NJ: Prentice-Hall.

Kotler, P., & Clarke, R. N. (1987). *Marketing for health care organizations.* Englewood Cliffs, NJ: Prentice-Hall.

Kumpfer, K., Turner, C., & Alvarado, R. (1991). A community change model for school health promotion. *Journal of Health Education, 22*(2), 94–96, 109–110.

Lefebvre, R. C., & Flora, J. A. (1988). Social marketing and public health intervention. *Health Education Quarterly, 15*(3), 299–315.

Leventhal, H., & Cleary, P. D. (1980). The smoking problem: A review of the research and theory in behavioral risk modification. *Psychological Bulletin, 88*(2), 370–405.

Lewin, K. (1935). *A dynamic theory of personality.* New York: McGraw-Hill.

Lewin, K. (1936). *Principles of topological psychology.* New York: McGraw-Hill.

Lewin, K., Dembo, T., Festinger, L., & Sears, P. S. (1944). Level of aspiration. In J. Hunt (Ed.), *Personality and the behavior disorders* (pp. 333–378). New York: Ronald Press.

Lindsay, G. B., & Edwards, G. (1988). Creating effective health coalitions. *Health Education, 19*(4), 35–36.

Maccoby, N., & Solomon, D. S. (1981). Heart disease prevention: Community studies. In R. E. Rice et al. (Eds.), *Public communication campaigns* (pp. 105–125). Beverly Hills, CA: Sage.

Marlatt, G. A. (1982). Relapse prevention: A self-control program for treatment of addictive behaviors. In R. B. Sturat (Ed.), *Adherence, compliance, and generalization in behavioral medicine* (pp. 329–377). New York: Brunner/Mazel.

Marlatt, G. A. (1985). Relapse prevention: Theoretical rationale and overview of the model. In G. A. Marlatt & J. R. Gordon (Eds.), *Relapse prevention* (pp. 3–70). New York: Guilford Press.

Marlatt, G. A., and Gordon, J. R. (1980). Determinants of relapse: Implications for maintenance of behavior change. In P. O. Davidson and S. M. Davidson (Eds.), *Behavioral medicine: Changing health lifestyles* (pp. 410–452). New York: Brunner/Mazel.

Mason, J. O., & McGinnis, J. M. (1990). "Healthy people 2000": An overview of the national health promotion and disease prevention objectives. *Public Health Reports, 105*(5), 441–446.

McAlister, A. L., Puska, P., Salonen, J. T., Tuomilehot, J., & Koskelia, A. (1982). Theory and action for health promotion: Illustrations from the North Karelia project. *American Journal of Public Health, 72*(1), 43–50.

McCarthy, E. J. (1978). *Basic marketing: A managerial approach* (6th ed.). Homewood, IL: Richard D. Irwin.

McConnaughy, E. A., Prochaska, J. O., & Velicer, W. F. (1983). Stages of change in psychotherapy: Measurement and sample profiles. *Psychotherapy: Theory, Research, and Practice, 20*(3), 368–375.

McGuire, W. J. (1981). Behavioral medicine, public health and communication theories. *Health Education, 12*(3), 8–13.

McKenzie, J. F. (1986). Cost-benefit and cost-effectiveness as a part of the evaluation of health promotion programs. *The Eta Sigma Gamman, 18*(2), 10–16.

McKenzie, J. F. (1988). Twelve steps in developing a schoolsite health education/promotion program for faculty and staff. *The Journal of School Health, 58*(4), 149–153.

McKenzie, J. F., & Dunn, S. (1984). Action-oriented health education. *Future Focus: Ohio Journal of Health Physical Education Recreation & Dance, 5*(4), 3–5.

McKenzie, J. F., Luebke, J., & Romas, J. A. (1992). Incentives: A means of getting and keeping workers involved in health promotion programs. *Journal of Health Education.*

Minter, S. G. (1986). Occupational health professionals control health care costs. *Occupational Hazards,* (April), 63–66.

Monahan, J. L., & Scheirer, M. A. (1988). The role of linking agents in the diffusion of health promotion programs. *Health Education Quarterly, 15*(4), 417–433.

Morris, L. L., Fitz-Gibbon, C. T., & Freeman, M. E. (1987). *How to communicate evaluation findings.* Newbury Park, CA: Sage.

Moskowitz, J. M. (1989). Preliminary guidelines for reporting outcome evaluation studies of health promotion and disease prevention programs. In M. Braverman (Ed.), *New directions for program evaluation* (pp. 59–74). San Francisco: Jossey-Bass.

Murphy, W. G., & Brubaker, R. G. (1990). Effects of a theory-based intervention on the practice of testicular self-examination by high school males. *Journal of School Health, 60*(9), 459–462.

National Task Force for the Preparation and Practice of Health Educators, Inc. (1985). *A framework for the development of competency-based curricula for entry-level health educators.* New York: Author.

Novelli, W. D., & Ziska, D. (1982). Health promotion in the workplace: An overview. *Health Education Quarterly, 9*(suppl.), 20–26.

Nye, R. D. (1979). *What is B. F. Skinner really saying?* Englewood Cliffs, NJ: Prentice-Hall.

Orlaldi, M. A. (1986). The diffusion and adoption of worksite health promotion innovations: An analysis of barriers. *Preventive Medicine, 15*(5), 522–536.

O'Rourke, T. W., & Macrina, D. M. (1989). Beyond victim blaming: Examining the micro-macro issues in health promotion. *Wellness Perspectives: Research, Theory and Practice, 6*(1), 7–17.

Parcel, G. S. (1983). Theoretical models for application in school health education research. *Health Education, 15*(4), 39–49.

Parcel, G. S., & Baranowski, T. (1981). Social learning theory and health education. *Health Education, 12*(3), 14–18.

Parcel, G. S., Ericksen, M. P., Lovato, C. Y., Gottlieb, N. H., Brink, S. G., & Green, L. W. (1989). The diffusion of school-based tobacco-use prevention programs: Project description and baseline data. *Health Education Research, 4*(1), 111–124.

Parkinson, R. S., & Associates. (1982). *Managing health promotion in the workplace: Guidelines for implementation and evaluation.* Palo Alto. CA: Mayfield.

Patton, M. Q. (1986). *Utilization-focused evaluation.* Beverly Hills, CA: Sage.

Patton, M. Q. (1988). *How to use qualitative methods in evaluation.* Newbury Park, CA: Sage.

Patton, R. W., Corry, J. M., Gettman, L. R., & Graf, J. S. (1986). *Implementing health/fitness programs.* Champaign, IL: Human Kinetics.

Pavlov, I. (1927). *Conditional reflexes.* Oxford: Oxford University Press.

Penner, M. (1989). Economic incentives to reduce employee smoking: A health insurance surcharge for tobacco using state of Kansas employees. *American Journal of Health Promotion, 4*(1), 5–11.

Pentz, M. A., Johnson, C. A., Dwyer, J. H., MacKinnon, D. M., Hansen, W. B., & Flay, B. R. (1989). A comprehensive community approach to adolescent drug abuse prevention: Effects on cardiovascular disease risk behaviors. *Annals of Medicine, 21*(3), 382–388.

Perlman, J. (1978). Grassroots participation from neighborhood to nation. In S. Langton (Ed.), *Citizen participation in America* (pp. 65–79). Lexington, MA: Lexington Books.

Perlman, R., & Gurin, A. (1972). *Community organization and social planning.* New York: John Wiley & Sons.

Pickett, G. E., & Hanlon, J. J. (1990). *Public health: Administration and practice.* St. Louis: Times Mirror/Mosby.

Piniat, A. J. (1984). How to put spirit in an incentive program. *National Safety News,* (January), 46–49.

Pollock, M. L., Foster, C., Salisburg, R., & Smith, R. (1982). Effects of a YMCA starter fitness program. *The Physician and Sportsmedicine, 10*(1), 89–91, 95–99, 120.

Popham, W. J. (1988). *Educational evaluation.* Englewood Cliffs, NJ: Prentice Hall.

Prochaska, J. O. (1979). *Systems of psychotherapy: A transtheoretical analysis.* Homewood, IL: Dorsey Press.

Prochaska, J. O. (1989, August). *What causes people to change from unhealthy to health-enhancing behavior?* Paper presented at the American Cancer Society's Human Behavior and Cancer Risk Reduction Conference, Bloomington, IN.

Prochaska, J. O., & DiClemente, C. C. (1982). Transtheoretical therapy: Toward a more integrative model of change. *Psychotherapy: Theory, Research, and Practice, 19*(3), 276–288.

Prochaska, J. O., & DiClemente, C. C. (1983). Stages and processes of self-change of smoking: Toward an integrative model of change. *Journal of Consulting and Clinical Psychology, 51*(3), 390–395.

Prochaska, J. O., DiClemente, C. C., Velicer, W. F., Ginpil, S., & Norcross, J. C. (1985). Predicting change in smoking status for self-changers. *Addictive Behaviors, 10*(4), 395–406.

Rakich, J. S., Longest, B. B., & O'Donovan, T. R. (1977). *Managing health care organizations.* Philadelphia: W. B. Saunders.

Rich, R. F., & Sugrue, N. M. (1989). Health promotion, disease prevention, and public policy. *Wellness Perspectives: Research, Theory and Practice, 6*(1), 27–35.

Rifkin, S. B. (1986). Lessons from community participation in health programmes. *Health Policy and Planning, 1*(3), 240–249.

Rogers, E. M. (1962). *Diffusion of innovations.* New York: Free Press of Glencoe.

Rogers, E. M. (1983). *Diffusion of innovations* (3rd ed.). New York: Free Press.

Rokeach, M. (1969). *Beliefs, attitudes and values: A theory of organization and change.* San Francisco: Jossey-Bass.

Rosenstock, I. M. (1966). Why people use health services. *Milbank Memorial Fund Quarterly, 44,* 94–124.

Rosenstock, I. M., Strecher, V. J., & Becker, M. H. (1988). Social learning theory and the health belief model. *Health Education Quarterly, 15*(2), 175–183.

Ross, H. S., & Mico, P. R. (1980). *Theory and practice in health education.* Palo Alto, CA: Mayfield.

Ross, M. G. (1967). *Community organization: Theory, principles, and practice.* New York: Harper & Row.

Rothman, J., & Tropman, J. E. (1987). Models of community organization and macro practice perspectives: Their mixing and phasing. In F. M. Cox, J. L. Erlich, J. Rothman, & J. E. Tropman (Eds.), *Strategies of community organization: Macro practice* (pp. 3–26). Itasca, IL: F. E. Peacock.

Rotter, J. B. (1954). *Social learning and clinical psychology.* New York: Prentice Hall.

Rotter, J. B. (1966). Generalized expectancies for internal versus external control of reinforcement. *Psychological Monographs, 80*(1).

Sachs, J. J., Krushat, W. M., & Newman, J. (1980). Reliability of the health hazard appraisal. *American Journal of Public Health, 70,* 730–732.

Schechter, C., Vanchieri, C., & Crofton, C. (1990). Evaluating women's attitudes and perceptions in developing mammography promotion messages. *Public Health Reports, 105*(3), 253–257.

Scriven, M. (1973). Goal-free evaluation. In E. House (Ed.), *School evaluation: The politics and procedures* (pp. 319–328). Berkeley, CA: McCutchan.

Shea, S., & Basch, C. E. (1990). A review of five major community-based cardiovascular disease prevention programs: Part I, rationale, design and theoretical framework. *American Journal of Health Promotion, 4*(3), 203–213.

Shepard, M. (1985). Motivation: The key to fitness compliance. *The Physician and Sportsmedicine, 13*(7), 88–101.

Shepard, R. J., Corey, P., Renzland, P., & Cox, M. (1982). The influence of an employee fitness and lifestyle modification program upon medical care costs. *Canadian Journal of Public Health, 73*(4), 259–263.

Sherwood, S. (Ed.). (1987). *Alcohol programs and policies on campus* (NASPA Monograph No. 7). Washington, DC: National Association of Student Personnel Administrators.

Shirreffs, J., Odom, J., McLeroy, K., Cryer, D., & Fors, S. (1990, April). *Incorporating ethics in the health education curriculum.* Papers presented at the meeting of the Association for the Advancement of Health Education, New Orleans, LA.

Skinner, B. F. (1953). *Science and human behavior.* New York: Free Press.

Smith, K. W., McKinlay, S. M., & McKinlay, J. B. (1989). The reliability of health risk appraisals: A field trial of four instruments. *American Journal of Public Health, 79*(12), 1603–1606.

Solomon, D. D. (1987), Evaluating community programs. In F. M. Cox, J. L. Erlich, J. Rolhman, & J. E. Tropman (Eds.), *Strategies of community organization: Macro practices* (pp. 366–368). Itasca, IL: F. E. Peacock.

Sorensen, G., Rigotti, N., Rosen, A., Pinney, J., and Prible, R. (1991). Effects of a worksite nonsmoking policy: Evidence for increased cessation. *American Journal of Public Health, 81*(2), 202–204.

Spilman, M. A., Goetz, A., Schultz, J., Bellingham, R., & Johnson, D. (1986). Effects of a corporate health promotion program. *Journal of Occupational Medicine, 28*(4), 285–289.

Stacy, R. D. (1987). Instrument evaluation guides for survey research in health education and health promotion. *Health Education, 18*(5), 65–67.

Stake, R. E. (1983). Program evaluation, particularly responsive evaluation. In G. F. Madaus, M. Scriven, & D. L. Stufflebeam (Eds.), *Evaluation models* (pp. 287–310). Boston: Kluwer-Nijhoff.

Strecher, V. J., DeVellis, B. M., Becker, M. H., & Rosenstock, I. M. (1986). The role of self-efficacy in achieving health behavior change. *Health Education Quarterly, 13*(1), 73–91.

Stufflebeam, D. L., & Members of the National Study Committee on Evaluation of Phi Delta Kappa (1971). *Educational evaluation and decision making.* Itasca, IL: F. E. Peacock.

Stunkard, A. J., & Braunwell, K. D. (1980). Worksite treatment for obesity. *American Journal of Psychiatry, 137,* 252–253.

Suchman, E. A. (1967). *Evaluative Research.* New York: Russell Sage Foundation.

Sullivan, D. (1973). Model for comprehensive, systematic program development in health education. *Health Education Report, 1*(1) (November-December), 4–5.

Syre, T. R., & Wilson, R. W. (1990). Health care marketing: Role evolution of the community health educator. *Health Education, 21*(1), 6–8.

Task Force of the Society of Prospective Medicine. (1981). *Guidelines for health risk appraisal/reduction systems.* (Available from Society of Prospective Medicine, 4405 East-West Hwy., Bethesda, MD, 20814.)

Thorndike, E. L. (1898). Animal intelligence: An experimental study of the associative processes in animals. *Psychological Monographs, 2*(8).

Toufexis, A. (1985). Giving goodies to the good. *Time,* (November 18), 98.

Udinsky, B. F., Osterlind, S. J., & Lynch, S. W. (1981). *Evaluation resource handbook: Gathering, analyzing, reporting data.* San Diego: EdITS.

United Nations. (1955). *Social progress through community development.* New York: United Nations.

U.S. Department of Health and Human Services (USDHHS). (1980). *Promoting health/preventing disease: Objectives for the nation.* Washington, DC: U.S. Government Printing Office.

U.S. Department of Health and Human Services (USDHHS). (1985). *No smoking: A decision maker's guide to reducing smoking at the worksite.* Washington, DC: U.S. Government Printing Office.

U.S. Department of Health and Human Services (USDHHS). (1986a). *Integration of risk factor interventions.* Washington, DC: U.S. Government Printing Office.

U.S. Department of Health and Human Services (USDHHS). (1986b). *The 1990 health objectives for the nation: A midcourse review.* Washington, DC: U.S. Government Printing Office.

U.S. Department of Health and Human Services (USDHHS). (1987). *Strategies for diffusing health information to minority populations: Executive summary.* Washington, DC: U.S. Government Printing Office.

U.S. Department of Health and Human Services (USDHHS). (1989). *Making health communication programs work: A planner's guide* (NIH Publication No. 89-1493). Washington, DC: U.S. Government Printing Office.

U.S. Department of Health and Human Services (USDHHS). (1990a). *Healthy people 2000: National health promotion disease prevention objectives* (DHHS Publication No. [PHS] 90-50212). Washington, DC: U.S. Government Printing Office.

U.S. Department of Health and Human Services (USDHHS). (1990b). *Prevention '89/'90.* Washington, DC: U.S. Government Printing Office.

U.S. Department of Health and Human Services (USDHHS). (No date). *Health style: A self test* (DHHS Publication No. [PHS] 81-50155). Washington, DC: U.S. Government Printing Office.

Wagner, E. H., & Guild, P. A. (1989). Choosing an evaluation strategy. *American Journal of Health Promotion, 4*(2), 134–139.

Walker, R. A., & Bibeau, D. (1985/1986). Health education as freeing—Part II. *Health Education, 16*(6), (December/January), 4–8.

Wallston, K. A., Wallston, B. S., & DeVellis, R. (1978). Development of the multi-dimensional health locus of control (mhlc) scales. *Health Education Monographs, 6,* 160–170.

Washington, R. (1987). Alternative frameworks for program evaluation. In F. M. Cox, J. L. Erlich, J. Rolhman, & J. E. Tropman (Eds.), *Strategies of community organization: Macro practices* (pp. 373–374). Itasca, IL: F. E. Peacock.

Watson, J. B. (1925). *Behaviorism.* New York: W. W. Norton.

Weiss, C. H. (1984). Increasing the likelihood of influencing decisions. In L. Rutman (Ed.), *Evaluation research methods: A basic guide* (2nd ed.) (pp. 159–190). Beverly Hills, CA: Sage.

Wilson, M. G. (1990). Factors associated with, issues related to, and suggestions for increasing participation in workplace health promotion programs. *Health Values, 14*(4), 29–36.

Wilson, M. G., and Olds, S. (1991). Application of the marketing mix to health promotion marketing. *Journal of Health Education, 22*(4), 254–259.

Windsor, R. A., Baranowski, T., Clark, N., & Cutter, G. (1984). *Evaluation of health promotion and education programs.* Palo Alto, CA: Mayfield.

Woolf, H. B. (Ed.). (1979). *Webster's new collegiate dictionary.* Springfield, MA: G. & C. Merriam.

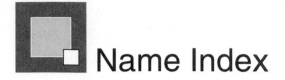

Name Index

Adcock, A. G., 101
Adcock, A. S., 101
Ajzen, I., 74–76
Alexy, B. J., 42
Alinsky, S. D., 124
Allen, F., 99
Alvarado, R., 125
Amler, R. W., 41
Anderson, D. M., 157
Andreasen, A. R., 159, 162
Archer, S. E., 122, 129, 130
Arkin, E. B., 100

Bandura, Albert, 72, 74
Baranowski, T., 38–40, 48, 70, 73, 215,
    227, 229, 249
Barnett, L. W., 165
Bartlett, E. E., 106
Basch, C., 157
Basch, C. E., 70, 89, 157
Bates, I. J., 6, 19, 22–23, 24
Becker, B. L., 12, 30, 40
Becker, M. H., 70–73, 79–81, 102,
    107–109
Behrens, R., 28, 103
Bellicha, T., 99
Bellingham, R., 29
Bensley, L. B., 163
Berkman, L. F., 102
Bernard, Amy Lynn, 44
Best, J. A., 42
Beyrer, M. K., 185
Bibeau, D., 77
Bisch, S. A., 122

Blackburn, H., 125
Blair, S. N., 29
Blitz, C. C., 168
Bloomquist, K., 170
Blumenthal, D. S., 125, 127
Bly, L., 29
Borg, W. R., 176, 178–179, 187
Bowne, D. W., 29
Brager, G., 122–124, 127–128, 131
Braithwaite, R. L., 125, 127
Branch, L. G., 165
Braunwell, K. D., 112, 165
Breckon, D. J., 7, 28
Brennan, Andrew J. J., 30
Brink, S. G., 157
Brownell, K., 102
Brubaker, R. G., 76

Campbell, D. T., 218, 220
Campbell, M. D., 12, 30, 40
Carr, P. A., 38
Cassell, J., 102
Chaplin, J. P., 68
Checkoway, B., 98, 122, 124
Chenoweth, D. H., 29, 102
Chess, C., 99
Cinelli, B., 168–170
Clark, N., 38–40, 48, 215, 227, 249
Clarke, A. E., 29
Clarke, R. N., 152, 160, 162
Cleary, P. D., 112, 165
Clinton, J., 148
Colletti, G., 102
Collingwood, T. C., 29

Conner, R. F., 214
Connor, D. M., 122
Cook, T. D., 218, 220
Corey, P., 29
Corry, J. M., 22–24, 102, 170, 182–183
Covello, V. T., 99
Cox, M., 29
Crofton, C., 45
Cryer, D., 106
Cummings, C., 112
Cummings, K., 102, 107–109
Cummings, K. M., 96
Cutter, G., 38–40, 48, 215, 227, 249

Deeds, S. G., 3, 12, 14, 24, 38–39, 96,
    108–110, 115
Dembo, T., 80
Dennison, D., 108, 111
DeVellis, B. M., 73
DeVellis, R., 109
DiBlase, D., 169
DiClemente, C. C., 162
Dignan, M. B., 38, 222
Dishman, R. K., 73, 112, 157, 165
Dole, Elizabeth, 97
Drachman, R. H., 80–81
Dunbar, J. M., 168
Dunn, S., 108
Dunton, S., 42
Dwyer, J. H., 125

Edwards, G., 129
Eggen, P., 55
Elias, W. S., 42

Emont, S. L., 96
Erfurt, J. C., 89
Ericksen, M. P., 157
Erickson, A. C., 99

Feldman, R. H. L., 102, 166, 168
Fennell, R., 185
Festinger, L., 80
Fink, A., 194, 246
Fishbein, M., 74–75
Fitz-Gibbon, C. T., 248
Flay, B. R., 125
Fleshman, R. P., 129, 130
Flora, J. A., 153, 159, 162
Foote, A., 89
Fors, S., 106
Forster, J., 170
Foster, C., 169
Frederiksen, L., 168
Freeman, M. E., 248
Freimuth, V. S., 160
Freire, P., 77

Gall, M. D., 176, 178–179, 187
Geer, J. H., 34–35
Gettman, L. R., 22–24, 102, 170,
    182–183
Gilmore, G., 12, 30, 40
Ginpil, S., 162
Goetz, A., 29
Gordon, J. R., 112–114, 165
Gottlieb, N. H., 157
Graf, J. S., 22–24, 102, 170, 182–183
Graves, T. D., 77
Green, L. W., 3, 12, 14–15, 24, 38–39,
    96, 102, 108–110, 115, 123, 127,
    156–157, 214, 221, 236–237
Greenberg, J., 77
Gregg, W., 89
Guild, P. A., 214
Gurin, A., 122

Hagen, R. D., 29
Hall, C. L., 70
Hanlon, J. J., 153
Hansen, W. B., 125
Hanson, R. C., 77
Harris, J. H., 137
Harvey, J. R., 7, 28
Hayes, D. M., 168–170
Heirich, M. A., 89
Hempel, C., 68
Horman, S., 102
Horne, W. M., 112, 165
Hosokawa, M. C., 169

Hottois, J., 34–35
House, E. R., 202–204
Howell, M. F., 168
Hunt, W. A., 165
Hutchins, E. B., 41

Iverson, D. C., 157

Jacobsen, D., 55
Janz, N. K., 80
Jason, L. A., 168
Jayaraj, S., 168
Jeffery, R., 170
Jessor, R., 70, 77–79
Jessor, S. L., 70, 77–79
Johnson, C. A., 125
Johnson, D., 29
Jones, R. C., 29

Kaplan, B., 102
Kauchak, D., 55
Kelly, C. D., 122
Kendall, R., 168–170
Kickbusch, I., 122
Kirscht, J. P., 80–81
Klett, L. E., 168
Kolbe, L. J., 157
Kosecoff, J., 194, 246
Koskelia, A., 125
Kotler, P., 152, 159–160, 162
Krawiec, T. S., 68
Kreuter, M. W., 3, 12, 14–15, 24,
    38–39, 96, 108–110, 115
Krushat, W. M., 42
Kumpfer, K., 125

Lancaster, R. B., 7, 28
Lefebvre, R. C., 153, 159, 162
Leventhal, H., 112, 165
Lewin, K., 80
Lewis, F. M., 214, 221, 236–237
Lindsay, G. B., 129
Longest, B. B., 166
Lovato, C. Y., 157
Lowe, J. B., 106
Luebke, J., 168
Lynch, S. W., 227–228
Lythcott, N., 125, 127

Maccoby, N., 125
MacKinnon, D. M., 125
Macrina, D. M., 90
Maile, M., 102, 108, 109
Maiman, L., 79
Marlatt, G. A., 108, 112–114, 165

Marshall, G. D., 168
Mason, J. O., 62–63
McAlister, A. L., 125
McCallum, D., 99
McCarthy, E. J., 162, 165
McConnaughy, E. A., 109
McGinnis, J. M., 62–63
McGrath, J., 99
McGuire, W. J., 100
McKenna, J. W., 99
McKenzie, J. F., 30–32, 108, 137, 168,
    209
McKinlay, J. B., 42
McKinlay, S. M., 42
McLeroy, K., 106
Mettger, W., 160
Michaels, M. H., 168
Mico, P. R., 16, 18, 24, 55–56, 176,
    180–181
Milner, N. A., 35
Milsum, J. H., 42
Minter, S. G., 29
Monahan, J. L., 157
Morgan, J. L., 29
Moriarty, D. G., 41
Morris, L. L., 248
Moskowitz, J. M., 242
Murphy, F., 125, 127
Murphy, W. G., 76

Nagy, S., 101
Nelson, G., 106
Newman, J., 42
Nickels, Cathy, 35
Norcross, J. C., 162
Novelli, W. D., 30
Nye, R. D., 71

Odom, J., 106
O'Donohue, W. T., 34–35
O'Donovan, T. R., 166
Olds, S., 162
Optenberg, S. A., 29
Orenstein, D. R., 73, 112, 165
Orlaldi, M. A., 157
O'Rourke, T. W., 90
Osterlind, S. J., 227–228

Parcel, G. S., 69–70, 72–73, 75, 157
Parkinson, R. S., 56, 176, 187
Partridge, K. B., 3, 12, 14, 24, 38–39,
    96, 108–110, 115
Patton, M. Q., 213, 245
Patton, R. W., 22–24, 102, 170,
    182–183

Pavlov, I., 70
Pavlova, M., 99
Penner, M., 102
Pentz, M. A., 125
Perlman, J., 122, 124–125
Perlman, R., 122
Pickett, G. E., 153
Piniat, A. J., 169
Pinney, J., 96
Pollock, M. L., 169
Popham, W. J., 203, 207
Portnoy, B., 157
Prible, R., 96
Prochaska, J. O., 81–82, 109, 162
Puska, P., 125

Rakich, J. S., 166
Renzland, P., 29
Reynolds, R., 29
Rich, R. F., 96
Richardson, J. E., 29
Rifkin, S. B., 122
Rigotti, N., 96
Rogers, E. M., 154–157
Rokeach, M., 109
Romano, R. M., 99
Romas, J. A., 168
Rose-Colley, M., 168–170
Rosen, A., 96
Rosenstock, I. M., 70–74, 80
Ross, H. S., 16, 18, 24, 55–56, 176,
        180–181
Ross, M. G., 122–123
Rothman, J., 123–125
Rotter, J. B., 72, 109
Russell, M. L., 29

Sachs, J. J., 42
Salisburg, R., 169
Sallis, J. F., 73, 112, 165
Salomone, K. L., 99
Salonen, J. T., 125
Sandman, P. M., 99
Schechter, C., 45
Scheirer, M. A., 157
Schultz, J., 29
Scriven, M., 207
Sears, P. S., 80
Shea, S., 70, 89
Shepard, M., 168
Shepard, R. J., 29
Sherwood, S., 97
Shirreffs, J., 106
Skinner, B. F., 70–72
Sliepcevich, E. M., 157
Smith, K. W., 42
Smith, M., 29
Smith, R., 169
Snell, M., 170
Solomon, D. D., 196, 245
Solomon, D. S., 125
Sorensen, G., 96
Specht, H., 122–124, 127–128, 131
Spilman, M. A., 29
Stacy, R. D., 238
Stake, R. E., 209
Sterling, C. L., 29
Strecher, V. J., 70–73, 80
Stufflebeam, D. L., 208
Stunkard, A. J., 112, 165
Suchman, E. A., 205–206
Sugrue, N. M., 96
Sullivan, D., 18, 20, 24

Sullivan, S., 170
Syme, S. L., 102
Syre, T. R., 156, 162

Thorndike, E. L., 70
Torczyner, J. L., 122–124, 127–128,
        131
Toufexis, A., 169
Tropman, J. E., 123–125
Tuomilehot, J., 125
Turner, C., 125

Udinsky, B. F., 227–228

Vanchieri, C., 45
Van Til, J., 122
Velicer, W. F., 109, 162

Wagner, E. H., 214
Walker, R. A., 77
Wallston, B. S., 109
Wallston, K. A., 109
Washington, R., 202, 206
Watson, J. B., 70
Weiss, C. H., 249
Wilson, M. G., 162, 168, 170–171
Wilson, R. W., 156, 162
Winder, A. E., 6, 19, 22–24
Windsor, R. A., 38–40, 48, 106, 215,
        227, 249
Woolf, H. B., 88, 184

Ziska, D., 30
Zuti, W. B., 137

Subject Index

Acceptability, standards of, 193, 245
Accreditation, 5
Action stage, 162
Active participants, 128
Ad Hoc Work Group, 91, 104
Administrative diagnosis, 14, 16–17
Advertising, 164–165, 180. *See also*
    Marketing
Advisory committee, 32
AIDS, 100, 185
Alcoholics Anonymous, 103, 167
Alcohol policy, 97, 267
Alpha level, 244–245
Alternative hypothesis, 244
American Cancer Society, 82, 106,
    147
American College of Obstetricians
    and Gynecologists, 105
American College of Sports
    Medicine, 105
American Health Foundation, 106
American Heart Association, 106
American Journal of Public Health, 81
American Lung Association, 106
American Public Health Association
    (APHA), 63, 98, 104
Americans for Nonsmokers' Rights,
    97
American Society of State and
    Territorial Health Officers, 63
Analysis of variance (ANOVA), 245
Anonymity, 226, 231
Art criticism, 203

Assessment. *See* Needs assessment
Assessment scales, 109
Association for the Advancement of
    Health Education (AAHE), 5
Association of Schools of Public
    Health, 63
Associations, 128–129
Attitude questions, 229
Attitudes, 56–57, 92
Attitudes, Personality, and Behavior
    (Ajzen), 75, 76
Audience segmentation, 39, 158–162,
    164
Autonomy, 106, 185–186
Aversive stimulus, 71–72
Awareness building, 56–57, 92, 108

Baseline data, 197
Behavior, 56–57, 77–79, 111
Behavioral capability, 73
Behavioral change theories, 70–79
    problem-behavior theory (PBT),
    69, 77–79, 83
    social cognitive theory (SCT),
    72–74, 83, 112
    stimulus response (SR) theory,
    70–72, 83, 93, 101–102
    theory of freeing (TF), 77, 83
    theory of planned behavior (TPB),
    75–76, 83
    theory of reasoned action (TRA),
    69, 74–75, 83
Behavioral diagnosis, 13, 15

Behavioral objectives model, 202,
    204–207
Behavior modification activities,
    93–95
    smoking cessation programs and,
    94–97
Beneficence, 186
Bias, 227
Blind study, 220
Bottom-up action, 125
Budget, 184–185. *See also* Financial
    resources

Canned programs, 139–145, 171
    for smoking cessation programs,
    139–142
Cardiovascular health programs,
    60–62, 69
Case study, 203
Census, 234
Centers for Disease Control (CDC),
    41, 63, 104, 131
Certification, 5
Certified Health Education Specialist
    (CHES), 5
CHEM (Comprehensive Health
    Education Model), 18–21, 24
Chi square, 245
Citizen initiated action, 125
Citizen participation, 122, 124. *See*
    also Community organization
Classical conditioning, 70
Client needs, 156–162, 165–171

Coalitions, 128–129
Code of Ethics, 184
Codes of practice, 105–106
Cognitive-behavioral model, 112
Combination health behavior
    models, 79–84
    health belief model (HBM), 80–81,
        83
    transtheoretical model (TTM),
        81–84
Commission, acts of, 183
Communication activities, 99–101
Communication-persuasion model,
    69
Community, 122
    entry into, 125–127
Community advocacy, 98
Community analysis, 38. See also
    Needs assessment
Community development, 69,
    122–124
Community diagnosis, 38. See also
    Needs assessment
Community education, 98
Community forum, 43–44, 234
Community opinion leaders, 125–127
Community organization, 126
    assumptions, 122–124
    Planned Approach to Community
        Health (PATCH), 131
    process, 124–131
        community entry, 125–127
        goals, 130
        organizing people, 127–129
        priorities, 130
        problem identification, 129
        problem recognition, 125
        solutions, 130–131
Community organization model, 69
Community participation, 122–124
Community participation activities,
    98
Community planning, 98
Community services development,
    98
Comparison group, 214, 216
Compensatory equalization of
    treatments, 219
Compensatory rivalry, 219
Competition, 103, 170–171
Comprehensive Health Education
    Model (CHEM), 18–21, 24
Concurrent validity, 218
Conditioning theories, 70
Conditions, 59

Conference of Local Health Officers,
    U. S., 63
Confidentiality, 186, 226
Constructs, 72–75
Construct validity, 218
Contemplation stage, 162
Content validity, 217
Context evaluation, 208
Contracts, 103, 166–167, 170
Control group, 213–214, 216
Correlation, 244
Cost-benefit analysis, 209
Cost-effectiveness analysis, 209
Cost sharing, 169
Cover letter, 227–228, 231
Criteria
    intervention design, 104–106
    program objectives, 59–60
Criterion-based validity, 217–218
Curriculum resources, 138–145

Data
    organizing, 242–243
    presenting, 248
Data analysis, 196, 242
    interpreting results, 245–246
    for needs assessment, 48–49
    types, 243–245
        descriptive, 243–244
        inferential, 244–245
Data collection, 40, 46, 196, 226–227
    form for, 44
    methods, 227–235
        direct observation, 233
        existing records, 233–235
        meetings, 234, 235
        self-report, 227–233, 235
    for needs assessment, 40–47
    pilot test, 177, 237–238
    sampling, 234–237
Decision facilitation model, 203
Decision makers, 249–250
    gaining support of, 28–30
Decision-making model, 202, 208
Deductive approach, 212
Dependent variables, 243
Descriptive data analysis, 243–244
Descriptive statistics, 243
Diffusion of Innovations (Rogers),
    154–155, 157
Diffusion of treatments, 219
Diffusion theory, 154–156
    smoking cessation programs and,
        156
Direct observation, 233

Directory of Research Grants, 148
Disease prevention, 3
Distal variables, 79
Double blind study, 220

Early adopters, 154–157
Early majority, 155–157
Economic incentives, 101–102,
    169–170
Educational activities, 92–93
Educational diagnosis, 13–14
Educational Research (Borg and Gall),
    179
Education component, 108
Efficacy expectations, 74
Emotional-coping responses, 74
Enabling factors, 14, 16, 110, 115
Endorsements, 165
Entry-level health educator, 5
Environmental change activities, 95
Environmental diagnosis, 15
Epidemiological data, 40–41
Epidemiological diagnosis, 13–15
Equipment resources, 146
Ethics, 96–97, 104, 106–107, 184–186,
    213–214
Evaluating with Validity (House), 204
Evaluation, 14, 17–18, 177, 192. See
    also Data analysis; Data
    collection; Evaluation design;
    Evaluation models
    application, 196
    approaches, 202–203
    planning, 195, 197
    problems, 196–197
    process, 195–196
    program evaluator, 198
    in program-planning stages, 197
    rationale, 194–195
    reporting, 196, 246–249
    results, 198, 249–250
    terminology, 193–194
Evaluation design, 212, 214–217
    control group, 213–214, 216
    experimental group, 213–214, 216
    qualitative approach, 212–213
    quantitative approach, 212–213
    reliability, 220–221
    selection of, 221–222
    validity, 217–218
        external, 219–220
        internal, 218–219
Evaluation models, 202–209
    approaches, 202–203

Evaluation models, *continued*
  behavioral objectives model, 202,
      204 207
  classification, 203
  decision-making model, 202, 208
  goal-attainment model, 203–208
  goal-based model, 202, 204–207
  goal-free model, 203, 207–208
  naturalistic models, 203, 209
  systems analysis model, 202, 209
Evaluation report, 196, 246–249
Evaluation Research (Suchman), 206
Evaluation Resource Handbook
      (Udinsky, Osterlind, and
      Lynch), 228
Executive participants, 127–129
Executives, gaining support of, 28–30
Exercise programs, 105, 112, 165–167,
      183
Existing records, 233–235
Expectancies, 73
Expectancy effect, 220
Expectations, 72–74
Experimental design, 215–216
Experimental group, 213–214, 216
External advertising, 164
External evaluation, 198
External money, 147–149
External program personnel, 137–138
External validity, 219–220

Face-to-face interviews, 46, 232–233
Facilitator training, 187
Fee collection, 183
Felt needs. *See* Perceived needs
Field test, 108. *See also* Pilot test
Fieldwork, 46–47
Financial resources, 146–149
  gifts, 147–149
  grants, 147–149
  organizational sponsorship, 147
  participant fee, 146–147
  third-party support, 147
Five-Day Plan to Stop Smoking, 106
Flex time, 136, 170
Focus group, 44–45, 234
Formative evaluation, 194, 197
Freeing, theory of (TF), 77, 83

Gamblers Anonymous, 103
Gatekeepers, 125–127
Generalizability, 219–220
Generic Health/Fitness Delivery
      System (GHFDS), 22–24
Gifts, 147–149

Goal-attainment model, 203–207
  compared with goal-free model,
      208
Goal-based model, 202, 204–207
Goal-free model, 203, 207–208
  compared with goal-attainment
      model, 208
Goals, 18
  community organization, 130
  examples, 60–62
  health promotion programs, 55–56
  intervention, 109–110, 115
  national health, 30, 62–64
  for participants, 115
Government involvement, 30, 62–64
Grants, 147–149
Grass-roots participation, 122,
      124–125. *See also* Community
      organization

Hard money, 147
Hawthorne effect, 220
Health and Human Services, U. S.
      Department of (USDHHS),
      2–3, 30, 41–42, 62–63, 97,
      100–101, 158
Health behavior, 2, 287
Health belief model (HBM), 80–81,
      83
Health care records, 41, 233–235
Health education, 3–4
  assumptions, 6
Health Education, 129
Health education program
  merits, 29
  rationale, 29–30, 34–35
Health Education Report, 19
Health educators, 4–6
  responsibilities and competencies
      of, 254–259
Health hazard appraisal (HHA),
      41–42
Healthier People, 41
Health insurance, 169
Health Insurance Association of
      America, 169
Health promotion, 3–4
  assumptions, 6
Health promotion materials, 140–142
Health Promotion Planning (Green and
      Kreuter), 15
Health promotion programs. *See also*
      Program goals; Program
      objectives
  cost benefit, 292–298

Health promotion programs,
      continued
  marketing process, 156–171
  statement of purpose, 54–55
Health risk appraisal (HRA), 41–42,
      108
Health screening, 108
Health Style: A Self-Test, 42, 260–266
Healthy People, 2, 62, 63
History effect, 218
HIV (human immunodeficiency
      virus), 43
Homogeneous group, 231
*How to Communicate Evaluation
      Findings* (Morris, Fitz-Gibbon,
      and Freeman), 248
Human immunodeficiency virus
      (HIV), 43

Imitation of treatments, 219
Impact evaluation, 193
Implementation, 17, 18, 176
  documentation, 181
  first day, 180
  models, 176–179
  planning, 182–187
  problems, 180–181
  reporting, 181
  strategies, 176–181
    phasing in, 178
    pilot test, 177
    total implementation, 178
  timetable, 180–181
Implementing Health/Fitness Programs
      (Patton, Corry, Gettman and
      Graf), 22–23
Incentives, 101 102, 164 165,
      168–170
Independent variables, 243
Indiana Bell Telephone Company,
      97, 269
Indiana Board of Health, 100
Inductive method, 213
Inferential data analysis, 244–245
Inferential statistics, 243
Informed consent, 106, 182, 186, 288
In-house materials, 139–142
Innovation diffusion, model of, 69
Innovators, 154
Input evaluation, 208
Institutionalization, 32
Instructional resources, 138–145
Instrumental conditioning, 70
Instrumentation effect, 218
Intangible products, 153

Integration of Risk Factor Interventions, 158
Internal advertising, 164
Internal consistency, 221
Internal evaluation, 198
Internal program personnel, 137–138
Internal validity, 218–219
Interrater reliability, 221, 233
Intervention, 88–89. *See also*
    Intervention activities
  designing, 104–115
    criteria, 104–106
    ethics, 106–107
    guidelines, 104–106
    model for, 107–115
  macro versus micro, 89–90
  model, 107–115
    awareness building, 108
    goals, 109–110, 115
    monitoring progress, 114–115
    personal assessment, 108–109
    practicing new behavior, 111
    relapse prevention, 111–114
    skill development, 110
Intervention activities, 89, 92–104
  organizational culture and, 99
  selection, 90–91
  types, 92–104
    behavior modification activities, 93–95
    communication activities, 99–101
    community participation activities, 98
    economic incentives, 101–102, 169–170
    educational activities, 92–93
    environmental change activities, 95
    regulatory activities, 95–97
    social intervention activities, 102–104
Interviews, 46, 232–233
Introduction to Health Education (Bates and Winder), 19
IOX Assessment Associates, 109

Joint Committee on Health
    Education Terminology, 3

Knowledge, 56–57, 92, 110
Knowledge questions, 229

Laggards, 155
Late adopters, 157
Late majority, 155

Legal concerns, 182–183
  informed consent, 106, 182, 186
  liability, 183
  negligence, 182–183
Letter-writing campaign, 98, 275–276
Level of significance, 244
Liability, 183
Liability insurance, 182
Literature, 43
Locality development, 124
Locus of control, 109
Logistics, 181, 184

Macro interventions, 89–90
Macro practice, 122–124
Maintenance stage, 162
*Making Health Communication
    Programs Work*, 101
Mandated activities, 95–97
Manuals, 186
Market, 152
Marketing, 152–153
  diffusion theory, 154–156
  health promotion programs and, 156–171
Marketing mix, 162–165
  person, 165
  placement, 163
  price, 162–163
  product, 162
  promotion, 164–165, 180
Marketing research, 156–158
Market segmentation, 39, 158–162, 164
Mass media, 99–101, 164, 167–168
Mass mobilization, 98
Material reinforcers, 168–169
Maturation effect, 218
Mean, 244
Measurement, 214–217
*Measurements and Evaluation of Health
    Education* (Dignan), 222
Measures of central tendency, 244
Measures of spread, 244
Measures of variation, 244
Median, 244
Medical clearance form, 289
Medical concerns, 183
Meetings, 234, 235
MHEP (Model for Health Education
    Planning), 16–18, 24
MHEPRD (Model for Health
    Education Planning and
    Resource Development),
    19–24
Micro interventions, 89–90

Minnesota Heart Health Program, 69, 70
Mode, 244
Model for Health Education
    Planning (MHEP), 16–18, 24
Model for Health Education
    Planning and Resource
    Development (MHEPRD),
    19–24
Model of innovation diffusion, 69
Models, 12, 24, 68–70, 83, 202. *See also*
    Theories
  behavioral objectives model, 202, 204–207
  cognitive-behavioral model, 112
  combination health behavior
    models, 79–84
  communication-persuasion model, 69
  community organization model, 69
  decision facilitation model, 203
  decision-making model, 202, 208
  for evaluation, 202–209
  goal-attainment model, 203–208
  goal-based model, 202, 204–207
  goal-free model, 203, 207–208
  health belief model (HBM), 80–81, 83
  for implementation, 176–179
  for intervention design, 107–115
  Model for Health Education
    Planning (MHEP), 16–18, 24
  Model for Health Education
    Planning and Resource
    Development (MHEPRD),
    19–24
  model of innovation diffusion, 69
  naturalistic models, 203, 209
  PRECEDE model, 12–14, 24, 39
  PRECEDE/PROCEED model,
    12–18, 24
  responsive model, 209
  systems analysis model, 202, 209
  transtheoretical model (TTM),
    81–84
Monetary incentives, 101–102, 169–170
Moral concerns. *See* Ethics
Mortality effect, 218–219
Motivation, 165–171
  using competition, 170–171
  using contracts, 166–167
  using incentives, 168–170
  using mass media, 167–168
  using social support, 167

Multi-dimensional Health Locus of Control (MHLC) Scales, 109

National Association of County Health Officers, 63
National Cancer Institute, 100, 160
National Commission for Health Education Credentialing, Inc. (NCHEC), 5
National Council for the Accreditation of Teacher Education (NCATE), 5
National Guide to Foundation Funding in Health, 148
National health goals, 30, 62–64
National Task Force on the Preparation and Practice of Health Educators, Inc., 5, 70
Naturalistic models, 203, 209
Needs assessment, 18, 29, 102, 129, 166
  conducting, 39–49
    data analysis, 48–49
    data collection, 40–47
    determining available health programs, 47–48
    determining health of target population, 40–47
    problems, 49
    validating need, 49
  defined, 38–39
  marketing research and, 156–158
  for smoking cessation programs, 38
Negative punishment, 72
Negative reinforcement, 71–72
Negligence, 182–183
Networking, 48, 104, 129
Nonexperimental design, 215–216
Nonmaleficence, 186
Nonprobability sample, 237
North Karelia Project, 69, 70
Null hypothesis, 244

Objectives. *See* Program objectives
Observation, 46–47, 233, 235
Observer bias, 233
Occasional participants, 128
Occupational Safety and Health Administration (OSHA), 97
Omission, acts of, 183
Open-ended questions, 229
Operant behaviors, 70
Opinion leaders, 46
Optifast, 103
Organizational culture, 32

Organizational culture, *continued*
  intervention activities and, 99
Organizational sponsorship, 147
Outcome evaluation, 194
Outcome expectations, 74
Outcomes. *See* Program objectives
Overeaters Anonymous, 103
Ownership, 31, 98, 136–137, 146–147

Parameters, 32
Parent Teacher Association (PTA), 43
Parent Teacher Organization (PTO), 43
Participant fee, 146–147
Participant goals, 115
Participant manual, 186
PATCH (Planned Approach to Community Health), 131
Pawtucket Heart Health Program, 69–70
Peace Corps, 124
Peer education, 137
Penetration rate, 99
Perceived barriers, 80
Perceived behavioral control, 76
Perceived benefits, 80
Perceived environment, 77–79
Perceived needs, 39
  determining, 43–47
    community forum, 43–44, 234
    fieldwork, 46–47
    focus group, 44–45, 234
    observation, 46–47, 233, 235
    opinion leaders' survey, 46
    target population survey, 46
Perceived seriousness, 80
Perceived susceptibility, 80
Perceived threat, 80
Person, marketing and, 165
Personal assessment, 108–109
Personality system, 77–79
Personnel, 136–138, 187
Phasing in, 178
Physical price, 163
Pilot program, 32
Pilot test, 177, 237–238
Placebo effect, 220
Placement, 163
Planned Approach to Community Health (PATCH), 131
Planned behavior, theory of (TPB), 75–76, 83
Planning, 7, 28–30
  ethical concerns, 184–186
  for evaluation, 195, 197
  facilitator training, 187

Planning, *continued*
  fee collection, 183
  for implementation, 182–187
  legal concerns, 182–183
  medical concerns, 183
  parameters for, 32
  participant manual, 186
  procedural manual, 186
  program budget, 184–185
  program logistics, 184
  program registration, 183
  program safety, 187
  recordkeeping, 184
Planning committee, 30–32
Policy development, 95–97
Policy diagnosis, 16–17
Positive punishment, 72
Positive reinforcement, 71–72
Posttest, 214
Practical significance, 245
PRECEDE model, 12–14, 24, 39
PRECEDE/PROCEED model, 12–18, 24
Precontemplation stage, 162
Predictive validity, 218
Predisposing factors, 13–14, 16
Pretest, 214, 216
Price, 162–163
Primary caregivers, 4
Primary data, 40
Primary prevention, 4
Priorities
  community organization, 130
  needs assessment, 49
Privacy, 186
Probability sample, 236–237
Problem Behavior and Psychosocial Development (Jessor and Jessor), 78
Problem-behavior theory (PBT), 69, 77–79, 83
Procedural manual, 186
Process evaluation, 193, 208
Product, 162
Product evaluation, 208
Product position, 159
Professional review, 203
Program aim, 54–55
Program budget, 184–185
Program cost sharing, 169
Program evaluator, 198
Program goals, 55–56
  examples, 60–62
  national, 62–64
Program logistics, 181, 184
Program need, ranking of, 44

Program objectives, 54
    criteria, 59–60
    development of, 57
    elements of, 58–60
    examples, 60–62
    levels of, 56–57
    national, 62–64
    for smoking cessation programs,
        57
Program overview, 54–55
Program ownership, 31, 136–137,
    146–147
Program planning. See Planning
Program registration, 183
Program safety, 187
Program significance, 245
Promoting Health/Preventing Disease:
    Objectives for the Nation, 62
Promotion, 164–165, 180
Proposal writing, 148–149
Proximal variables, 79
Prudence, 182
Psychotherapy, 81
Public health, national goals for, 30,
    62–64
Public Health Service, 100
Public policy, 98
Public service announcement (PSA),
    100
Punishment, 71–72
Purpose, statement of, 54–55

Qualitative approach, 212–213
Quantitative approach, 212–213
Quasi-experimental design, 215–216
Quasi-legal evaluation, 203
Questionnaires, 46, 229, 231–232
Questions for self-report, 227–231

Random assignment, 216
Random-digit dialing, 232
Randomization, 214, 219, 236
Random sample, 236–237
Rationale
    for evaluation, 194–195
    for health education programs,
        29–30, 34–35
    for sex education program, 34–35
Reactive effects, 219–220
Real needs. See Service needs
Reasoned action, theory of (TRA), 69,
    74–75, 83
Recidivism, 111–114, 165
Reciprocal determinism, 74

Recordkeeping, 93–95, 108, 114–115,
    184
    using existing records, 233–235
Registration procedures, 183
Regulatory activities, 95–97
Reinforcement, 71–73. See also
    Incentives
Reinforcing factors, 14, 16
Relapse prevention, 111–114, 165
Relapse Prevention, 112, 113, 114
Release of liability, 182
Reliability, 220–221, 233
Reporting, 242
    evaluation, 196, 246–249
    implementation, 181
Representativeness, 46
Request for proposals (RFP), 148
Research and development cycle,
    178–179
Resentful demoralization of
    respondents, 219
Resources, 136
    curriculum, 138–145
    equipment, 146
    financial, 146–149
    instructional, 138–145
    personnel, 136–138
    space, 145
    supplies, 146
Respondents, 227
Response rate, 226, 231
Responsive model, 209
Risk appraisal, 108
Risk appraisal program, 105
Risk reduction, 56–57
Risk reduction program, 105
Role Delineation Project, 4–5
Rotter Internal-External Locus of
    Control Scale, 109

Safety, 187
Safety belt policy, 97
Sample, 234
Sample size, 237
Sampling, 234–237
    nonprobability sample, 237
    probability sample, 236–237
    sample size, 237
Sampling bias, 236
Seat belt policy, 269
Secondary data, 40
Secondary prevention, 4
Segmentation, 39, 158–162, 164
Selection effect, 218

Self-control, 73
Self-efficacy, 73–74, 109
Self-management, 73
Self-report, 227–233, 235
    face-to-face interviews, 46, 232–233
    questionnaires, 46, 229, 231–232
    questions for, 227–231
    telephone interviews, 46, 232
Service demands, 39, 47
    community forum, 43–44, 234
    fieldwork, 46–47
    focus group, 44–45, 234
    observation, 46–47, 233, 235
    opinion leaders' survey, 46
    target population survey, 46
Service needs, 39
    current literature, 43
    epidemiological data, 40–41
    health care records, 41, 233–235
    health hazard appraisal (HHA),
        41–42
    health risk appraisal (HRA), 41–42,
        108
    significant others, 43
Service wants. See Service demands
Sex education program, rationale for,
    34–35
Significant others, 43
Simple random sample, 236
Skill development, 56–57, 92, 110
SmokEnders, 106
Smoking cessation programs,
        105–106, 112, 165, 270–274
    behavior modification activities
        and, 94–97
    canned program for, 139–142
    code of practice, 280–281
    diffusion theory and, 156
    needs assessment and, 38
    program objectives for, 57
    stimulus response (SR) theory and,
        71–72
Social action, 98, 125
Social activities, 103–104
Social behavioral community
    psychology theory, 69
Social cognitive theory (SCT), 72–74,
    83, 112
Social desirability, 219–220
Social diagnosis, 13–14
Social intervention activities, 102–104
    social activities, 103–104
    social network, 104
    support group, 103

Social Learning Theory (Bandura), 74
Social learning theory (SLT), 69
Social marketing, 153
Social modeling, 73
Social network, 104
Social planning, 124–125
Social price, 163
Social reinforcers, 102, 168
Social support, 167
Society for Public Health Education
    (SOPHE), 5, 184, 290–291
Society of Prospective Medicine, 105
Soft money, 147
SOPHE/AAHE Baccalaureate
    Program Approval
    Committee (SABPAC), 5
Space resources, 145
Speaker's bureaus, 137–138
Sponsorship, 147
Stability reliability, 221
Stages of change, 109
Staggered treatment design, 217
Stakeholders, 30, 130, 192
Standardized questionnaires, 229
Standard of practice, 184
Standards of acceptability, 193, 245
Stanford Five-City Project, 69–70
Stanford Three Community Study,
    69–70
Statement of purpose, 54–55
Statistical interaction effects, 220
Statistical regression, 218
Statistical significance, 245–246
Steering committee, 30–32
Stimulus response (SR) theory,
    70–72, 83, 93, 101–102
    smoking cessation programs and,
        71–72
*Strategic Marketing for Nonprofit
    Organizations* (Kotler and
    Andreasen), 159
Stratified random sample, 236–237
Subjective norm, 75
Substance abuse, 165
Summative evaluation, 194, 197
Supplies resources, 146
Support group, 103
Supporting participants, 128
Survey population, 234–235
Systematic sample, 236
Systems analysis model, 202, 209

Tangible products, 153
Target marketing, 159

Target population, 3, 38, 60. *See also*
    Segmentation
    determining present state of
        health, 40–47
    monitoring progress, 114–115
    surveying, 46
Task force, 128–129
Telephone interviews, 46, 232
Terminal values, 109
Testing effect, 218
Test-retest reliability, 221
Theories, 68–70, 83. *See also* Models
    behavioral change theories, 70–79
    conditioning theories, 70
    diffusion theory, 154–156
    problem-behavior theory (PBT),
        69, 77–79, 83
    social behavioral community
        psychology theory, 69
    social cognitive theory (SCT),
        72–74, 83, 112
    social learning theory (SLT), 69
    stimulus response (SR) theory,
        70–72, 83, 93, 101–102
    theory of freeing (TF), 77, 83
    theory of planned behavior (TPB),
        75–76, 83
    theory of reasoned action (TRA),
        69, 74–75, 83
    value-expectancy theories, 72
*Theory and Practice in Health
    Education* (Ross and Mico),
    16–17
Theory of freeing (TF), 77, 83
Theory of planned behavior (TPB),
    75–76, 83
Theory of reasoned action (TRA), 69,
    74–75, 83
Third-party support, 147
Time series evaluation design, 216
Top down action, 125
Total implementation, 178
Training for facilitators, 187
Training manual, 186
Transtheoretical model (TTM), 81–84
Treatment. *See* Intervention
Triple blind study, 220
Twelve-step programs, 103
Type I error, 244–245
Type II error, 244–245

United Nations, 123
United Way, 124
Unstructured questions, 229

USDHHS (U. S. Department of
    Health and Human Services),
    2–3, 30, 41–42, 62–63, 97,
    100–101, 158

Validity
    concurrent validity, 218
    construct validity, 218
    content validity, 217
    criterion-based validity, 217–218
    external validity, 219–220
    internal validity, 218–219
    predictive validity, 218
Value-expectancy theories, 72
Value Survey, 109
Variables, 79, 243
Vendors, 28, 137, 282–286
Vicarious reinforcement, 73
Voluntary health organizations,
    137–138

Waiver of liability, 182
Weight loss programs, 112, 165
Weight Watchers, 103, 167
Well pay, 169